NUTRITION AND HEALTH
Topics and Controversies

Edited by
FELIX BRONNER

Department of Biostructure and Function
The University of Connecticut Health Center
Farmington, Connecticut

CRC Press
Boca Raton   New York   London   Tokyo

Library of Congress Cataloging-in-Publication Data

Nutrition and health: topics and controversies / edited by Felix
Bronner
     p.   cm. -- (CRC series on modern nutrition)
    Includes bibliographical references and index.
    ISBN 0-8493-7849-4 (alk. paper)
    1. Nutrition. 2. Health. 3. Medicine, Preventive. I. Bronner,
Felix. II. Series: Modern nutrition (Boca Raton, Fla.)
QP141.N7765   1995
613.2--dc20   95-16297
                                                          CIP

MODERN NUTRITION

Edited by Ira Wolinsky and James F. Hickson, Jr.

Published Titles

Manganese in Health and Disease, Dorothy Klimis-Tavantzis
Nutrition and AIDS: Effects and Treatment, Ronald R. Watson

Forthcoming Titles

Calcium and Phosphorus in Health and Disease, John B. Anderson and
    Sanford Garner
Zinc in Health and Disease, Mary E. Mohs

Edited by Ira Wolinsky

Published Titles

Advanced Nutrition: Macronutrients, Carolyn D. Berdanier
Childhood Nutrition, Fima Lifshitz
Handbook of Dairy Foods and Nutrition, Gregory D. Miller, Judith K. Jarvis and
    Lois D. McBean
Nutrition and Health: Topics and Controversies, Felix Bronner
*Nutritional Care for HIV-Positive Persons: A Manual for Individuals and
    Their Caregivers*, Saroj M. Bahl and James F. Hickson, Jr.
Practical Handbook of Nutrition in Clinical Practice, Donald F. Kirby and
    Stanley J. Dudrick

Forthcoming Titles

Laboratory Tests for the Assessment of Nutritional Status, 2nd Edition,
    H. E. Sauberlich
Nutrition and Cancer Prevention, Ronald R. Watson and Siraj I. Mufti
Nutrition and Hypertension, Michael B. Zemel
Nutrition: Chemistry and Biology, 2nd Edition, Julian E. Spallholz and
    L. Mallory Boylan
Nutritional Concerns of Women, Ira Wolinsky and Dorothy Klimis-Tavantzis

SERIES PREFACE FOR MODERN NUTRITION

The CRC Series in Modern Nutrition is dedicated to providing the widest possible coverage to topics in nutrition. Nutrition is an interdisciplinary, interprofessional field par excellence. It is noted by its broad range and diversity. We trust that the titles and authorship in this series will reflect that range and diversity.

Published for a scholarly audience, the volumes in the CRC Series in Modern Nutrition are designed to explain, review, and explore present knowledge and recent trends, developments, and advances in nutrition. As such, they will also appeal to the educated layman. The format for the series will vary with the needs of the author and the topic, including, but not limited to, edited volumes, monographs, handbooks, and texts.

Contributors from any bona fide area of nutrition, including the controversial, are welcome.

Ira Wolinsky, Ph.D
Series Editor

PREFACE

Recent decades have seen a shift in public attitude and concern away from worrying about acute infectious diseases to caring about chronic diseases and long-lasting health impairment. In part, this is because means are available to recognize and combat microbial infections, causing them to be of relatively short duration. These are, moreover, conditions where host resistance, though important, plays a minor and not well-understood role. In chronic diseases and health compromising conditions, the prior status of the individual seems to matter much more. Nutrition and nutritional status are recognized factors in influencing susceptibility and the ability to overcome a chronic condition. For this reason, it seemed logical to explore in greater detail the relationship between diet, nutritional status, and disease, and to evaluate nutritional practices intended to minimize the incidence and slow the progress of major chronic illnesses.

Concern in the American populace with the relationship between diet and disease is widespread, and has given rise to many health food outlets and to a variety of regulations and provisions regarding food labeling. It therefore is logical to inquire whether American dietary patterns have undergone change. Marion Nestle and Catherine Woteki have examined this question, emphasizing methodological problems. They point out that no single measurement has been found sufficient to reflect nutritional status. Instead, a variety of approaches is needed to define nutritional risk. In identifying fat intake as one crucial index, Nestle and Woteki report that while fat intake from meat and dairy products has gone down in the last three generations, the intake of fats and oils has gone up, with a marked increase in the consumption of salad and cooking oils. Moreover, although it appears the public has become more aware of links between nutrition and health, it has been difficult to demonstrate a direct relationship between education and behavior change.

It is this topic that Deborah Bowen and Lesley Tinker address in their chapter, Controversies in Changing Dietary Behavior. Drawing on their experiences in the Women's Health Trial, they analyze whether and how extensively people can change their dietary intake behavior, how such changes can be maintained, whether one or several food elements can and should be changed, how to tailor changes for individuals, and what the role of the behavior and nutritional expert can and should be. Both groups of authors, Nestle and Woteki in the first, and Bowen and Tinker in the second chapter, emphasize the need for research to develop appropriate methodologies for surveys and intervention studies.

In the third chapter, Maryce Jacobs summarizes the role nutrition can and might play in cancer prevention. She deals with macro- and micronutrients, as well as nonnutrients, like catechins or sulfur compounds. Catechins may function as antioxidants, whereas sulfur compounds inhibit carcinogen activation. Some amino acids suppress melanoma growth and metastasis, whereas other tumors avidly utilize some amino acids. The application of these insights to actual tumor therapy is as yet uncertain.

Cardiovascular disease is one of the major causes of death in the U.S., and the role played by nutrition in preventing or aggravating the disease is discussed by David Kritchevsky. Notwithstanding the general concern with cholesterol, Kritchevsky points out that most studies have shown that dietary cholesterol plays a relatively limited role in cholesterolemia. Moreover, from a number of studies it is apparent that dietary cholesterol has only a minor effect on the blood cholesterol level. On the other hand, the type and amount of fat significantly affect plasma cholesterol levels. Interestingly, protein of animal origin is also relatively cholesterolemic. But the major risk factor for cardiovascular disease may turn out to be obesity. Hence, maintaining a desirable body weight can be a principal means for controlling cardiovascular disease.

As people age, their skeletons lose mass, with the loss of trabecular bone occurring first, particularly in the decade after the menopause. Felix Bronner and Wilfred Stein in their chapter, Calcium Nutrition and Osteoporosis, discuss the importance of gonadal hormones for maintenance of a positive calcium and bone balance and how hormone replacement can minimize bone loss. Since calcium is one of two principal mineral components of bone, adequate calcium intake throughout life is needed if the skeleton is to attain its genetically programmed maximum size.

Recent work has attributed an important role to calcium in cardiovascular function and health. While the role of intracellular calcium in muscle contraction has been appreciated for some time, possible beneficial effects of a relatively high calcium intake in lowering systolic and possibly also diastolic pressures are examined by Chandana Saha and colleagues in their chapter, Calcium and Heart Disease. Both effects and mechanisms are controversial, but it is intriguing to speculate that elevated calcium intakes (e.g., 1.5 grams per day) may be beneficial for both heart and bone.

The last three chapters each deal with the need for antioxidants in our bodies. The possible role of two nutrients, vitamin E and selenium, in assuring adequate antioxidant levels, are reviewed by Lloyd Witting (Chapter 7) and John Milner (Chapter 8). In the chapter, Vitamin E: Do We Need It?, Witting reviews in detail the biochemistry and nutritional role of vitamin E in combating free radical formation in both aqueous and lipid phases of cells. The controversy arises as to whether vitamin E supplementation actually helps combat free radical formation.

In his chapter, Milner analyzes the role selenium plays in mitigating free radical formation. Selenium is effectively an oligonutrient and its primary function may be as selenoprotein or other seleno compounds. Whether increasing selenium intake is useful in combating free radical formation is as yet unclear. Moreover, as pointed out by Milner, at certain intake levels, selenium becomes toxic. Consequently, the question of what constitutes practical selenium nutrition in still unanswered.

In the last chapter, Ishwarlal Jialal and Scott Grundy return to the question of low density lipoprotein cholesterol — LDL, the "bad" molecule — and its role in the genesis of atherosclerotic lesions. There is increasing evidence that oxidative modification of LDL is a key step in the production of atherosclerotic lesions. The question then arises how to prevent this oxidative modification and whether ingestion of dietary antioxidants such as vitamin C or vitamin A can have a protective effect.

Perhaps the overall lesson that emerges from the chapters in this book is the need to carry out careful, statistically valid intervention studies to determine whether insights concerning molecular and cellular events can be applied to the organism as a whole. Ultimately such studies should enable us to develop nutrition policies that are scientifically sound and fruitful.

I want to thank the authors and the publishers for the opportunity to begin a process that may ultimately benefit many.

Felix Bronner, Ph.D.

THE EDITOR

Felix Bronner, Ph.D., is Professor Emeritus of BioStructure and Function and of Nutritional Sciences at the University of Connecticut. A graduate of the University of California at Berkeley and Davis and of the Massachusetts Institute of Technology, Dr. Bronner has worked in the general area of calcium nutrition and metabolism for the past 40 years. He was among the first to study the kinetics of ^{45}Ca in humans, did detailed kinetic and balance studies in rats, and then proceeded to an analysis of calcium transport in the intestines and kidneys. In recent years, he has returned to the problems of calcium homeostasis and calcium nutrition and developed a course in nutrition policy. Throughout his career he has attempted to describe in quantitative fashion the events by which calcium moves in the body at the subcellular, cellular, and organ levels, aiming for a conceptual synthesis.

Dr. Bronner has published 86 research articles, has contributed 60 chapters to texts and symposia volumes, and has edited 50 volumes of texts and symposia. He was founding editor of *Current Topics in Membranes and Transport* and first chair of the Gordon Research Conference on Bones and Teeth. He is currently on the editorial boards of the *Journal of Nutrition* and *The American Journal of Physiology*.

A member of numerous scientific societies, including fellowship in the American Association for the Advancement of Science and the American Institute of Nutrition, he was the 1974 recipient of the André Lichtwitz prize, awarded by the French National Institutes of Medical Research (INSERM) for outstanding work in calcium and phosphorus metabolism, and the honoree of the 4th International Workshop on Calcium and Phosphate Transport Across BioMembranes, held in Lyon in 1989 under NATO sponsorship. He has organized and chaired national and international symposia and workshops and trained graduate students and many postdoctoral fellows.

CONTRIBUTORS

Deborah J. Bowen, Ph.D.
Fred Hutchinson Cancer Research
  Center
Seattle, Washington

Felix Bronner, Ph.D.
University of Connecticut Health
  Center
Farmington, Connecticut

S. Deveraj, Ph.D.
Center for Human Nutrition
University of Texas Southwestern
  Medical Center
Dallas, Texas

Scott M. Grundy
Center for Human Nutrition
University of Texas Southwestern
  Medical Center
Dallas, Texas

Judith K. Gwathmey, V.M.D., Ph.D.
Harvard Medical School
Boston, Massachussetts

Maryce M. Jacobs, Ph.D.
McLean, Virginia

I. Jialal, M.D., F.A.C.N., D.A.B.C.C.
Center for Human Nutrition
University of Texas Southwestern
  Medical Center
Dallas, Texas

David Kritchevsky, Ph.D.
Wistar Institute
Philadelphia, Pennsylvania

Ronglih Liao, Ph.D.
Harvard Medical School
Boston, Massachussetts

John A. Milner, Ph.D.
Department of Nutrition
Pennsylvania State University
University Park, Pennsylvania

Marion Nestle, Ph.D., M.P.H.
Nutrition and Food Studies
New York University
New York, New York

Chandana Saha, Ph.D.
Harvard Medical School
Boston, Massachussetts

Wilfred D. Stein, Ph.D.
Institute of Life Sciences
The Hebrew University
Jerusalem, Israel

Gowriharan Thaiyananthan
Harvard Medical School
Boston, Massachussetts

Lesley F. Tinker, Ph.D.
Fred Hutchinson Cancer Research
  Center
Seattle, Washington

Lloyd A. Whitting, Ph.D.
Department of Nutrition
Penn State University
University Park, Pennsylvania

Catherine E. Woteki
Office of Science and Technology
  Policy
Washington, D.C.

TABLE OF CONTENTS

Chapter 1

TRENDS IN AMERICAN DIETARY PATTERNS: RESEARCH ISSUES AND POLICY IMPLICATIONS

Marion Nestle and Catherine Woteki

CONTENTS

0-8493-7849-4/95/$0.00+$.50

I. INTRODUCTION

Accurate information about trends in American dietary patterns is critical to the development of rational policies, programs, and resource allocations designed to improve the nutritional intake and health status of the population. The importance of this information is illustrated, for example, by its use to establish dietary recommendations to reduce intake of fat from one level to another, to assess progress toward achieving national nutrition objectives, and to identify changes in the proportion of the population requiring food assistance.[97] Although assessing changes in the dietary intake of individuals or population groups might appear to be a simple task, it is in fact exceedingly difficult to accomplish with any acceptable degree of scientific rigor. The determination of usual dietary intake at any one point in time presents formidable difficulties that are further complicated when it is necessary to determine time trends. Indeed, the assessment of dietary changes over time constitutes one of the most intellectually challenging problems in the field of nutrition, and is currently the focus of intense professional interest.[17]

As many authorities have noted, no "gold standard" exists for dietary intake measurement.[72,86] Each of the methods commonly used to assess dietary intake is limited in its ability to produce reliable information, and results obtained by any one method are not necessarily comparable to those obtained by another. Therefore, inferences about time trends can only be made with many caveats, especially when the measures used to assess dietary intake and nutritional status differ from one survey period to another. Such problems impair the differentiation of genuine trends from apparent changes that are artifacts of alterations in methods or interpretations.

Despite such difficulties, much useful information can be obtained through careful analysis and interpretation of existing survey data, especially when methodologic limitations are taken into account. In this chapter, we review current methods for assessing the dietary intake of individuals and populations, review the strengths and limitations of these methods, and describe the ways they are used to determine trends in food and nutrient intake. We use this information to draw inferences about time trends in the intake of certain dietary factors selected for their relevance to current public health concerns. Because nutrition policy objectives are designed to improve the health of the population, we examine the ways in which societal trends influence dietary intake from one point in time to another. Finally, we suggest directions for policy and research initiatives designed to promote more favorable dietary trends among American population groups.

II. BACKGROUND

A. HISTORICAL TRENDS

Current dietary practices reflect thousands of years of an almost Darwinian process of natural selection: the foods that have survived and are still consumed by modern cultures are those that have been grown successfully and enjoyed throughout history, and existing dietary patterns are those that have evolved over the ages in response to food availability, biologic need, and taste preferences.[46,134] Interactions between eating behavior and food availability, as modified by cultural, social, economic, and agricultural practices and trends, at least in part explain the wide variation in the ways the world's many populations successfully achieve nutritional needs.[117]

As much as can be determined, prehistoric humans obtained food by hunting, fishing, and collecting plants. Life expectancy was short, and people suffered from the consequences of vitamin deficiencies, seasonal malnutrition, plant poisons, and microbial contamination. With the development of agriculture, thought to have taken place some 10,000 years ago, diets became increasingly based on plants cultivated for food.[28] The domestication of crop plants permitted their increased storage and consumption, and reliance on plant foods as the principal energy source continues to be typical of nonindustrialized populations today.[49]

In the early years of the United States, foods were obtained through farming, gathering, hunting, fishing, and — to some extent — internal and external trade. Diets varied according to season, climate, and geographical location and, as trade became more extensive, according to social status.[149,150] By 1800, meat had become the focus of the main meal, accompanied by fruit, vegetables, grains, dairy foods, sweets, and alcohol. This pattern reflected the Northern European origin of early immigrants to this country.[68] Increasing industrialization and urbanization throughout the 19th century fostered improvements in the ability to preserve, store, and distribute foods.[63] By the mid-1800s, the diet typically included relatively large amounts of beef, pork, and other meats; potatoes, cabbage, onions, and seasonal vegetables and fruit; bread, rolls, and pastries made with white flour; butter, milk, and eggs used primarily for baking; and coffee and tea.[150] Toward the end of the century, W.O. Atwater, the first director of nutrition research at the U.S. Department of Agriculture (USDA), noted that the American diet contained "a relative excess of the fat of meat, of starch, and of sugar..." and recommended that Americans reduce consumption of fatty meats as a means to improve health.[4]

Atwater's primary dietary concerns focused on the relationship between food intake and *deficiencies* of essential nutrients, however. Coronary heart disease was virtually unknown at the end of the 19th century, and leading causes of death were infectious diseases such as tuberculosis, pneumonia, and diarrheal diseases related to poor nutrition and lack of sanitation. In 1900, life expectancy at birth was 46.3 years for men, but had increased to 71.3 years by 1986; at age 40, life expectancy was 27.7 years in 1900, but had increased to 34.5 years in 1986.[56]

With improvements in economic status, dietary patterns in the U.S. and elsewhere began to shift toward an even greater reliance on foods from animal sources that are high in fat, saturated fat, and cholesterol. This shift was accompanied by a decline in the prevalence of health problems related to undernutrition and a rapid increase in the prevalence of diet-related chronic diseases. Since the 1940s, chronic diseases such as coronary heart disease, certain cancers, diabetes, and stroke increasingly have replaced infectious diseases and conditions related to undernutrition as leading causes of death among adults in the U.S.[84] The role of diet in chronic disease prevention is well established, and substantial evidence indicates that the typical American diet — high in energy, fat, saturated fat, cholesterol, salt, sugar, and alcohol, but low in starch and fiber — contributes to chronic disease incidence and severity.[93,144,157]

B. EARLY FEDERAL MONITORING ACTIVITIES

These historical trends in diet and disease patterns have been reflected in federal activities designed to monitor such changes. The U.S. government first began to collect information about dietary patterns and practices in the late 1890s when it granted funds for this purpose to the USDA.[104] The USDA collected its first data on the disappearance or use of commodities from the food supply in 1909, and has continued to collect such data on an annual basis ever since. In the 1930s, the Agency began collecting data on food disappearance at the retail level. Since the 1940s, the USDA has produced annual estimates of the per capita nutrient content of the food supply.

The USDA first obtained data on household food purchases through a Nationwide Food Consumption Survey (NFCS) in 1936–1937; since that time, it has conducted such surveys at approximately ten-year intervals, most recently in 1987–1988. The USDA began collecting data on the food consumption of individuals in those households in 1965, and repeated such measurements in the 1977–1978 and 1987–1988 NFCS, and in Continuing Surveys of Food Intakes by Individuals (CSFII) conducted in 1985–1986 and 1989–1991[45] and in process for 1994–1996.

The Department of Health, Education and Welfare (DHEW), now the Department of Health and Human Services (DHHS), conducted dietary interviews as part of the National Center for Health Statistics' first National Health and Nutrition Examination Survey in 1971–1974 (NHANES I). This survey was followed by NHANES II in 1976–1980, the Hispanic HANES in 1982–1984, and NHANES III in 1988–1991 (phase 1) and 1991–1994 (phase 2). The various NHANES surveys have collected data from dietary interviews, physical examinations, and biochemical and hematological tests conducted on a large, highly stratified, probability sample of the civilian, noninstitionalized U.S. population.[152]

C. NATIONAL NUTRITION MONITORING SYSTEM

Today, the prevalence of conditions related to malnutrition, and of dietary and other risk factors for these conditions, is assessed in the U.S. through a series of national surveys known collectively as the National Nutrition Monitoring and Related Research Program. This system presently includes more than 70 separate surveys, conducted by more than 20 federal agencies, which measure health and nutritional status, food and nutrient consumption, dietary knowledge and attitudes, foods available for purchase, and sociodemographic and economic indicators related to dietary intake. By far, the most important of these surveys are conducted by just two agencies, DHHS (NHANES) and USDA (NFCS, CSFII, and food supply).[45,60] Information derived from these surveys is published regularly in comprehensive reports[61,78,146] and in numerous articles in professional journals.

Such activities were mandated by Congress when it passed the National Nutrition Monitoring and Related Research Act in 1990. This Act required federal agencies to coordinate their monitoring activities, establish and follow a ten-year plan for data collection and reporting, and use comparable methods for collecting and reporting data. It also required the agencies to establish an Interagency Board to develop and oversee implementation of the plan, and to appoint a National Nutrition Monitoring Advisory Council to evaluate its scientific and technical quality and implementation.[146]

These Congressional directives were developed, in part, in response to concerns that the existing monitoring surveys were incapable of identifying time trends in dietary intake patterns, and that the overall system failed to provide adequate data on changes in dietary intake patterns, the prevalence of hunger, and the specific dietary patterns of minority groups.[97] The system also had been criticized for delays in coordinating data collection and in reporting results.[153]

These concerns derived from observations that the two principal agencies conducting monitoring surveys, DHHS and USDA, were using different methods to collect different kinds of information from different groups of people.[92] The results of their surveys, therefore, were not comparable and often yielded widely divergent estimates of trends in nutrient intake.[24] For example, the USDA published household dietary data in different formats from the 1977–1978 and 1987–1988 NFCS,[125] but the CSFII was limited to just three population sub-groups: children ages 1 through 5 years, and adult men and women ages 19 through 50 years.[136,137] Because these USDA surveys differed in sample populations, food composition databases, and methods of data collection, it was not possible to draw reliable conclusions about dietary changes between 1977 and 1988.[50] The methods used in these surveys also differed from those used in the various NHANES. Although some of these problems have been corrected or are in the process of being corrected, others have not. The overall monitoring system is still considered to be poorly integrated, lacking in priorities, insufficiently comprehensive and continuous, and in general, inadequately planned.[45] Specific details related to such issues will be reviewed in later sections.

III. RESEARCH ISSUES

A. ANALYTICAL APPROACHES

For this chapter, we are defining trends in dietary patterns as changes in a populations's food and nutrient intake over time. Such changes are influenced by a great many factors such as food availability, lifestyle, and educational level. As we will discuss later, the availability of food from which individuals can select diets is determined by agricultural production, marketing trends, new products introduced through innovation and trade, and food advertising. Among lifestyle factors, income is one of the primary determinants of food intake. Other important contributors are family structure, work patterns, meals eaten at home and away from home, and taste preferences. Nutrition knowledge and information provided through food labeling and other educational routes are also important determinants.

For the purposes of analysis, however, trends are a function of three variables: age, cohort, and time. Differentiation of these variables requires different data sources and analytical approaches, as each addresses a different aspect of change.[30] These distinctions lead to three types of questions:

- Do food and nutrient intakes vary with *age* within a population observed at a given point in time?
- Do food and nutrient intakes vary as a *cohort* ages?
- Do food and nutrient intakes vary over *time* among people of the same age?

These three general approaches to analysis depend on different sets of data. An examination of age variation requires a cross-sectional approach based on population surveys that provide a picture of dietary patterns at one point in time. Cohort analyses require a longitudinal approach that follows a cohort's dietary patterns through time as the group ages. The time series approach is usually based on multiple cross-sectional surveys performed at different points in time.[156]

In addition to these population-based methods, trend analyses can also take advantage of the historical series of data that the USDA has maintained on the overall availability of food. Called the "food supply" series, this important source of time series data reports the per capita availability of food and nutrients beginning in 1909 and continuing to the present.[108]

One further approach to assessing change in dietary patterns is to apply the techniques of meta-analysis to multiple smaller studies conducted over time. This approach is used less often than the population-based methods, but can provide valuable insights when a sufficient number of studies of high quality can be found in the literature and when certain statistical pitfalls are avoided.[132]

As we will discuss, the ability to assess trends is dependent on the availability, reliability, and validity of the data. Among the various methods, cross-sectional surveys and the food supply series have provided the most data; few data are available from longitudinal studies or meta-analyses. In the sections that follow, therefore, we concentrate on the cross-sectional survey and food supply data, the inferences that can be drawn from these approaches, the sources of survey bias, and the strengths and limitations of the methods used to assess dietary intake.

B. INFERENCES

To draw conclusions about trends in food and nutrient intake from available data, it is necessary to consider the multiple data sources together, and to recognize the sources of error that confound dietary intake measurements. The level of confidence in any conclusion about the direction and magnitude of a trend will increase to the extent that the following conditions are met: the multiple data sources point in the same direction, are of comparable magnitude, and are in accord with other indicators external to the data.

In attempting to draw inferences, we ask the following kinds of questions:

- What is the direction and magnitude of the change in the food supply data?
- Is the direction and magnitude of the change in population surveys concordant with the food supply data?
- Is the trend consistent among sex and age categories within the population survey data?
- Are there any other studies of different designs that indicate a similar trend (e.g., meta-analyses)?
- Could an error in measurement account for the observed change? Were the same methods used to study dietary intake at each point in time?
- Do external data substantiate the plausibility of the trend? For example, are observed changes in intake of dietary fat consistent with data on trends in blood cholesterol levels and coronary heart disease mortality?

C. BIAS ISSUES

From 1970–1990, federal agencies conducted nine separate national surveys. The principal features of these surveys are displayed in Table 1. Most of these surveys employed cross-sectional designs and were designed to provide a "snapshot" of the dietary practices of the sample population at one point in time. Two of the surveys employed longitudinal designs: the follow-up to the NHANES I (the NHEFS), and the NHANES III. NHANES III was the first national nutrition survey to be designed as a longitudinal study from its inception. One of the surveys listed in Table 1 used a panel design: the USDA's 1985–1986 CSFII, in which a new panel was selected for interview six times during the year.[136,137]

All nine of these surveys used either a daily food consumption method or a food frequency questionnaire to obtain information about food consumption. Most of the surveys used 24-hour dietary recalls. The USDA supplemented this method with a two-day food diary to provide a better description of "usual" food intake patterns. The NHANES surveys used food frequency questionnaires to provide estimates of usual food intake. The NHEFS and the 1987 NHIS relied exclusively on food frequency questionnaires. The USDA obtained 24-hour recalls in the CSFII, and conducted five follow-up interviews by telephone to obtain additional recall information.

These various surveys would seem to provide sufficient information on which to base inferences about changes in food consumption patterns during this 20-year period. Unfortunately, several sources of sampling and nonsampling errors complicate interpretation of the data. In particular, the surveys are

TABLE 1
National Dietary Surveys, 1970–1990

Design Method	Years	Dietary Intake Method	
		Daily	Food Frequency
Cross-Sectional			
NHANES I	1971–1974	24-hr recall	X
NHANES II	1976–1980	24-hr recall	X
NFCS	1977–1978	Recall + diary	
NFCS	1987–1988	Recall + diary	
NHIS	1987		X
CSFII	1989–1990	Recall + diary	
Longitudinal			
NHEFS	1982		X
NHANES III	1988–1994	24-hr recall	X
Panel			
CSFII	1985–1986	24-hr recall	

susceptible to bias as well as variable errors. Bias refers to the systematic errors that may affect all of the samples drawn under a specified survey design, whereas variable errors occur randomly in sampling or measurement.

Biases may be introduced into the design or implementation of surveys. Biases can occur in sampling frames that are developed when the "actual physical listing of all sampling units in the population is too difficult."[67] Such frame biases become evident, for example, in situations in which a telephone book is used to draw a survey sample. The sample would only be able to include households with telephones and would be biased in two directions: households without telephones would be missing, and so would households with unlisted telephone numbers. Thus, the sample would be likely to underrepresent low-income households as well as those of wealthier individuals who guard their privacy.

Consistent sampling biases can be introduced by mechanical procedures used to select units from the frame into the sample. Such a bias might arise if all telephone calls to the sample households were made during normal business hours. Employed persons would be unlikely to be at home during those hours, and the sample would underrepresent them.

Nonsampling biases arise from systematic errors related to noncoverage, nonresponse, measurement, or data processing errors. Noncoverage is the failure to include all appropriate elements in the sample — the exclusion of areas with few Hispanic residents from the Hispanic HANES, for example, an error that might result in underrepresentation of more affluent Hispanic individuals. Nonresponse bias is the failure to obtain observations on some of the elements selected and designated for the sample. The greater the nonresponse, the greater is the potential for bias. This error occurs when people are not at home, refuse to participate, or are incapacitated and unable to participate. It also occurs when interview or laboratory data are inadvertently lost. Such biases affect the ability to draw inferences about trends in dietary intake in ways that are discussed below.

D. ASSESSMENT METHODS

At the present time, no single, independent measurement of dietary, biochemical, or clinical status has been found sufficient to indicate the nutritional status of individuals or populations. Instead, nutritional risk usually is defined by a combination of methods: nutritional history, medical history and physical examination, anthropometric measurements, and laboratory tests. In practice, surveys rarely use the full range of nutritional assessment methods; many are too imprecise, inconvenient, or expensive for frequent use.[3]

Two distinct classes of data are used to evaluate dietary trends: food supply and dietary intake. In both methods, information about the supply or consumption of foods must be converted to information about the supply or consumption of energy and nutrients. In practice, this conversion is performed through reference to a database on food composition, corrected for serving size. The development and use of this database produce many opportunities for random and systematic error.

1. Food Composition Data

The basis of all determinations of energy and nutrient intake is the comprehensive collection of data on food composition maintained by the USDA, and published in print and computer formats. The print format is known collectively as Agriculture Handbook No. 8; to date, it comprises 21 volumes published between 1977 and 1992, annual supplements and corrections issued since 1989, and another 2 volumes in preparation (see, for example, ref. 138). The volumes are organized by food group — dairy, beef, legumes and legume products, snacks and sweets, for example — and contain data on about 70 nutrient components of approximately 5,300 food items. For each food item, data are presented on a single page, either for 100 g of the product, its common serving size, or for the edible portion of one pound as purchased. The data are also available on computer disk from the USDA's National Nutrient Data Bank Electronic Bulletin Board.[44]

The challenge faced by the USDA in establishing this database can best be understood by considering a specific food item such as, for example, a carrot. Carrots grown on different soils in differing climates, and transported, stored, prepared, and consumed under different conditions, will not necessarily contain identical amounts of carbohydrate, calcium, or vitamin A. Similar problems of variability apply to any other naturally grown food item, and immediately suggest the need for careful attention to sampling methods. To be scientifically valid, food composition data must be obtained under standardized conditions governing sample selection, the number of samples to be analyzed, the protection and treatment of the sample before it is analyzed (e.g., refrigeration), the methods of analysis, and the laboratory procedures used to verify the accuracy of analytical results.

In practice, however, such standardized conditions are rarely obtained. The USDA collects its data through cooperation with food manufacturers and other government agencies, or through contracts with academic and other research institutions. The responsible USDA agency, the Human Nutrition Information Service, maintains the database on an annual budget of under one million dollars, of which just $200,000 is available for food analyses obtained by contract. This limited budget in part explains why many values in the database are missing or imputed. Thus, it is not surprising that authorities question the reliability of these data, with concerns specifically focused on the adequacy of the sampling methods, the reliability of the analytical methods, and the overall lack of oversight, particularly of data contributed by the food industry.[44]

Changes in the food composition database also influence interpretation of dietary trends. The USDA's 1988 Bridging Study, an investigation of methodologic artifacts that might have been responsible for differences in the results of the 1977–1978 and 1987–1988 NFCS, concluded that changes in food composition data used in those surveys were responsible for both the degree and direction of trends identified for certain nutrients and should have led to a revision of the results of the earlier survey.[50]

2. Serving Size Estimations

The USDA food composition data display energy and nutrient content by serving size as well as by weight. An accurate summation of total dietary intake is entirely dependent on the accuracy of estimating serving size, yet these estimates are difficult to obtain for foods that are not prepackaged. Dietary intake surveys often use food models, photographs, or cardboard shapes to improve the accuracy of estimating serving sizes.[72] Even so, the process is difficult. There is great variation in the amounts of food consumed by individuals from day to day; this within-person variation has been found to exceed between-person variation.[59] Individuals often underestimate the serving sizes of foods thought to be high in calories.[77]

The Nutrition Labeling and Education Act of 1990 (NLEA) defined serving size as the amount of food customarily consumed. In response, the Food and Drug Administration (FDA) established standard serving sizes based on the mean amounts reported consumed in the 1977–1978 NFCS.[35] These standard portion sizes are often much smaller than those commonly consumed by the population, however.[16] Underestimation of serving sizes is sufficient to account for the relatively low caloric intakes frequently reported in population surveys, such as the 1985 CSFII which reported an average intake of 1,500 kcal/day among women aged 35 to 50 years.[136]

3. Food Supply Surveys

The USDA compiles information on food availability from annual estimates of the quantities of food commodities produced and marketed in the U.S. and has been doing so since 1909. The agency published these data as an historical series in the mid-1960s.[135] Currently, it publishes annual reports of data for the most recent 20 years.[108] These data describe the amounts of food that are available at the wholesale and retail level, without correction for waste, losses, inedible components, or amounts fed to pets. For this reason, they are assumed to overestimate dietary intake. Because the data do not include information about foods grown and consumed at home, they may underestimate dietary intake for certain fruits and vegetables. The data also are uncorrected for variations in use by population subgroups. Thus, food supply data provide only an indirect indication of dietary intake and are limited in the ways they reveal dietary trends. They are, however, often the only data source available to examine long-term dietary trends in the U.S. or internationally,[34] and they are used frequently for such purposes.

4. Dietary Intake Surveys

Short of duplicate meal analysis, no ideal method exists to determine the usual dietary intake of individuals. Standard techniques produce approximations that cannot be interpreted too literally; they include a record of foods consumed during a specified time period (food record), retrospective recall of foods consumed within a recent time period (24-hour recall, or longer), measures of the frequency of consumption of specific index foods (food frequencies), and measures or reports of the amounts of food used by households. The nutrient content of diets described by these methods is obtained from tables of food composition and compared to standards of nutrient intake such as the Recommended Dietary Allowances (RDAs) or to patterns of food consumption described by dietary goals and guidelines.

Each of these methods, used singly or in combination, has strengths and weaknesses. All yield useful, if imprecise, information. Demographic and socioeconomic data are especially useful as indirect indicators of nutritional risk in community surveys where detailed diet histories, physical examinations, and laboratory tests would be impractical. The strengths and limitations of methods for assessment of dietary intake have been described in detail elsewhere.[17,19,27,72,156]

a. 24-Hour Recalls

In this method, an interviewer asks respondents to list the foods and beverages consumed on the previous day, and to estimate serving sizes associated with each food item. Subsequent data processing requires conversion of the interview information to estimates of nutrient intake through assignment of each food item to a code in a nutrient database, conversion of each serving size estimate to gram weights, multiplication of the gram weights by the nutrient composition, and summation of the nutrients contributed by each food item. For group estimates, these steps must be performed for each respondent, followed by calculation of the appropriate population statistic. These steps present multiple opportunities for errors with respect to recall, measurement, or calculation, as well as for errors due to inaccuracies in food composition tables.

b. Food Records or Diaries

In this method, the subject self-records all foods or drinks at the time of consumption, and estimates serving sizes at the same time, either by direct measurement or by comparison to models (estimated food records) or by weighing each item (weighed food record). In either case, subsequent data processing requires the same steps as those for 24-hour recalls. This method relies less on memory, but requires more effort and may perturb usual eating patterns.[72]

c. Food Frequency Questionnaires (FFQs)

These are list-based recalls in which subjects are asked to check how often they have consumed a specified food item during the past day, week, or month. Because FFQs can be filled out rapidly, do not require an interviewer, and can be scanned by computers, they are often — and increasingly — used in large population surveys. The reliability of this method in comparison to diet recalls or records, or to actual dietary intake, is a matter of great current interest. Some evaluations of the method have found its results to be highly correlated to those obtained by other methods,[32,158] whereas others have raised questions about the loss of information that occurs when food lists are predetermined,[121] and about biases resulting from measurement errors.[79]

d. Household Food Consumption

This method, used by the USDA in its various NFCS assessments, consists of an assessment of the amounts of foods reported as brought into a household from the store, garden, or farm during a given time period. Household food use is computed as the difference between amounts present at the beginning of the survey period, plus foods brought in, minus those that have disappeared during the period.[101] This information is converted to daily average consumption of foods and nutrients per person, based on the total amount of food reported as used and the number of individuals in the household. Household food accounts permit monitoring of food consumption over relatively long time periods, but the method may not identify food fed to animals or discarded for other reasons, and the data only describe family — not individual — consumption patterns.[72]

5. Questions of Comparability

At issue are the reliability and validity of self-reported measures of dietary intake. Reliability refers to whether similar responses have been given to the same questions over time. Validity refers to the degree to which a method measures what it is supposed to be measuring.[27,72] As is evident from the previous discussion, determination of dietary intake is a philosophical problem of challenging complexity. If each method for measuring dietary intake is imperfect, and asking questions about diet perturbs normal intake patterns, the issue of standards becomes critical. Validation studies can only compare data obtained by one imperfect method to those obtained by another; it is not surprising, therefore, that results obtained by different methods are sometimes poorly correlated with one another.[14,25,126] These problems also help to explain why no "gold standard" of dietary intake measurement has yet been identified.[86]

Of particular concern is the number of days of dietary intake measurements necessary to achieve an acceptable approximation of usual dietary intake. A careful examination of this question in a study that collected food records for 29 individuals for 365 days, found that the day-to-day variation in the dietary intake of any one individual exceeded the variation between members of the group.[85] The data from this study permitted calculation of the number of days of records that would be required to provide an estimate of usual dietary intake, defined in this case as within 10% of the average intake for the year. The number of records needed to predict usual intake varied greatly within and between individuals. For any one individual, the number of days required varied from 31 for energy to 433 for vitamin A intake. For the group as a whole, the number of days required was much smaller, and varied from 3 for energy to 41 for vitamin A.[6] Therefore, one-day dietary intake measurements are unlikely to provide information on usual intake patterns.

IV. STANDARDS OF DIETARY ADEQUACY

In order to know whether dietary intake is adequate, it must be measured against an appropriate standard. An ideal diet should provide food energy and essential nutrients within ranges that are optimal for health. Because nutritional problems involve conditions of undernutrition as well as overnutrition, several types of standards are used to assess dietary adequacy.

A. RECOMMENDED DIETARY ALLOWANCES

In the U.S., estimates of levels of nutrient intake "adequate to meet the known nutritional needs of practically all healthy persons" are published at approximately five-year intervals by the National Research Council as RDA. The 1989 edition recommends specific levels of intake for protein, 11 vitamins, and 7 minerals according to age, body size, gender, and developmental stage. The 1989 edition also presents estimates of "safe and adequate" intake ranges for seven additional nutrients for which research is too limited to define an RDA. Allowances for energy, however, reflect average needs of individuals of varying heights and weights, ages, and activity levels.[94] These standards are similar to those of other industrialized countries, but typically exceed standards for populations of developing nations.[23]

Because RDAs are used in the U.S. to assess dietary adequacy, to interpret food consumption records, and to evaluate the nutritional status of individuals and populations, their limitations require careful attention.[51,112] In interpreting comparisons to RDAs, it is useful to understand that the research on which they are based is rarely complete and often uncertain. Moreover, the RDAs are established at levels that exceed the requirements of 97% of the population; most individuals can meet nutrient requirements at lower levels of intake. Because they are designed to prevent deficiencies, the RDAs do not address issues of overconsumption or of risks for chronic disease.

B. QUANTITATIVE DIETARY GOALS

Until the mid-1970s, federal and health agencies in the U.S. advised the public to select diets from specific groups of foods (e.g., dairy; meat; fruits and vegetables; grains) in order to assure adequate intake of nutrients most likely to be consumed at below-standard levels.[58] As recognition that the role of diet in chronic diseases has increased,[93,144] the focus of recommendations has shifted to the prevention of these conditions.[84]

The first U.S. report to reflect this new focus established percentage targets for dietary changes to reduce chronic disease risks. The report, *Dietary Goals for the U.S.,* called for reduced intake of fat (to 30% or less of total energy), saturated fat (to 10%), sugar (to 10%), cholesterol (to 300 mg/day or less), and salt (to 5 g/day); it also called for increased intake of foods containing starch, fiber, and naturally-occurring sugars (to 48% of energy). In addition, the Dietary Goals report included calls to moderate alcohol intake, and to maintain appropriate body weight by balancing energy intake and expenditure. To achieve these goals, the public was advised to consume more fruits, vegetables, and grains, and to select meat and dairy foods low in fat.[120] Since publication of that report, similar percentage targets have been adopted by health associations and government agencies throughout the world.[20] Moreover, these goals have remained remarkably unchanged over time and are considered universal in the sense that they apply equally well to prevention of virtually all diet-related chronic conditions.[93,144]

C. QUALITATIVE DIETARY GUIDELINES

To help the public translate the numerical targets of dietary goals into diets that provide sufficient energy and nutrients, yet minimize dietary risks for chronic disease, federal agencies have developed the *Dietary Guidelines for Americans.* The current guidelines, which represent a statement of federal nutrition policy, are to "eat a variety of foods; maintain healthy weight; choose a diet low in fat, saturated fat, and cholesterol; choose a diet with plenty of vegetables, fruits, and grain products; use sugars in moderation; use salt and sodium in moderation; if you drink alcoholic beverages, do so in moderation."[141]

To help individuals translate these recommendations into appropriate food choices, the USDA developed the *Food Guide Pyramid.* This guide recommends that the daily diet contain 6 to 11 portions of cereal foods, 2 to 4 of fruits,

3 to 5 of vegetables, 2 to 3 of meats or meat substitutes, and 2 to 3 of dairy foods.[139]

Thus, assessment of the adequacy of current and past diets can be measured against nutrient standards (the RDAs); macronutrient intake as a percent of energy (Dietary Goals); dietary patterns of energy, fat, saturated fat, cholesterol, carbohydrate, sugar, salt, and alcohol consumption (Dietary Guidelines); or the number of daily servings of foods from various groups (the Pyramid).

V. TRENDS IN FAT CONSUMPTION

In July 1988, the *Surgeon General's Report on Nutrition and Health* identified overconsumption of fat as a national priority for dietary change.[144] The report, however, provided no information on trends in fat consumption that could be used to confirm the need for dietary change or to serve as a basis for the evaluation of intervention strategies. This omission was the result of a decision by the report's oversight committee that existing survey methods did not provide sufficient information from which to draw scientifically valid conclusions about time trends in fat consumption.[97] When published, the report described the major monitoring surveys but drew no inferences for either long- or short-term trends in intake of fat or other nutrients. Discrepancies among trends that emerged from food supply, dietary intake, and meta-analysis data are among the reasons that led to that omission.

A. FOOD SUPPLY

Food supply data for the past 20 years document an overall increase in the availability of total fat, nearly all of which can be accounted for by increased use of polyunsaturated vegetable oils and their partial substitution for fats from animal sources. From 1970 to 1990, total fat availability fluctuated from 155 to 171 g/capita/day;[108] it increased by 4 g/capita/day from 1980 to 1990.[107] Use of saturated fats has fluctuated around 60 g/capita/day, and monounsaturated at about 66 g/capita/day during this entire period. The availability of polyunsaturated fat, however, rose from 27 to 32 g/capita/day, reflecting an increase in the supply of salad and cooking oils from 15.4 lbs/capita/year in 1970 to 25.6 lbs/capita/year in 1992.[108]

Another USDA study used food supply data to examine trends in the types of foods that were major contributors to total fat and to various fatty acids during the period from 1909–1914 to 1988.[109] These data are summarized in Table 2. In 1909–1914, the most important food sources of total fat were meat (36.1%), dairy foods (14.9%), and fats and oils (38.2%). By 1988, the proportion from meat and dairy foods had dropped to 31.7% and 11.7%, respectively, while that from fats and oils had increased to 46.5%. Within these categories, the proportion of total fat from beef, pork, and lamb dropped, as did that from whole milk, butter, and lard and beef tallow. On the other hand, the proportion from cheese, margarine, shortening, and salad and cooking oils increased. The most profound shifts occurred in the supply of butter (a decrease from 14.4 to 2.7%), margarine (an increase from 1.2 to 6.2%), and salad and cooking oils (an increase from 1.9 to 20.0%). Taken together, the data indicate that foods of animal origin — meat, dairy, butter, lard, and beef tallow — accounted for 75.2% of the total fat in the 1909–1914 food supply, but for only 48.0% of the supply in 1988.

Sources of saturated fat also changed to some extent during that period. The proportion from whole milk, butter, and lard and beef tallow decreased, while the proportion from cheese, margarine, shortening, and salad and cooking oils increased. Overall, foods from animal sources constituted 86.7% of the saturated fat in the 1909–1914 food supply, but only 67% in 1988.

The largest shifts in sources of monounsaturated fatty acids during that period also occurred as a result of decreased use of meat, whole milk, butter, and lard, and increased use of cheese, margarine, shortening, and salad and cooking oils. These changes, especially a sharply increased contribution from salad and cooking oils from 7.5 to 48.0%, also accounted for shifts in sources of polyunsaturated fatty acids.

Taken together, food supply data indicate an overall increase in availability of total fat, nearly all of which can be accounted for by the increasing avail-

TABLE 2
Principle Food Contributors to Total Fat and to Various Fatty
Acids in the U.S. Food Supply, 1909–1988

	Percentage of Total in Food Supply							
			Fatty Acids					
	Total Fat		**Saturated**		**Monounsaturated**		**Polyunsaturated**	
	1909–1914	**1988**	**1909–1914**	**1988**	**1909–1914**	**1988**	**1909–1914**	**1988**
Meat, total	36.1	31.7	37.8	39.9	40.9	35.1	31.8	17.2
Beef, pork lamb	33.5	25.4	36.3	35.0	38.2	28.8	26.5	10.2
Dairy, total	14.9	11.7	20.2	20.2	10.7	8.2	5.0	1.9
Milk, whole	8.8	2.6	12.0	4.5	6.4	1.9	3.0	0.5
Cheese	1.3	4.8	1.9	8.6	0.9	3.4	0.4	0.2
Fats & Oils, t.	38.2	46.5	36.5	32.4	40.9	47.5	31.9	68.7
Butter	14.4	2.7	19.6	4.7	10.4	1.9	5.0	0.5
Margarine	1.2	6.2	0.9	3.3	1.6	6.5	1.5	10.4
Shortening	8.9	15.8	4.9	13.4	14.1	21.5	5.6	9.0
Hard beef tallow	11.8	1.9	10.1	2.2	13.3	2.1	12.3	0.8
Salad and cooking oils	1.9	20.0	1.1	8.8	1.3	15.5	7.5	48.0

From Raper, N. R., Zizza, C., and Rourke, M., *Home Econ. Res. Rep.,* 50, 1992.[109]

TABLE 3
Percent of Calories from Fat, Saturated Fat, and Polyunsaturated
Fat from Five Surveys of Women Ages 19–50 Years,
United States 1971–1986

Variable	Age Group	% of Total kcal[1]				
		NHANES I 1971–1974	NHANES II 1976–1980	NFCS 1977	CSFII 1985	CSFII 1986
Fat	19–34	36.1	35.9	40.4	36.2	36.1
	35–50	37.0	36.8	41.3	37.2	36.7
	All	36.5	36.3	40.8	36.6	36.4
Saturated fat	19–34	12.9	12.6	—[2]	13.1	13.4
	35–50	13.3	12.8	—	13.4	13.1
	All	13.1	12.7	—	13.2	13.3
Polyunsaturated	19–34	4.2[3]	5.3[3]	—	7.2	6.9
fat	35–50	4.1[3]	5.5[3]	—	7.5	7.4
	All	4.2[3]	5.4[3]	—	7.3	7.1

Method	Response Rates %				
Interview	95	91	68[4]	58[4]	64[4]
Examination	74	73	—	—	—
Nonresponse bias assessment	Yes	Yes	No	No	Yes

[1]   Energy provided by fat was calculated using the general factor of 9 kcal/g.
[2]   Not reported.
[3]   Linoleic acid only.
[4]   Rates for first 24-hour recall.

From Life Sciences Research Office, Federation of American Societies for Experimental Biology, DHHS Publ. No. (PHS) 89-1255, 1989.[78]

ability of vegetable oils. At issue, is whether these oils are consumed. They have been used increasingly for frying foods served in fast food outlets, which discard an estimated 50% after use. Discarded fat is rendered for further use in animal feeds and pet foods, for industrial purposes, and for export. At least one study has estimated that these uses account for 9% of the total amount of fat in the food supply.[107]

B. DIETARY INTAKE
1. Method Comparisons
   Five national dietary surveys were conducted in the 1970s and 1980s (Table 3). Two of these surveys were conducted in overlapping years — the NHANES II in 1976–1980 and the NFCS in 1977. Although somewhat different sampling approaches were used, the intent of each survey was to produce nationally representative data on food and nutrient intake by the civilian, noninstitutionalized population.

Table 3 demonstrates a remarkable consistency in survey results related to consumption of fat, saturated fat, and polyunsaturated fat during the 15-year period. The single greatest deviation was the higher 1977 NFCS estimate for fat intake as a percent of energy. Because they provided data only for linoleic acid, NHANES I and II necessarily underestimated the percent of energy from polyunsaturated fatty acids. In contrast, the CSFII estimates reflected total intake of polyunsaturated fatty acids.

Table 3 also illustrates potential problems of nonresponse bias. Response rates for the interview and examination components of NHANES traditionally have exceeded those of the interview surveys conducted by USDA. The Table indicates that nearly one-fourth of the NHANES I and II subjects who appeared for interview did not participate in the examination components of the surveys. Because the NHANES dietary interviews were conducted in conjunction with the physical examination, the examination response rate is the appropriate comparison with the USDA household interview response rate.

NCHS investigators performed nonresponse bias analyses to determine whether there were systematic differences between responses of subjects who were interviewed and examined and those who only were interviewed; they found no evidence of bias. The USDA, however, did not perform nonresponse analyses for either the 1977 NFCS or the 1985 CSFII, even though the data could have been adjusted appropriately through sample weighting techniques. The USDA did compare the 1986 CSFII data to that from the 1986 population survey, and it conducted a follow-up survey of nonrespondents. This study identified differences that might be related to food intake patterns. With the exception of an overestimate of food stamp usage, the differences disappeared when adjusted for sample weights. The low response rate of the survey sample in the 1987–1988 NFCS, and the failure to correct for this problem, was the subject of a General Accounting Office conclusion that the integrity of USDA data was questionable.[43] Therefore, 1987–1988 NFCS data are not included in this discussion.

In all five surveys, estimates of fat and cholesterol intakes were obtained from 24-hour recalls. Table 4 illustrates sources of measurement error in the NHANES II of 1976–1980 and the NFCS of 1977–1978. Whereas NHANES II reported that 23% of respondents consumed less than 30% of energy from fat, the NFCS identified only 6% of respondents consuming this level of intake. An analysis of the possible contributions of measurement errors to this discrepancy identified five possible sources of such errors.[154] The most apparent difference between the two surveys was that the NHANES II was based on a single 24-hour recall, while the NFCS data represented the average of three days of observation drawn from one 24-hour recall, and two follow-up days of diet diaries. Because of these differences, the analysis was based solely on comparisons of 24-hour recalls in the two surveys. It revealed differences in the food composition database, in the contribution of certain foods to fat intake, in the ways interviews and coding were performed, in performance of interviews

TABLE 4
Comparisons of Fat Intakes for Persons 1–74 Years,
NHANES II and NFCS

	Mean Fat Intake, g	% kcal From Fat	% Respondents Below 30% kcal From Fat
NHANES II, 24-hour	80	36	23
NFCS, 3-day	86	41	6

on weekends, and in reports of alcoholic beverage consumption. For example, for NHANES II, NCHS developed its own food composition database from various USDA handbooks and from information provided by the food industry. For the NFCS, the USDA developed its own food composition database using one of its handbooks and food industry information.

The effects of adjustments of these differences on energy, fat, and percent energy from fat in NHANES II and NFCS are illustrated in Table 5. In NHANES II, respondents were probed as to whether they trimmed visible fat from meat or consumed poultry skin. In NFCS, if respondents did not specify whether they trimmed fat or ate poultry skin, they were assigned a code that assumed that they consumed a certain amount of visible fat. The result of this difference was that the majority of NHANES II respondents reported that they avoided visible fat, whereas the majority of NFCS respondents were assumed to eat visible fat. Since some of the respondents were likely to have avoided visible fat, but were not reported as doing so, the NFCS estimate is most probably too low. NHANES II did not interview or examine respondents on weekends, whereas NFCS conducted daily interviews and probed differences in food habits between weekends and weekdays. Adjusting the NFCS data for weekend consumption reduces both the mean fat intake and the percent energy from fat.

Finally, NHANES II reported higher alcoholic beverage consumption than did the NFCS. Alcohol intake contributed to the higher energy estimates for

TABLE 5
Effects of Adjustments on Energy, Fat and % kcal
from Fat for Persons 1–74 Years

	kcal	Fat, g	% kcal From Fat
NFCS, original	1,884	86	41
Convert all meat and poultry to lean only or without skin	−84	−11	38
Remove data for weekends	−13	−1	38
Remove kcal from alcoholic beverages	−23	0	38
NFCS, adjusted	1,764	74	38
NHANES II, adjusted	1,969	80	37

NHANES and to the difference in percent energy from fat. When the results are also adjusted for the energy contributed by alcohol, almost all of the differences disappear; the adjusted surveys differ only by about 200 kcal and 6 g of fat, and produce nearly identical estimates of percent energy from fat.

2. NHANES I to NHANES II

Investigators have used data from NHANES I and II to estimate changes in fat and energy intake from 1971–1974 to 1976–1980.[122] For white and black men and women, they compared energy intake in kilocalories; total fat, saturated fat, and linoleic acid as percent of energy; and cholesterol intake in milligrams. Data from this study indicated little change in any of these measures, except for an approximately 10% decline in cholesterol intake among the groups. This study also examined changes in food groups during that period, and reported consistent decreases in intake of dairy products, meats, eggs, and fats and oils. Food composition data for vegetables in NHANES I, however, assumed the addition of saturated fat from butter when respondents did not specify how vegetables were prepared; those from NHANES II assumed the addition of margarine. This change suggests the need for caution in interpretation of the apparent increase in linoleic acid and decrease in saturated fat observed in Table 3.[78]

Because serum cholesterol values were also obtained in the survey, the investigators were able to calculate the change in serum cholesterol that would be predicted by the equations of Keys et al.[66] and Hegsted et al.[54] The direction and magnitude of the observed changes were similar to those predicted from these equations. From these data, therefore, the investigators concluded that intake of energy, total fat, and saturated fat had not changed significantly during that period, and that changes in mean consumption of fat and cholesterol do indeed influence serum cholesterol levels in predictable ways.

3. NHANES II to NHANES III

The first phase of NHANES III was conducted from October 1988 to October 1991. Originally designed to sample 30,000 persons,[152] this phase eventually included interviews of 86% of an original sample of about 20,000 persons (17,467 individuals), and physical examination of 77% (15,630 persons). Of those examined, 14,801 individuals completed 24-hour recalls that were considered complete and reliable. These data were analyzed for total energy, total dietary fat, and saturated fat as a basis for drawing inferences about levels of consumption of these items for the entire U.S. population, by age group, from 2 to 11 months to more than 80 years old.[73]

For the adult population over the age of 2 (13,314 persons), daily energy intake averaged 2,095 kcal. Of this amount, 33.9% was derived from total fat, and 11.9% from saturated fat. These results did not differ significantly by sex, and represent a decrease from the levels observed in NHANES I and II and in the NFCS.

In the report of these findings, the investigators implied that the data for NHANES III were likely to be more reliable than those of the previous surveys. They cited three changes in dietary methods to substantiate this view: the use of automated data collection to improve data standardization, specific design of the protocol to probe for food sources of fat, and inclusion in the interview of additional questions to ensure more complete dietary recall. The survey used a different food composition database from that used in NHANES II, however, thereby impairing comparability. This study found energy intakes to be 100 to 300 kcal higher for persons above age 12, as compared with the results of NHANES II. Whether this increase is a true trend, consistent with increasing rates of obesity in the U.S.,[89] or an artifact resulting from methodologic improvements, is uncertain at this time.

4. Meta-Analysis

One meta-analysis of assessments of energy and fat intake identified 171 studies drawn from more than 300 publications between 1920 and 1984. These studies had collected information on the dietary intake of nearly 118,000 individuals of various age groups, occupations, physical conditions, and ethnic backgrounds, by means of a variety of recall, record, and duplicate meal methods. In analyzing these studies, the investigators identified levels of energy and fat intake, computed the percent of energy from fat, and plotted these data by year, after applying a number of correction factors to make the data more comparable.

The result of this analysis was a plot of percent energy intake from fat as a function of time. The graph indicated a gradual rise in fat intake from 32% kcal in 1920 to a peak of 40 to 42% in the mid-1950s followed by a gradual decline to about 36% in 1984.[128] The investigators cited this trend as associated with the fall in coronary heart disease rates that has been evident since the mid-1950s. They predicted that the percentage would be in the range of 30 to 35% kcal by 1990, as indeed was found in NHANES III.[73]

Because the dietary intake methods and sample populations differed so widely among the 171 studies, it is difficult to know whether this trend is real or a result of random or systematic errors in data collection, reporting, or analysis.

C. SUMMARY: DIETARY FAT

This discussion illustrates the difficulties involved in drawing conclusions about trends in dietary intake. Food supply data indicate that the per capita availability of fat has increased. Some proportion of this fat may not be eaten, however, and the data reflect a decrease in contribution to total fat from animal fats, and an increase from vegetable oils. Survey data and the meta-analysis indicate that fat intakes remained fairly constant during the 1970s, and may have been decreasing slowly since that time. The survey data are generally consistent in direction of change within sex and age categories. As illustrated by the comparisons between NFCS and NHANES data, measurement of dietary fat intake is particularly problematic, but the dietary trend can be validated by examination of concurrent external trends in blood cholesterol levels and in cardiovascular disease mortality. Blood cholesterol levels have declined significantly since the 1970s,[88] and both the magnitude and direction of that change can be predicted on the basis of the small observed changes in dietary fat and cholesterol. Cardiovascular disease mortality also has declined steadily during that period of time.[89] Therefore, our overall conclusion is that the data support a weak trend toward lower intake of dietary fat.

VI. TRENDS IN ANTIOXIDANT CONSUMPTION

As noted earlier, dietary recommendations for disease prevention and health promotion emphasize the importance of consuming large proportions of energy from fruits, vegetables, and grains. In recent years, in response to numerous research studies identifying protective effects of plant antioxidants against cancer and other chronic diseases, increasing attention has focused on the need to increase overall intake of these substances among the general population. As might be expected, manufacturers of dietary supplements have led this effort, but they have been strongly supported by many researchers impressed by the weight of the evidence supporting a wide range of health benefits stemming from adequate antioxidant consumption.[69]

At issue in these efforts is whether typical diets supply amounts of antioxidants sufficient to produce protective benefits. During the 1970s, a milestone of sorts was passed in the evolution of the U.S. food supply. At some point during that decade, more than half the foods purchased shifted from fresh agricultural products to processed foods.[145] This shift has had only a minor influence on the types and sources of antioxidants in the food supply, however, mainly because a significant proportion of the population takes nutrient supplements.

Despite the high level of academic and commercial interest in these substances, information about the levels of antioxidants in foods, and the resulting population exposure to these substances is surprisingly scanty. Multiple sources of data provide information about nutrient and nonnutrient antioxidants in the food supply: USDA food supply data, the FDA's Food Additives Survey, the NCHS's Health Interview Survey, the various USDA and DHHS dietary intake surveys, and data derived from these surveys on dietary patterns. Because data are most readily available for vitamins C and E and the carotenoids, this discussion focuses on those nutrients.

A. FOOD SUPPLY DATA

Table 6 presents data on the food supply of antioxidant vitamins from 1970 to 1990,[108] as compared to the most recent RDA.[94] These data suggest that the per capita annual availability of antioxidant nutrients changed very little during

TABLE 6
Antioxident Vitamins in the U. S. Food Supply,
1970–1990, as Compared to the 1989 RDA

Antioxidant Vitamin	1970	1990	RDA 1989
Vitamin A, R.E.[a]	1,550	1,480	800–1000[b]
Carotenes, R.E.	500	620	—[c]
Vitamin E., mg alpha-TE	13.4	15.7	8–10
Vitamin C, mg	108	105	60

[a]   Given in μg R.E.: 1 R.E. is equivalent to 1 μg retinol or 6 μg beta-carotene.
[b]   The lower figure is for adult females, the higher for adult males; see reference 94.
[c]   Not established.

From Putnam, J. J. and Allshouse, J. E., *Stat. Bull.*, 867, 1993.[108]

that 20-year period. The slight decline in vitamin A (preformed retinol) availability, which can be attributed to a decrease in the supply of meat (see Table 2), has been offset by an increase in beta-carotene due to an increase in the supply of dark green and deep yellow vegetables. Vitamin E availability has increased steadily since the early 1900s, a trend that can be entirely attributed to increased availability of vegetable oils, especially during the past decades as illustrated in Table 2. Because oils used for frying foods are not necessarily consumed, it is uncertain whether the apparent increase in vitamin E intake represents increased consumption. The slight decrease in availability of vitamin C is due to an overall decline in the use of vegetables, particularly potatoes, although the decline is almost completely offset by the increased supply of citrus fruit.[109] For all of these nutrients, the per capita supply of antioxidant nutrients is much higher than RDA levels.[94]

B. FOOD ADDITIVES SURVEY

The Food Additives Survey is conducted by the National Research Council's Food and Nutrition Board, under a contract from the FDA, to monitor use of substances Generally Recognized as Safe (GRAS).[33] It was conducted six times since 1970, most recently in 1987. The survey has two components; it assesses poundage and level of use. In the poundage survey, companies report the total pounds of each additive used within a calendar year.[22] In the level-of-use surveys, the Food and Nutrition Board estimates consumer exposure to food additives by food categories, as well as by total pounds used.

The 1987 Food Additives Survey reported that 46 different substances were added to the food supply to achieve "antioxidant technical effects." Of these, eight were nutrient antioxidants derived from vitamin C or vitamin E. Table 7 lists the number of pounds of nutrients used in 1987, pounds of derivatives, and the pounds of two nonnutrient antioxidants used that year. As shown in Table

7, the number of pounds of antioxidants varied from as little as 35 lbs of alpha-tocopherol to 3,900,000 lbs of ascorbic acid. Beta-carotene is also a food additive, but is used mainly as a colorant, as in margarine. In 1987, 3,660,000 lbs of beta-carotene were added to the food supply.

When converted to amounts per capita per day, however, nutrient antioxidants added to the food supply made only a negligible contribution. For example, the 3,900,000 lbs of ascorbic acid added per year translate into only an additional 0.02 mg/capita/day. The addition of this substance, however, plays a very important role in combating oxidative degradation of food and in reducing the ingestion of oxidized lipids.

Most (38 of the 46) antioxidants added to food were nonnutrients. The chemical composition of these substances is highly diverse, and the amounts available per capita are relatively small. The amounts of butylated hydroxyanisole (BHA) and butylated hydroxytoluene (BHT) used in 1987 (Table 7) contributed only 0.000044 mg and 0.002 mg, respectively, per person per day.

Table 8 displays changes in the use of antioxidant food additives for nutrient and technical purposes between 1982 and 1987.[151] These data indicate a large increase in the use of vitamin A, mainly for technical purposes; the use of vitamin A as a nutrient additive declined by 79% during that period. The overall decline in use of vitamin A and C has been attributed to substitution during this period of unenriched soft drinks for vitamin-fortified milk or fruit juices. The reason for the decline in use of vitamin E for both nutrient and antioxidant purposes is uncertain.

C. NATIONAL HEALTH INTERVIEW SURVEY

The 1986 Health Interview Survey, conducted by the NCHS, provided the most recent and complete information on the use of nutrient supplements by the

TABLE 7
Food Additive Antioxidents in 1987

	Pounds Used
Nutrient	
Ascorbic Acid	3,900,000
Ascorbyl Palmitate	330
Sodium Ascorbate	1,300,000
D-a-Tocopherol	55
D-a-Tocopherol Acetate	119,000
DL-a-Tocopherol	231,000
Tocopherals Concentrated, Mixed	6,100
Nonnutrient	
Butylated Hydroxyanisole	86,000
Butylated Hydroxytoluene	402,000

From Committee on Food Additives Survey Data, 1987 Poundage and technical effects update of substances added to food, 1989.[22]

TABLE 8
Commercial Use of Antioxident Food
Additives, 1982–1987

Antioxidant	Pounds × 1000		
	1982	1987	% Change
Vitamin A	2,621	4,087	+156
Vitamin E	1,320	497	−62
Vitamin C	6,691	3,548	−46

From Waslien, C. I. and Rehwoldt, R. E., Nutr. Today, July/August, 36, 1990.[151]

U.S. population.[61,87] It sampled nearly 12,000 adults.[8] Its questions and procedures on vitamin and mineral supplement use were designed to be similar to those used in the 1980 FDA Vitamin and Mineral Supplement Use Survey, thereby permitting comparisons.[8,61] From 1980 to 1986, overall use of supplements dropped slightly from 42 to 38%, although the proportion of individuals who were considered "light" users of supplements (those who take one-a-day, broad-spectrum types) increased from 42 to 57%. Table 9 displays changes in intake levels of antioxidant nutrients during that period, expressed as percent RDA. Among respondents who took broad-spectrum supplements, intake levels rose from 170 to 219% of the RDA, an overall increase of 29%. The amounts of vitamin E and C taken as specialized supplements, however, dropped by 28 and 18%, respectively. The number of supplements reported taken also decreased from an average of 2.15 per day to 1.77.[8]

The 1986 survey found that more women (41%) used supplements than men (31%). Women of ages 45 to 64 were found to be the highest users. Approximately 43% of children two to six years of age were reported as regular supplement users. More than 70% of all vitamin and mineral products used by

TABLE 9
Change in Intake of Antioxidant Supplements, 1980–1986

	1980	1986	% Change
Broad-spectrum supplements			
Vitamin A, % RDA	170	219	29
Specialized supplements			
Vitamin E, % RDA	1,198	862	−28
Vitamin C, % RDA	757	622	−18
Products used, number/day	2.15	1.77	−18
Broad-spectrum	0.75	0.63	−16
Specialized	1.40	1.14	−19

From Bender, M. M., Levy, A. S., Schucker, R. E., and Yetley, E. A., *J. Am. Diet Assoc.*, 92, 1096, 1992.[8]

adults and young children were taken every day. Most users (24% of adults and 38% of children) were reported to take broad-spectrum supplements;[87] only 15% of adults and 6% of children in the U.S. had taken a specialized product during the 2 weeks prior to their interview.

Approximately 30% of adults and 40% of children were found to take supplements that contained vitamin C, and 26% of adults and 37% of children were taking products containing vitamin E.[87] For adults, the median amount of vitamin C was 250% of the RDA, and the 95th percentile was more than 2,000% of the RDA. The median amount of vitamin E was 200% of the RDA, and the 95th percentile was more than 2,800% of the RDA. For children, the median percent RDA was 167% for vitamin E and 133% for vitamin C, with 95th percentiles of 400% and 769%, respectively. Thus, dietary supplements make a major contribution to intakes of vitamins C and E among users of these products.

One study has compared data from the 1987 NHIS to those from previous studies of supplement usage. Although the methods used in those studies differed, their results suggest that levels of supplement use did not change substantially during the previous 20 years. This study found that 23.1% of respondents took a daily supplement, a result comparable to that found in both NHANES I (21.4%) and NHANES II (22.8%), using the same definition. The higher levels reported in the 1986 NHIS could well have resulted from its broader definition of use as at least once in the previous 14 days. Response rates to a similar definition in the 1987 NHIS were similar to those of the 1986 survey. These differences in definition resulted in an increase of nearly 16% in the proportion of respondents classified as regular supplement users.[129]

D. DIETARY INTAKE SURVEYS

Dietary intake of vitamin E was first assessed in the CSFII of 1985. This study found that the mean intake by women 20 to 49 years of age was 7.0 mg of alpha-tocopherol equivalents, and by children 1 to 5 years of age, 5.5 mg — both barely at RDA levels. The same survey first estimated carotenoid intakes: mean intakes by women were estimated at 353 RE, and children 252 RE, substantially below RDA levels.[94]

As shown in Table 10, four surveys since 1971 have estimated vitamin C intakes. These surveys indicate a slight upward trend in intake of vitamin C from the early 1970s through the mid-1980s, but the increase is not consistent among all age groups. The mean intakes, however, exceed the RDAs for all of the age and sex groups examined. These same surveys indicate that intake of vitamin A increased from the early 1970s to the late 1980s among all of the age and sex groups.[78]

E. DIETARY PATTERNS

In general, intakes of vitamins C and E and of carotenoids increase with income and education levels, and are higher among whites than blacks, reflecting higher intakes of fruits and vegetables. Similarly, supplement users tend to

TABLE 10
Vitamin C Intakes, 1971–1986

Age (yr)	NHANES I 1971–1974	NFCS 1977–1978	NHANES II 1976–1980	CSFII 1985–1986
1–2	71	66	88	81
3–5	82	71	100	81
Male				
20–29	102	89	118	107
30–39	78	84	102	104
40–49	84	86	98	124
Female				
20–29	80	74	95	86
30–39	76	73	86	86
40–49	79	78	91	81

From Life Sciences Research Office, Federation of American Societies for Experimental Biology, DHHS Publ. No. (PHS) 89-1255, 1989.[78]

be white and to reside in households with incomes above $40,000 in which at least one adult has some college education.

Despite current recommendations to increase fruit and vegetable consumption, the majority of the population consumes far less than the recommended number of daily servings. One analysis of data from NHANES II found that 83% of adults reported consuming vegetables and 59% reported consuming fruits on the day before their survey interview.[99] Only 21%, however, reported eating fruits or vegetables high in vitamin A (presumably, carotenoids), and 28% reported eating foods high in vitamin C. When these data were examined by tertile of the poverty index ratio, whites and blacks in the lowest tertile had lower intakes of fruits and vegetables high in vitamins A and C. Individuals in the highest income tertiles reported the highest intakes, but even then, the proportion consuming fruits and vegetables was below 50%. These results were similar to those of reported in the 1977–1978 NFCS.[26]

1. Serum Antioxidant Levels

Dietary patterns, use of supplements, and other lifestyle variables can affect serum levels of antioxidant nutrients.[155] NHANES II, for example, examined serum levels of vitamin C and reported that levels differed by age and sex. For children, mean levels decreased with age from a peak of about 1.5 mg/dl for those 3 to 5 years of age, to 1.1 mg/dl for those 15 to 17 years of age. Adult values remained fairly stable, with some increases observed in older groups. Males were found to have lower mean serum levels than females throughout adulthood.

The prevalence of very low vitamin C levels in serum (<0.25 mg/dl) was less than 3%, but it varied considerably among subpopulations. Rates of low serum vitamin C were much higher among adults who smoked cigarettes and did not take nutrient supplements than might be expected from their representation in the population. For males, 34% were current cigarette smokers who did not regularly use supplements. Among this group, 71% exhibited low serum vitamin C. The comparable figures for women were 25% and 61%. In contrast, regular supplement users consituted approximately 20% of the population, but less than 2% of the low serum vitamin C group. For women, regular supplement users constituted 28% of the population, and less than 8% of the low serum vitamin C group. Dietary intakes of vitamin C-containing foods, as well as serum vitamin C levels, were higher among the supplement users and the nonsmokers.[155]

2. Variables Affecting Intake

Additional variables, such as age, living alone, or poverty, have been found to influence intake of vitamin C. For example, the elderly living alone are at risk of poor dietary patterns. One study of older adults found that the best dietary patterns were associated with living with a spouse, especially for men. Living alone, or in some arrangement other than with a spouse, was related to lower intakes of fruits and vegetables. Poverty increased the likelihood of poor fruit and vegetable intake regardless of living arrangement. As shown in Table 11, 5 to 10% of older women with incomes above the poverty level consumed fewer than one fruit or vegetable per day as compared to 20 to 40% of older men living in poverty.[116]

F. SUMMARY: ANTIOXIDANT TRENDS

Gaps in the data make it difficult to generalize about trends in antioxidant consumption. Food supply data and the limited data on dietary intake and supplement use suggest that levels of vitamins E and the carotenoids have increased since the 1970s. The increase in vitamin E levels in the food supply is directly attributable to the steady increase in use of vegetable oils since the

TABLE 11
Fruit and Vegetable Intakes of Older Adults

	Living Arrangement		
	Alone	**With Spouse**	**Other**
Men below poverty	38.7	21.8	40.8
Men above poverty	26.6	12.2	22.4
Women below poverty	14.4	12.1	23.7
Women above poverty	5.9	5.3	9.8

From Ryan, A. S., Martinez, G. A., Wysong, J. L., and Davis, M. A., *Am. J. Human Biol.,* 1, 321, 1989.[116]

early 1900s, but there is some question as to whether this change is reflected in dietary intake, and data on this point are unavailable. The food supply data indicate a slight decrease in availability of vitamin C since the 1970s, but surveys of dietary intake indicate that vitamin C levels have increased since the 1970s as a result of greater use of supplements, vitamin-C rich foods, and food fortification. The increased intake is not consistent among all age and sex groups, however. Unfortunately, trend data on blood levels of vitamins E, C, or carotenoids are not available, and there are no meta-analyses. Beyond these surveys, there are no other reliable trend indicators that can be used for external validation. Therefore, we conclude that there has been a weak upward trend in the intake of antioxidant nutrients.

VII. FACTORS THAT AFFECT DIETARY TRENDS

Although food selection might appear to be a simple matter of personal choice, trends in the ways foods have been produced, distributed, and marketed throughout this century have greatly affected dietary intake patterns; individuals make food choices within the context of the social, economic, and cultural environment in which they live.[5] As a general rule, adults prefer foods that taste, look, and smell good,[115] are familiar,[103] and provide variety,[111] but these preferences are influenced strongly by family and ethnic background, levels of education, and factors related to income, age, and gender. Food availability, advertising, and the demand for convenience also affect dietary intake. The many factors that help to determine food choices have been reviewed recently.[131] Because many of these factors are subjective, the precise nature and extent of their influence has proven difficult to measure or to evaluate.

A. FOOD SYSTEM ECONOMICS
In 1991, the U.S. food marketing system had almost $750 billion in sales, with nearly $570 billion in retail food sales and $85 billion in sales of alcoholic beverages.[40] In 1989, only 24 cents out of every food dollar was spent for the food's farm value — the food itself. The rest went for added value such as service, packaging, transportation, fuel, rents, repairs, advertising, and profit. The profit share amounted to 2.5 cents.[13] By 1992, the farm value had dropped to 22 cents on the dollar. Increased labor costs and an increase in before-tax profits to 3.5 cents accounted for the relative increase in marketing costs.[31]

1. Agricultural Production
The system of food production in the United States has changed markedly since the early years of the century. In the mid-1930s, there were 6.5 million farms throughout the country, but only 2.3 million in 1985. The average size of farms, however, increased from 155 to 437 acres during this period.[82] In 1970, 4% of all employed persons worked in farming and agricultural services,

but this figure had declined to 2% by 1985.[142] Changes in the structure of agricultural markets have occurred in parallel with those in farming. In 1919, there were 68,000 food manufacturing companies in the U.S., but their number declined to 36,000 in 1947, and to 19,000 in 1985; this consolidation has occurred in parallel with the growth of large corporations and the disappearance of many local milk dealers and bakeries.

Such changes have led to greater efficiency in production. Output per farm worker, for example, doubled between 1810 and 1880 and again by the early 1940s; it has risen sixfold since 1950. These production increases have resulted from expansion of agricultural lands and shifts among crops; improvements in farm management, and pest control; and advances in applied genetics. Genetic advances alone are thought be responsible for 65- to 450-fold increases in yields per acre of corn, tomatoes, and other crops.[142]

These changes have resulted in massive overproduction of food in the U.S. By the early 1900s, Americans already had enough food to eat, and could not be persuaded to eat more. This meant that the choice of any one food commodity would have to occur at the expense of another.[74] Today, the U.S. food system supplies an average of 3,700 kcal per capita per day,[108] an amount nearly twice that required by the average woman, and a third higher than that required by the average man.[94] This overabundance has created intense marketing competition for consumer food dollars.

2. Marketing Trends

In 1939, 67% of foods for home use were purchased in grocery or other food stores and only 6% were purchased in supermarkets. By 1982, only 20% were purchased in grocery and food stores, and supermarkets accounted for 67% of food purchases for home use.[82] From 1978 to 1986, the average number of items in a supermarket rose from under 12,000 to over 20,000.[36] Today, most large supermarkets stock 25,000 to 35,000 separate food items.[41]

3. New Product Introductions

In this highly competitive retail environment, manufacturers have produced increasing numbers of packaged, prepared, and convenience foods in efforts to increase their market share of consumer food purchases.[41] Many of these products were designed to take advantage of the reduction in preparation time accomplished by microwave cooking,[106] and other products have been packaged to increase shelf life as well as to be convenient. The number of dry-packaged dinner items, for example, increased by 19% between 1982 and 1987, with sales that increased from $470 to $783 million during that time.[9]

From 1982 to 1991, food processors introduced more than 90,000 new food products, most of them extensions of existing lines. In 1991 alone, food processors introduced nearly 12,400 new grocery products, an increase of nearly 20% over the previous year. Among new product introductions, condiments, candy and snacks, baked goods, soft drinks, and dairy products (mostly cheese and ice cream) accounted for 70%.

Many of these new products were developed in response to consumer concerns about health. In 1991, nearly 6,000 new food products advertised health claims, a threefold increase over 1988; most of these claims were for foods labeled as reduced in energy, fat, cholesterol, or salt.[41] By 1993, however, the number of such products had dropped nearly by half, for reasons that are uncertain.[2]

4. Food Advertising

Food advertising accounted for 4.5 cents on every food dollar in 1990.[130] Advertising has been shown to enhance the sales of food products to adults and to influence the eating habits of children.[21] It also has been shown to promote consumption of entire categories of foods, and to stimulate the production, processing, and marketing of new food products.[39,130] In 1991, food marketing firms spent nearly $12 billion in direct consumer advertising, and an additional $24 billion on retail promotion through trade shows, market promotions, discounts, coupons, and other incentives.[40] Expenditures on media advertising alone for food rose 230% from $2.3 to $7.6 billion in the decade from 1980 to 1990. The largest increase occurred in advertising for food consumed away from home; such expenditures rose from $121 million in 1980 to $2.6 billion in 1990.[130]

B. LIFESTYLE ISSUES

1. Work and Family Structure

From 1975 to 1988, the proportion of married women with children under six years of age who worked outside the home increased from 37 to 57%. In 1988, 52% of all mothers — and 72% of black mothers — of infants aged one year or under were in the labor force.[143] In addition, people are working longer and longer hours.[118] The traditional American family, consisting of husband, wife, and two children, now describes only a fourth of families in this country.[98] Such trends explain in part why convenience and speed in preparation have become principal driving forces for new product development as well as for food selection.[41,106]

Today, an increasing proportion of families is headed by a single, working parent, and that parent is more likely to be female. From 1970 to 1988, the number of female-headed households grew from 12 to 24% of all families with children under age 18. Up to 60% of all children born today are expected to spend some of their childhood in households headed by a single female.[38] In 1993, 27% of children under the age of 18 lived with a single parent who had never married, an increase of nearly 3 million children in this situation since 1983. The median family income in two-parent households was $43,578 that year; in contrast, in one-parent families where the mother was divorced, the median income was $17,014, and where the mother had never married, it was

$9,272.[57] Low-income households spend less money on food, although food expenses account for a greater share of their income.[38]

2. Meals Away from Home

Such trends also explain why increasing numbers of adults and children are consuming meals prepared outside the home in worksites, restaurants, and schools.[13] In 1962, 28% of every food dollar was spent on food eaten away from home; the share grew to over 37% in 1982,[15] and to 46% in 1989.[13] In 1939, 47% of meals consumed out of the home were eaten in restaurants, lunchrooms, and cafeterias and only 7% in fast food places. By 1982, 40% were eaten in restaurants, and meals in fast food places comprised 30%.[82] In the 1985 CSFII, meals consumed away from home accounted for 25 to 30% of food energy and nutrient intake by women aged 19 to 50 and 13 to 18% by their children aged 1 to 5 — an increase over the percentages observed in 1977.[136] This trend, which was similar for men,[137] has raised concerns about its effects on the nutritional quality of American diets,[15] particularly since sales of fast food alone accounted for 34% of meals consumed outside the home in 1990.[81]

Given this trend, the nutritional quality of institutional food service takes on increasing importance. Because of this trend, it will be necessary to focus educational and other interventions away from consumers, to whom they have been traditionally addressed, to food providers in restaurants, schools, worksites, hospitals, nursing homes, child care centers, and other institutions. Food service industry officials have noted that meals served in restaurants are increasingly reflecting health concerns and believe that customers will increasingly be demanding meals that meet dietary recommendations.[95]

3. Poverty

One in five children lives in a family with an income level below the federal poverty line.[91] Access to food and the nutritional quality of diets among such families are sources of great concern. Some studies have found reduced intakes of essential nutrients with decreasing income. For example, the 1985 CSFII survey reported that low income women consumed lower amounts of energy, vitamin B_6, calcium, magnesium, folacin, and vitamin E than women in higher income groups.[133] Understanding the effect of poverty on nutrient intake is made difficult by inconsistencies in the data; iron intake, for example, was not found to be related to poverty in women in the CSFII. The effect also is complicated by the relationship between food and nutrient intake. Although lower income households have less money to spend on food, and consume less food energy, they have been shown in at least one study to obtain more nutrients for each dollar spent than do higher income households.[100]

Because members of racial and ethnic minority groups are disproportionately poor in this country, they bear a disproportionate burden not only of undernutrition but also of chronic disease.[96] Their nutritional intake, therefore, is of special concern. The contribution of diet to chronic disease risk in these groups, however, is difficult to evaluate. Available data do not permit identification of consistent associations between dietary patterns and disease risk in minority populations; also, few consistent differences have been found in the dietary intake patterns of minority and majority populations.[70]

C. TASTE PREFERENCES

As might be expected, palatability, texture, and odor influence food selections,[113] as does the variety of foods available.[111] Exposure to foods, and the resulting familiarity with them affects the development of food preferences.[7,11,102,103,114] The food acceptance and preferences of children are affected by the eating behavior of their parents, other adults, siblings, and peers,[10] by positive reinforcement through praise, reward, recognition, or approval,[55] and by the social context in which foods are presented.[12,131] The food choices of adults also are influenced by peers.[127]

D. EDUCATION
1. Nutrition Knowledge

The U.S. public is increasingly well informed about the relationship between diet and health. In 1986, more than 90% of respondents to a telephone survey believed that reducing blood pressure, blood cholesterol levels, body weight, and intake of high-fat foods and salt might help prevent heart disease, and more than 60% believed that they could control high blood cholesterol by reducing intake of cholesterol, fat, luncheon meats, and eggs, by replacing meat with poultry and fish, and by substituting low-fat milk for whole milk.[119] In 1994, more than 90% of survey respondents agreed that balance, variety, and moderation were keys to healthy eating, and 80% agreed that eating fruits and vegetables could reduce cancer risk.[42]

2. Dietary Behavior

The translation of this knowledge into behavior, however, is less certain.[131] In 1992, 58% of shoppers reported that they had changed their diets during the past three years. Most likely to report such changes were women, individuals of middle age, and those who are most conscious of health. Of those who said they were making dietary changes, 44% said they were eating less fat, 32% said they were limiting sodium intake, and 27% reported reducing the amount of dietary cholesterol.[37] A 1993 survey reported that 64% of respondents said they were making an effort to consume fiber, 58% said they were limiting fat, 51% said they were limiting sodium, and 49% said they were limiting cholesterol.[105] Among respondents to a telephone survey in 1994, 71% said they were reducing dietary fat; among these, 36% reported eating more low-fat foods, and 23% reported reducing or eliminating meat.[42]

Although such surveys suggest that the public has become more aware of links between nutrition and health and that people increasingly report improvements in dietary choices, it has proven difficult to demonstrate a direct link between education and actual behavior change. Increases in nutrition knowledge are relatively easy to achieve and to document, but changes in attitudes and behavior are more resistant to change and more difficult to detect, especially in short-term studies. The difficulties of altering dietary behavior cannot be underestimated. Alterations in established dietary preferences may require deviations from accepted patterns of food intake and may be perceived as demanding increased skills, costs, or efforts in preparation.[47] The translation of knowledge into dietary practices takes place within an environment of food intake in the U.S. where convenience in eating takes precedence over nutritional quality; where meals are increasingly consumed from restaurant, fast food, and take-out establishments; and where the food industry actively produces, markets, and advertises alcohol and foods that are high in calories, fat, cholesterol, sugar, and salt.

3. Education Campaigns

Notwithstanding such problems, many studies that have examined the effectiveness of nutrition education have been able to demonstrate that nutrition education leads to increases in knowledge as well as to improvements in food choices.[64,131] Nutrition education has been shown to be an important factor in fostering dietary change in individuals with heart disease, hypertension, diabetes, and renal disease.[47] Small-scale public educational efforts also have proved successful; one supermarket campaign, for example, resulted in increased purchases of products containing reduced amounts of energy, fat, cholesterol, and sodium.[75] Health claims on the labels of such products promote sales.[76] In the U.S., broad public health campaigns such as the National High Blood Pressure Education Program have proven effective.[110] The National Cholesterol Education Program[90] and the National Cancer Institute's 5-A-Day campaign to increase fruit and vegetable consumption[53] also have the potential to reduce diet-related risks in large segments of the population.

Of special concern has been the need to address the dietary needs of pregnant women, infants, young children, and of elderly individuals — groups that are particularly vulnerable to nutritional deficiencies, especially when poor. Community-based, media-oriented public education ("social marketing") campaigns[62] that transmit culturally-sensitive messages[140] designed to address the needs and attitudes of specific target groups have been applied successfully to promote breastfeeding and other dietary improvements in developing countries.[83] In the U.S., these techniques have been used to improve the nutritional status of low-income homemakers,[1] to increase the prevalence of breastfeeding,[18] and to improve health and function in the elderly.[80] On the basis of preliminary results, dietary intervention studies that apply these techniques to chronic disease prevention among high-risk, minority groups also show promise.[48] In the long term, education methods that empower community members to determine their own dietary needs and decide on their own interventions are most likely to prove effective.[65]

4. Key Elements

One question that arises in these studies is whether education-induced dietary change is sustained over time. Research on this question has yielded inconsistent results. Most studies have suggested that long-term follow up is required to maintain dietary changes,[47] but some studies have reported continued improvements with time.[29]

Research on nutrition education has been limited by the lack of effective methods and theories.[29,124] Nevertheless, considerable information is available about the key elements that make educational interventions more effective. An analysis of 67 studies published between 1968 and 1983, for example, concluded that the most successful programs were those that designed strategies to change specific target behaviors, used specific instruments to measure such changes, used multiple methods to effect change, and allowed sufficient time for the changes to occur.[123] Other studies have defined the elements of effective nutrition intervention campaigns: they involve individuals and groups in the design, conduct, and evaluation of their own dietary plans, employ multiple strategies for conveying information, and use a team approach.[124] They also tend to base their information on previous investigation of issues, to adjust their activities in response to evaluation, to provide incentives for both educators and clients, and to include continuing support for implementation.[52] Consideration of these factors suggests the need for systematic, larger-scale studies to verify their impact on nutrition knowledge and attitudes.[64,131]

VIII. POLICY IMPLICATIONS

The quantity, strength, and consistency of evidence that relate dietary factors to chronic diseases, and the substantial impact of these conditions on health, are reasons enough to promote policies to improve consumption of recommended diets. Dietary factors related to the occurrence of chronic degenerative diseases are calories, fat, cholesterol, protein, sugar, salt, alcohol, and fiber. Trends in consumption of these factors would be expected to affect the prevalence of chronic disease in the U.S. Trends in consumption of vitamins and minerals would also be expected to affect health and nutritional status.

In order to establish a rational basis for policies to improve the diet and, therefore, the health of the American population, much more basic and applied research is needed to identify food consumption trends in the general population and in its subgroups, and the ways in which institutional, economic, and other environmental factors act to hinder or to promote desirable dietary changes. Table 12, therefore, provides suggestions for a research agenda that includes basic and applied projects grouped in key areas related to dietary trends: measurement of dietary intake, evaluation and correction of survey biases, and implementation of recommendations for dietary change.

Many of these suggestions emphasize the need to improve existing methods for obtaining information about dietary intake and for analyzing dietary data.

TABLE 12
Research Agenda for Improved Data Collection on Dietary Trends, and Development of Interventions to Improve Dietary Intake

Improved Methods for Dietary Intake Measurement

Coordination of the collection and analysis of data from existing population surveys of food and nutritional status.

Development of the most effective interview techniques and settings.

Development of a nutrient database that facilitates time-trend and longitudinal analysis.

Identification of common sample populations and sampling techniques for the various national nutrition monitoring surveys.

Statistical evaluation of the results of dietary intake surveys.

Internal and external validation of dietary survey results.

Identification of more accurate ways to estimate serving sizes.

Improved Methods for Evaluation and Correction of Survey Biases

Estimation of sampling and non-response biases in dietary intake surveys.

Measurement of the extent to which 24-hour recalls, food frequencies, food diaries, and history methods yield biased estimates of energy, fat, fatty acid, and cholesterol intake.

Measurement of the extent to which biases are consistent for age, sex, and racial groups, and for individuals of varying body weights.

Development of methods to evaluate the extent to which education programs bias survey responses.

Development of methods to measure the extent to which survey results are biased by different sets of probes or their uneven application.

Improved Methods for Implementing Desirable Dietary Changes

Identification of demographic, socioeconomic, and behavioral factors that affect food and nutrient intake and act as barriers to desirable dietary change.

Development of a coordinated nutrition education campaign that encourages the public to follow overall dietary recommendations and to increase daily levels of physical activity.

Identification of the most effective educational methods to help the public translate dietary messages into appropriate food choices.

The development of such methods will depend on the commitment and ingenuity of individual researchers. The achievement of some of the other research objectives, however, will require the federal government to develop new policies or to improve implementation of existing policies. As demonstrated in this chapter, there is much room to improve coordination of the federal dietary intake surveys. Efforts to develop a coordinated nutrition education campaign at the national level also will require more effective policies. The importance of information about dietary change underscores the need for development of such policies, especially at a time when health promotion and disease prevention are at the forefront of the national health agenda.

ACKNOWLEDGMENTS

The authors thank Lisa Young for assistance with organization of this project, and are particularly grateful to Jean-Naté Fonté for preparation of the Tables.

REFERENCES

1. Amstutz, M. K. and Dixon, D. L., Dietary changes resulting from the expanded food and nutrition education program, *J. Nutr. Educ.,* 18, 55, 1986.
2. Anon., The food industry discovered that nutrition information sells...but something happened in 1993, *Food Rev.,* 17(1), 35, 1994.
3. Anderson, S. A., Ed., Core indicators of nutritional state for difficult-to-sample populations, *J. Nutr.,* Suppl. 120, 1559, 1990.
4. Atwater, W. O., Food and diet, in *Yearbook of the United States Department of Agriculture,* 1894, U.S. Government Printing Office, Washington, D.C., 357, 1895.
5. Axelson, M. L., The impact of culture on food-related behavior, *Annu. Rev. Nutr.,* 6, 345, 1986.
6. Basiotis, P. P., Welsh, S. O., Cronin, F. J., Kelsay, J. L., and Mertz, W., Number of days of food intake records required to estimate individual and group nutrient intakes with defined confidence, *J. Nutr.,* 117, 1638, 1987.
7. Beauchamp, G. K. and Moran, M., Dietary experience and sweet taste preference in human infants, *Appetite,* 3(2), 139, 1982.
8. Bender, M. M., Levy, A. S., Schucker, R. E., and Yetley, E. A., Trends in prevalence and magnitude of vitamin and mineral supplement usage and correlation with health status, *J. Am. Diet. Assoc.,* 92, 1096, 1992.
9. Best, D., Shelf-stable dinner helpers, *Prepared Foods,* October, 152, 1987.
10. Birch, L. L., Effects of peer models' food choices and eating behaviors on preschoolers' food preferences, *Child Dev.,* 51(2), 489, 1980.
11. Birch, L. L. and Marlin, D. W., I don't like it; I never tried it: effects of exposure on two-year-old children's food preferences, *Appetite,* 3(4), 353, 1982.
12. Birch, L. L., Zimmerman, S. I., and Hind, H., The influence of social-affective context on the formation of children's food preference, *J. Nutr. Educ.,* 13, Suppl. 1, 115, 1981.
13. Blaylock, J., Elitzak, H., and Manchester, A., Food expenditures, *Natl. Food Rev.,* Jul-Oct, 17, 1990.
14. Block, G., A review of validations of dietary assessment methods, *Am. J. Epidemiol.,* 115, 492, 1982.
15. Bunch, K. L., Food away from home and the quality of the diet, *Natl. Food Rev.,* 25, 14, 1984.
16. Burros, M., Some bagels are hefty in calories, *New York Times,* July 6, 1994.
17. Buzzard, I. M. and Willett, W. C., Eds., First International Conference on Dietary Assessment Methods: assessing diets to improve world health, *Am. J. Clin. Nutr.,* 59, 143s, 1994.
18. Cadwallader, A. A. and Olson, C. M., Use of a breast feeding intervention by nutrition paraprofessionals, *J. Nutr. Educ.,* 18, 117, 1986.
19. Cameron, M. E. and Van Staveren, W. A., *Manual on Methodology for Food Consumption Studies,* Oxford University Press, Oxford, Great Britain, 1988.
20. Cannon, G., *Food and health: the experts agree,* Consumers' Association, London, 1992.
21. Clancy, K. L. and Helitzer, D. L., Food advertising, *Nutr. Update,* 1, 357, 1983.
22. Committee on Food Additives Survey Data, 1987 Poundage and technical effects update of substances added to food, Food and Nutrition Board, National Research Council, 1989.
23. Committee 1-5 of the International Union of Nutritional Sciences, Recommended dietary intakes around the world, *Nutr. Abstr. Rev.,* 53, 939 and 1075, 1983.
24. Crane, N. T., Lewis, C. J., and Yetley, E. A., Do time trends in food supply levels of macronutrients reflect survey estimates of macronutrient intake?, *Am. J. Public Health,* 82, 862, 1992.
25. Crawford, P. B., Obarzanek, E., Morrison, J., and Sabry, Z. I., Comparative advantage of 3-day food records over 24-hour recall and 5-day food frequency validated by observation of 9-and 10-year-old girls, *J. Am. Diet. Assoc.,* 94, 626, 1994.

26. Cronin, F. J., Krebs-Smith, S. M., Wyse, B., and Light, L., Characterizing food usage by demographic variables, *J. Am. Diet. Assoc.,* 81, 661, 1982.

27. Dwyer, J. T., Dietary Assessment, in *Modern Nutrition in Health and Disease,* 8th ed., Shils, M. E., Olson, J. A., and Shike, M., Eds., Lea and Febiger, New York, Vol. 1, 1994, 842.

28. Eaton, S. B. and Konner, M., Paleolithic nutrition: a consideration of its nature and implications, *N. Engl. J. Med.,* 312, 283, 1985.

29. Edwards, P. K., Acock, A. C., and Johnston, R. L., Nutrition behavior change: outcomes of an educational approach, *Eval. Rev.,* 9, 441, 1985.

30. Elahi, V. K., Elahi, D., Andres, R., et al., A longitudinal study of nutritional intake in men, *J. Gerontol.,* 38(2), 162, 1983.

31. Elitzak, H., Food marketing costs rose little in 1992, *Food Rev.,* 16(3), 28, 1993.

32. Feskanich, D., Rimm, E. B., Giovannucci, E. L., et al., Reproducibility and validity of food intake measurements from a semiquantitative food frequency questionnaire, *J. Am. Diet. Assoc.,* 93, 790, 1993.

33. Food Additives Survey Committee, Food and Nutrition Board, Estimating consumer exposure to food additives and monitoring trends in use, National Academy Press, Washington, D.C., 1992.

34. Food and Agriculture Organization of the United Nations, FAO food balance sheets, 1984–86 average, FAO, Rome, 1991.

35. Food and Drug Administration, Food labeling; serving sizes: proposed rule, *Federal Register,* 55(139), 29517, 1990.

36. Food Marketing Institute, Historical data, FMI, Washington, D.C., 1987, 207.

37. Food Marketing Institute and *Prevention* Magazine, Shopping for health: a Report on food and nutrition, FMI and *Prevention* Magazine, Washington D.C., Emmaeus, PA, 1992.

38. Frazao, E., Female-headed households spend less on food, *Food Review,* 16(2), 6, 1993.

39. Gallo, A. E. and Connor, J. M., How advertising affects U.S. food consumption, *CNI Weekly Rep.,* 12(42), 4, 1982.

40. Gallo, A. E., The food marketing system in 1991–92, Agric. Inform. Bull. 659, U.S. Department of Agriculture, Economic Research Service, Washington, D.C., 1992a.

41. Gallo, A. E., Record number of new products in 1991, *Food Rev.,* 15(2), 19, 1992.

42. Gallup Organization, How are Americans making food choices? — 1994 update, American Dietetic Association and International Food Information Council, Chicago, IL and Washington, D.C., 1994.

43. General Accounting Office, Nutrition monitoring: mismanagement of nutrition survey has resulted in questionable data, GAO/RCED-91-117, GAO, Washington, D.C., 1991.

44. General Accounting Office, Food nutrition: better guidance needed to improve reliability of USDA's food composition data, GAO/RCED-94-30, GAO, Washington, D.C., 1993.

45. General Accounting Office, Nutrition monitoring: progress in developing a coordinated program, GAO/PEMD-94-23, GAO, Washington, D.C., 1994.

46. Gifft, H. H., Washbon, M. B., and Harrison, G. G., *Nutrition, Behavior, and Change,* Prentice Hall, Englewood Cliffs, NJ, 1992, pp. 19–75, 231–246.

47. Glanz, K., Nutrition education for risk factor reduction and patient education: a review, *Prev. Med.,* 14, 721, 1985.

48. Glanz, K., Lewis, F. M., and Rimer, B. K., Eds., *Health Behavior and Health Education: Theory, Research, and Practice,* Jossey-Bass, San Francisco, CA, 1990.

49. Grivetti, L. E., Culture, diet, and nutrition: selected themes and topics, *Bioscience,* 28(3), 171, 1978.

50. Guenther, P. M., Perloff, B. P., and Vizioli, T. L., Separating fact from artifact in changes in nutrient intake over time, *J. Am. Diet. Assoc.,* 94, 270, 1994.

51. Gussow, J. D. and Thomas, P. R., *The Nutrition Debate: Sorting Out Some Answers,* Bull Publishing, Palo Alto, CA, 1986.

52. Gwatkin, D. R., Nutrition education: an overview of the issues, *Food Nutr. Bull.,* 7(6), 55, 1985.

53. Havas, S., Heimendinger J., Reynolds, K., et al., 5 a day for better health: a new research initiative, *J. Am. Diet. Assoc.,* 94, 32, 1994.

54. Hegsted, D. M., McGandy, R. B., Myers, M. L., and Stare, F. J., Quantitative effects of dietary fat on serum cholesterol in man, *Am. J. Clin. Nutr.,* 17, 281, 1965.

55. Hertzler, A. A., Children's food patterns: a review. II. Family and group behavior, *J. Am. Diet. Assoc.,* 83, 555, 1983.

56. Hinman, A. R., 1889 to 1989: a century of health and disease, *Public Health Rep.,* 105, 374, 1990.

57. Holmes, S. A., Birthrate for unwed women up 70% since '83, study says, *New York Times,* A2, July 20, 1994.

58. Houghton, B., Gussow, J. D., and Dodds, J. M., A historical study of the underlying assumptions for United States food guides from 1917 through the basic four food group guide, *J. Nutr. Educ.,* 19, 169, 1987.

59. Hunter, D. J., Sampson, L., Stampfer, M. J., et al., Variability in portion sizes of commonly consumed foods among a population of women in the United States, *Am. J. Epidemiol.,* 127, 1240, 1988.

60. Interagency Board for Nutrition Monitoring and Related Research, Nutrition monitoring in the United States: a directory of Federal and State nutrition monitoring activities, DHHS Publ. No. (PHS) 92-1255-1, Public Health Service, Hyattsville, MD, 1992.

61. Interagency Board for Nutrition Monitoring and Related Research, Nutrition monitoring in the United States. Chartbook I: selected findings from the National Nutrition Monitoring and Related Research Program, DHHS Publ. No. (PHS) 93-1255-2, Public Health Service, Hyattsville, MD, 1993.

62. Israel, R. C., Operational guidelines for social marketing projects in public health and nutrition, UNESCO, Paris, France, 1987.

63. Jerome, N. W., The U.S. dietary pattern from an anthropological perspective, *Food Technol.,* 35(2), 37, 1981.

64. Johnson, D. W. and Johnson, R. T., Nutrition education: a model for effectiveness, a synthesis of research, *J. Nutr. Educ.,* 17 Suppl. 2, s1, 1985.

65. Kent, G., Nutrition education as an instrument of empowerment, *J. Nutr. Educ.,* 20, 193, 1988.

66. Keys, A., Anderson, J. T. and Grande, F., Serum cholesterol response to changes in the diet. II. The effect of cholesterol in the diet, *Metabolism,* 14, 759, 1965.

67. Kish, L., *Survey Sampling,* John Wiley & Sons, New York, 1965.

68. Kittler, P. G. and Sucher, K., *Food and culture in America,* Van Nostrand Reinhold, New York, 1989.

69. Kritchevsky, D., Antioxidant vitamins in the prevention of cardiovascular disease, *Nutr. Today,* 27(1), 30, 1992.

70. Kumanyika, S., Diet and chronic disease issues for minority populations, *J. Nutr. Educ.,* 22, 89, 1990.

71. Kuczmarski, R. J., Flegal, K. M., Campbell, M. H. S., and Johnson, C. L., Increasing prevalence of overweight among U.S. adults: the National Health and Nutrition Examination Surveys, 1960 to 1991, *JAMA,* 272, 205, 1994.

72. Lee, R. D. and Nieman, D. C., *Nutritional Assessment,* Wm. C. Brown Publishers, Dubuque, IA, 1993.

73. Lenfant, C. and Ernst, N., Daily dietary fat and total food-energy intakes — third national health and nutrition examination survey, phase 1, 1988–91, *MMWR,* 43(7), 116, 1994.

74. Levenstein, H., *Revolution at the Table: the Transformation of the American Diet,* Oxford University Press, New York, 1988.

75. Levy, A. S., Mathews, O., Stephenson, M., et al., The impact of a nutrition information program on food purchases, *J. Publ. Pol. Market.,* 4(6), 1, 1985.

76. Levy, A. S. and Stokes, R. C., Effects of a health promotion advertising campaign on sales of ready-to-eat cereals, *Public Health Rep.,* 102, 398, 1987.

77. Lichtman, S. W., Pisarska, K., Berman, E. R., et al., Discrepancy between self-reported and actual caloric intake and exercise in obese subjects, *N. Engl. J. Med.,* 327, 1893, 1992.
78. Life Sciences Research Office, Federation of American Societies for Experimental Biology, Nutrition monitoring in the United States: an update report on nutrition monitoring, DHHS Publ. No. (PHS) 89-1255, Public Health Service, Washington, D.C., 1989.
79. Liu, K., Statistical issues related to semiquantitative food-frequency questionnaires, *Am. J. Clin. Nutr.,* 59 Suppl., 262s, 1994.
80. Maloney, S., Setting the pace in geriatric health promotion, in *Surgeon General's Workshop on Health Promotion and Aging,* Abdellah, F. G. and Moore, S. R., Eds., Office of the Surgeon General, Washington, D.C., 1988.
81. Manchester, A. C., The food marketing revolution, 1950–1990, Agric. Inform. Bull. 627, U.S. Department of Agriculture, Economic Research Service, Washington, D.C., 1991.
82. Manchester, A. and Lipton, K. L., The food system: a century of transition, *Natl. Food Rev.,* 28, 1, 1985.
83. Manoff, R. K., *Social Marketing: New Imperative for Public Health,* Praeger, New York, 1985.
84. McGinnis, J. M. and Foege, W. H., Actual causes of death in the United States, *JAMA,* 270, 2207, 1993.
85. Mertz, W., Ed., Beltsville one-year dietary intake study, *Am. J. Clin. Nutr.,* 40 Suppl., 1323, 1984.
86. Mertz, W., Food intake measurements: is there a "gold standard?", *J. Am. Diet. Assoc.,* 92, 1463, 1992.
87. Moss, A. J., Levy, A. S., Kim, I., and Park, Y. K., Use of vitamin and mineral supplements in the United States: current users, types of products, and nutrients. Advance data from vital and health statistics, No. 174, National Center for Health Statistics, Hyattsville, MD, 1989.
88. National Center for Health Statistics, Prevention Profile. Health, United States, 1991, Public Health Service, Hyattsville, MD, 1992.
89. National Center for Health Statistics, Health, United States, 1993, Public Health Service, Hyattsville, MD, 1994.
90. National Cholesterol Education Progam, Second report of the expert panel on detection, evaluation, and treatment of high blood cholesterol in adults, National Heart, Lung, and Blood Institute, Bethesda, MD, 1993.
91. National Commission on Children, Beyond Rhetoric: a New American Agenda for Children and Families, U.S. Government Printing Office, Washington, D.C., 1991.
92. National Research Council, National Survey Data on Food Consumption: Uses and Recommendations, National Academy Press, Washington, D.C., 1984.
93. National Research Council, Diet and Health: Implications for Reducing Chronic Disease Risk, National Academy Press, Washington, D.C., 1989.
94. National Research Council, Food and Nutrition Board, Recommended Dietary Allowances, 10th ed., National Academy of Sciences, Washington, D.C., 1989.
95. National Restaurant Association, 1990 National Restaurant Association Forecast. NRA, Washington, D.C., 1990.
96. Nestle, M. and Cowell, C., Health promotion for low-income minority groups: the challenge for nutrition education, *Health Educ. Res.,* 5, 527, 1990.
97. Nestle, M. and Porter, D., Federal nutrition policies: impact on dietetic practice, *J. Am. Diet. Assoc.,* 89, 944, 1989.
98. Only one U.S. family in four is "traditional.", *New York Times,* p. 8, January 30, 1991.
99. Patterson, B. H. and Block, G., Food choices and the cancer guidelines, *Am. J. Public Health,* 78, 282, 1988.
100. Peterkin, B. B. and Hama, M. Y., Food shopping skills of the rich and the poor, *Fam. Econ. Rev.,* 3, 8, 1983.
101. Peterkin, B. B., Rizek, R. L., and Tippett, K. S., Nationwide food consumption survey, 1987, *Nutr. Today,* Jan/Feb, 18, 1987.

102. Pliner, P., The effects of mere exposure on liking for edible substances, *Appetite,* 3(3), 283, 1982.
103. Pliner, P., Family resemblance in food preference, *J. Nutr. Educ.,* 15, 137, 1983.
104. Porter, D. M., A National Nutrition Monitoring System: brief background and bill comparison, updated July 18, 1986, Congressional Research Service, Library of Congress, Washington, D.C., 1986.
105. Prevention Index, *A Report Card on the Nation's Health,* Rodale Press, Emmaus, PA, 1993.
106. Przybyla, A. E., Driving forces behind 1986 new food introductions, *Food Engineer,* Apr, 61, 1987.
107. Putnam, J. J., American eating habits changing: part 1. Meat, dairy, and fats and oils, *Food Rev.,* 16(3), 2, 1993.
108. Putnam, J. J. and Allshouse, J. E., Food Consumption, Prices, and Expenditures, 1970–92, Stat. Bull. 867, U.S. Department of Agriculture, Economic Research Service, Washington, D.C., 1993.
109. Raper, N. R., Zizza, C., and Rourke, M., Nutrient content of the U.S. food supply, 1909–1988, Home Econ. Res. Rep. 50, U.S. Department of Agriculture, Washington, D.C., 1992.
110. Roccella, E. J., Bowler, A. E., Ames, M. V., and Horan, M. G., Hypertension Knowledge, Attitudes, and Behavior, 1985 NHIS Findings, Public Health Rep. 101, 599, 1986.
111. Rolls, B. J., Sensory-specific satiety, *Nutr. Rev.,* 44, 93, 1986.
112. Rosenberg, I. H., Ed., Minisymposium: behind and beyond the Recommended Dietary Allowances, *Am. J. Clin. Nutr.,* 41, 139, 1985.
113. Rozin, P. and Fallon, A., The acquisition of likes and dislikes for foods, in *What is America Eating,* National Academy Press, Washington, D.C., 1986, 58.
114. Rozin, P., Ebert, L., and Schull, J., Some like it hot: a temporal analysis of hedonic responses to chili pepper, *Appetite,* 3(1), 13, 1982.
115. Rozin, P. and Vollmecke, T. A., Food likes and dislikes, *Annu. Rev. Nutr.,* 4, 433, 1986.
116. Ryan, A. S., Martinez, G. A., Wysong, J. L., and Davis, M. A., Dietary patterns of older adults in the United States, NHANES II 1976-1980, *Am. J. Human Biol.,* 1, 321, 1989.
117. Sanjur, D., *Social and Cultural Perspectives in Nutrition,* Prentice Hall, Englewood Cliffs, NJ, 1982.
118. Schor, J. B., Americans work too hard, *New York Times,* p. A21, July 20, 1991.
119. Schucker, B., Bailey, K., Heimbach, J. T., et al., Change in public perspective on cholesterol and heart disease: results from two national surveys, *JAMA,* 258, 3527, 1987.
120. Select Committee on Nutrition and Human Needs, United States Senate, Dietary Goals for the United States, 2nd ed., U.S. Government Printing Office, Washington, D.C., 1977.
121. Sempos, C. T., Invited commentary: some limitations of semiquantitative food frequency questionnaires, *Am. J. Epidemiol.,* 135, 1127, 1992.
122. Sempos, C., Dresser, C., Carroll, M., et al., Recent trends in cholesterol and in the consumption of dietary fat and cholesterol, *Fed. Proc.,* 43, 1002, 1987.
123. Sims, L. S., Evaluating nutrition education programs in the community, in *Proc. 1983 Lilian Fountain Smith Conf. Nutr. Educ.,* Jansen G. R. and Anderson, J., Eds., Department of Food Science and Nutrition, University of Colorado, Fort Collins, CO, 1984, 62.
124. Sims, L. S., Nutrition education research: reaching toward the leading edge, *J. Am. Diet. Assoc.,* Suppl. 9, 87, 10, 1987.
125. Sims, L. S., Contributions of the U.S. Department of Agriculture, *Am. J. Clin. Nutr.,* 47, 329, 1988.
126. Sorenson, A. W., Calkins, B. M., Connolly, M. A., and Diamond, E., Comparison of nutrient intake determined by four dietary intake instruments, *J. Nutr. Educ.,* 17, 92, 1985.
127. Stalling, R. B. and Friedman, L., External social cues and obesity: the influence of others' food evaluations on eating, *Obesity and Metab.,* 1(2), 111, 1981.
128. Stephen, A. M. and Wald, N. J., Trends in individual consumption of dietary fat in the United States, 1920–1984, *Am. J. Clin. Nutr.,* 52, 457, 1990.

129. Subar, A. F. and Block, G., Use of vitamin and mineral supplements: demographics and amounts of nutrients consumed: the 1987 health interview survey, *Am. J. Epidemiol.,* 132, 1091, 1990.
130. Sun, T. Y., Blaylock, J. R., and Allshouse, J. E., Dramatic growth in mass media food advertising in the 1980s, *Food Rev.,* 16(3), 36, 1993.
131. Thomas, P. R., Ed., *Improving America's Diet and Health: From Recommendations to Action,* National Academy Press, Washington, D.C., 1991.
132. Thompson, S. G. and Pocock, S. J., Can meta-analyses be trusted?, *Lancet,* 338, 1127, 1991.
133. Tippett, K. S. and Riddick, H. A., Diets of American women by income, spring 1977 and spring 1985, *Fam. Econ. Rev.,* 1, 10, 1987.
134. Tannahill, R., *Food in History,* Stein and Day, New York, 1973.
135. U.S. Department of Agriculture, Food Consumption, Prices, and Expenditures, *Agric. Econ. Rep.,* 138, U.S. Government Printing Office, Washington, D.C., 1968.
136. U.S. Department of Agriculture, Nationwide Food Consumption Survey, Continuing Survey of Food Intakes by Individuals. Women 19–50 Years and Their Children 1–5 Years, 1 Day, NFCS, CSFII Report 85-1, U.S. Department of Agriculture, Hyattsville, MD, 1985.
137. U.S. Department of Agriculture, Nationwide Food Consumption Survey, Continuing Survey of Food Intakes by Individuals. Men 19–50 Years, 1 Day, NFCS, CSFII Report 85-3, NFCS, CSFII Report 85-1, U.S. Department of Agriculture, Hyattsville, MD, 1985.
138. U.S. Department of Agriculture, Composition of foods: baked products. Raw, processed, prepared, Ag. Handbook No. 8-18, U.S. Department of Agriculture Human Nutrition Information Service, Washington, D.C., 1992.
139. U.S. Department of Agriculture, The Food Guide Pyramid, HG 252, U.S. Department of Agriculture, Hyattsville, MD, 1992.
140. U.S. Department of Agriculture and U.S. Department of Health and Human Services, Cross-cultural Counseling: A Guide for Nutrition and Health Counselors, FNS-250. U.S. Department of Agriculture, Alexandria, VA, 1986.
141. U.S. Department of Agriculture and U.S. Department of Health and Human Services, Nutrition and Your Health: Dietary Guidelines for Americans, 3rd ed., H.G. 232, U.S. Government Printing Office, Washington, D.C., 1990.
142. U.S. Department of Commerce, Bureau of Census, Statistical Abstracts of the United States, 107th ed., U.S. Government Printing Office, Washington, D.C., 1986.
143. U.S. Department of Commerce, Bureau of Census, Statistical Abstracts of the United States, 109th ed., U.S. Government Printing Office, Washington, D.C., 1989.
144. U.S. Department of Health and Human Services, The Surgeon General's Report on Nutrition and Health, DHHS (PHS) Publ. No. 88-50210, Public Health Service, Washington, D.C., 1988.
145. U.S. Department of Health and Human Services, Public Health Service, Healthy people: the Surgeon General's report on health promotion and disease prevention, U.S. Government Printing Office, Washington, D.C., 1979.
146. U.S. Department of Health and Human Services and U.S. Department of Agriculture, Nutrition Monitoring in the United States: A Progress Report from the Joint Nutrition Monitoring Evaluation Committee. DHHS Publ. No. (PHS) 86-1255, Public Health Service, Washington, D.C., 1986.
147. U.S. Department of Health and Human Services and U.S. Department of Agriculture, Ten-Year Comprehensive Plan for the National Nutrition Monitoring and Related Research Program, *Fed. Reg.,* 58(111), 32752, 1993.
148. U.S. Preventive Services Task Force, *Guide to Clinical Preventive Services,* Williams and Wilkins, Baltimore, MD, 1989.
149. Van Sycle, C., Some pictures of food consumption in the United States. Part I. 1630 to 1680, *J. Am. Diet. Assoc.,* 21, 508, 1945.
150. Van Sycle, C., Some pictures of food consumption in the United States. Part II. 1860 to 1941, *J. Am. Diet. Assoc.,* 21, 690, 1945.

151. Waslien, C. I. and Rehwoldt, R. E., Micronutrients and antioxidants in processed foods — analysis of data from 1987 food additives survey, *Nutr. Today,* July/August, 36, 1990.

152. Woteki, C. E., Briefel, R. R., and Kuczmarski, R., Contributions of the National Center for Health Statistics, *Am. J. Clin. Nutr.,* 47, 320, 1988.

153. Woteki, C. E. and Fanelli-Kuczmarski, M. T., National Nutrition Monitoring System, in *Present Knowledge in Nutrition,* 6th ed., Brown, M. L., Ed., International Life Sciences Institute Nutrition Foundation, Washington, D.C., 1990, p. 415.

154. Woteki, C. E., Kovar, M. G., and Riddick, H. A., Sources of differences in estimates of fat intake in national surveys, *Fed. Proc.,* 43, 666, 1984.

155. Woteki, C. E., Johnson, C., and Murphy, R., Nutritional status of the U.S. population: iron, vitamin C, and zinc, in *What is America Eating?* National Academy Press, Washington, D.C., 1986.

156. Willett, W. C., *Nutritional Epidemiology,* Oxford University Press, New York, 1990.

157. Willett, W. C., Diet and health: what should we eat?, *Science,* 264, 532, 1994.

158. Willett, W. C., Reynolds, R. D., Cottrell-Hoehner, S., Sampson, L., and Browne, M. L., Validation of a semi-quantitative food frequency questionnaire: comparison with a 1-year diet record, *J. Am. Diet. Assoc.,* 87, 43, 1987.

Chapter 2

CONTROVERSIES IN CHANGING DIETARY BEHAVIOR

Deborah J. Bowen and Lesley F. Tinker

CONTENTS

I. INTRODUCTION

The past 10 to 15 years have seen a minor revolution in the field of nutrition intervention. First, the focus of nutrition has increasingly turned from one of only correcting nutritional problems and deficiencies to one of disease prevention and risk reduction. We are increasingly aware of specific nutrients and their role in the development of chronic diseases, such as cancer, heart disease, osteoporosis, and others. Large scale dietary behavior changes are called for in the population to change the disease risk in the United States. For example, national recommendations target a reduction of dietary fat and increases in fruits, vegetables, and grams in response to the high prevalence of nutrition related chronic disease in America.[1-5]

Many issues about implementing dietary behavior change remain to be identified and understood. These range from the best methods for delivering nutrition interventions within populations to changing individual dietary patterns. These issues must be identified, investigated, and ultimately resolved before the public's nutrient intake can be changed with a view toward an improvement in the public health. To move the nutrition intervention field forward, several leaders in the field of nutrition have called for a merger of nutritional and behavioral sciences.[6] This merger should include the use of sound behavioral principles and strategies in designing nutrition interventions and in counseling individuals and populations about dietary changes.

The purpose of this chapter is to identify and discuss several key topics in nutrition intervention and dietary behavior change that have remained largely unaddressed. To form a platform, we first discuss the classic behavior change controversies of making and maintaining dietary change. We then use the platform to discuss the questions crucial to successful dietary intervention. How many elements can be changed simultaneously? Should all people receive the same intervention? Does dietary change need an "expert?" Is a personalized goal best?

Some of the dietary change issues have received limited empirical investigation, whereas others have never been the subject of study or publication. Most individuals with experience in either research or practice will have opinions and judgments about these issues, as they are critical to the practical application of nutritional and behavioral science and to the activities of nutrition intervention and dietary change ultimately. However, research on each of these issues is needed to provide direction for these efforts. This is not an exhaustive review paper, but it represents our perspective on questions we ask as we design and evaluate nutrition interventions at the level of the individual or the population.

This chapter is written around a series of questions. Each discussion is presented in a similar fashion. First, the issue is defined, and where possible, illustrated with examples. Then, relevant research evidence is summarized. Finally, conclusions are proposed or drawn. The chapter ends with an outline for future research in this area. We thus hope this chapter will encourage nutritions and behaviorists to investigate these issues, thereby helping to gain increased understanding of dietary change.

II. THE POSSIBILITY OF DIETARY CHANGE

A. CAN PEOPLE MAKE INTENSIVE CHANGES TO THEIR DIETARY HABITS?

All acknowledge that changes in health behavior (as in all behavior) are difficult to make. Estimates of compliance with physician recommendations, for example, range from 10 to 75%.[7] Changing dietary behavior is thought to be particularly complicated, because of the multidimensional nature of dietary intake which encompasses social, cultural, and psychological factors in addition to the basic need for life sustenance. Traditionally, intensive behavioral changes should be made in small, slow increments.[8] Each small behavioral step should be reinforced and participants should proceed at their own pace and direction.[9] These behavioral principles have been integrated into nutritional counseling, and nutritionists have been using these principles to counsel people who need to change their dietary habit.[10]

The difficulty lies in the nature of the current dietary recommendations and the amount of change necessary to follow these recommendations. Making dietary changes in small, slow increments may not be sufficient to alter disease risk at the individual level. Many of the current recommendations require people to make large changes to many of their dietary habits. For example, current recommendations for dietary fat intake are that individuals should consume 30% or less of daily energy as fat,[2] yet current mean intake approximates 34%. Fifteen years ago daily energy from fat constituted 36%. Thus, the current average daily fat intake in the adult U.S. population has dropped only 2% in the 10 year span from 1976–1980 to 1988–1991.[11] Potentially, within the 2% are people who made large changes, people who didn't change or changed in the wrong direction, and people who made very small changes. These data show that many Americans may not achieve the 30% goal by the year 2000.[12] This relatively slow response will in turn slow the possible impact of nutritional changes on chronic disease incidence, such as cardiovascular disease or cancer.

There is some evidence, however, that motivated women can make large, rapid and long-lasting changes in their diet. The Women's Health Trial (WHT) feasibility studies have determined whether large numbers of women can be recruited to a dietary trial to prevent breast cancer and whether these women, aged 45 to 69, could reduce their daily fat intake by half (i.e., to 20% of energy).[13] Approximately 2,000 women were recruited and assigned, on a random basis, to a control or intervention group. In the latter, the women participated in group sessions led by a nutritionist trained in facilitation skills. Eighty percent of the women in the intervention group reduced their daily fat intake by half at the three month follow-up point, indicating that the dietary intervention was successful.[13,14]

At this point we cannot generalize beyond the group of individuals in the Women's Health Trial feasibility studies. The participants were white, middle class, and well educated women who were motivated to participate in the project. It is not known whether men or women of differing motivations and backgrounds can also make large dietary changes. For example, the Multiple Risk Factor Intervention Trial (MRFIT) utilized several thousand men in an effort to reduce the risk of heart disease by lowering the intake of saturated fat and cholesterol. The average reduction of saturated fat and cholesterol approximated 25 to 30%; this indicates that men can change dietary behavior.[15] However, the magnitude of the change for men in MRFIT was only about half of what the WHT intervention produced in women. Moreover, the husbands of the WHT participants reported dietary changes of a magnitude as similar or greater than that of men who had received direct intervention in MRFIT.[16]

Together, these studies indicate that people can make the changes needed to reduce the risk of chronic disease, but whether this applies to all people at any given timepoint is not clear. Perhaps the successful findings of the WHT can be explained by the fact that all participants were women and had been screened for willingness to come to group sessions and to attempt dietary changes. How intervention procedures may be adapted to men or to less motivated individuals should be the topic of future research projects.

The hypothesis that women change their dietary patterns more easily or effectively than do men holds promise for innovative intervention designs. In many of the studies we conducted in the Cancer Prevention Research Program, over 90% of primary food preparers in a family unit are women. If women are easier to reach with dietary change messages and if women can be convinced to pass these changes onto their family members through the preparation of healthful meals and foods, then the dietary patterns of other family members will be changed as well. As previously noted, this occurred in the WHT. For this reason, food preparers should be made an integral part of the intervention.

Targeting women in dietary change interventions has potential for changes beyond the family unit. Motivated women, such as those recruited into the WHT, can in turn, help other people change their dietary habits. The participant procedures and dietary intervention for the Breast Cancer Dietary Intervention (BCDI), which is led by trained volunteers, are modeled after the WHT intervention trial. Participants in the BCDI are postmenopausal women, recently diagnosed with breast cancer. Potential participants are screened using a telephone assessment and a series of screening visits. Once assigned to a group by random selection, intervention women participate in a series of six individual weekly dietary change sessions. After the six individual sessions are completed, intervention participants attend ten monthly group dietary change sessions with other BCDI intervention participants. Participants in the intervention group receive information on exercise and activity to assist them in meeting the exercise goal: 20 minutes of brisk walking 5 or more times per week, or the equivalent. Participants in the control group receive the American Cancer Society guidelines on consuming a diet containing 30% of energy from fat. Assessment visits for all participants occur at baseline and 3, 6, and 12 months after assignment to a group. Assessments include dietary intake as measured with a 4-day food record, quality of life, diet-related satisfaction variables, and social support. All of these activities are conducted by volunteers in their community settings.[17]

The BCDI has five types of volunteers, called volunteer adjunct researchers or VARs. One is a site coordinator who monitors and coordinates all study-related activities at one of nine local sites. Assessment VARs conduct screening and assessment visits, collecting 4-day food records and other trial-wide assessments from participants. There are two intervention VARs: Individual VARs who conduct the six individual intervention sessions with each new intervention participant, and the Group VAR who facilitates group sessions with participants after individual sessions are completed. Control VARs meet with control participants, providing them support and health information.

The antecedent stage of this project included volunteer identification, recruitment, and training. During this stage, VARs were recruited using a variety of approaches, including electronic media alerts, flyers in oncology clinics, and notices in the newsletters of state professional organizations. Each potential VAR was identified for a potential volunteer job and given a complete description of the project. After agreeing to participate, the volunteer read and signed a consent form detailing the study procedures. Each VAR was given a job description and background readings and exercises to prepare volunteers for training. All VARs attended a one-day training session with other VARs. Training consisted of background to the research, an overview of the BCDI study, and the general role of volunteers in research. VARs learned about their own role in the volunteer system and received a manual of operations containing detailed procedures for their use in conducting the study. During the training session, VARs reviewed the procedures relevant to their particular job and practiced the skills needed to perform their jobs well.

Preliminary data indicate that the volunteers have been successful and that participants have made the expected dietary changes. The use of volunteers thus yields high quality research findings at a lower cost. But, perhaps more importantly, the volunteer-conducted dietary change intervention model can be implemented in diverse public health settings, including religious organizations, community organizations, schools, and other settings where people gather, talk, and, especially, eat. Imagine a group of women who encourage others in their communities to choose carrots instead of cookies! These types of intervention studies should be the focus of future efforts.

B. CAN DIETARY CHANGES BE MAINTAINED?

Maintenance of health behavior that has resulted from change is often considered more difficult than the initial change. Behavioral theory offers explanations of relapse to prior behavioral patterns.[18] Reasons why changes in food intake might be particularly difficult to maintain rest on metabolic, behavioral, and cultural factors. For example, set point theory predicts that each individual's body weight fluctuates around a given value that is not readily altered. Accordingly, if someone loses or gains weight, the body will attempt to return to the original weight. Research on other metabolic adjustments that occur when people change food intake and thus body weight support the idea that changes in energy intake can alter weight but cannot easily be maintained.[19]

Several lines of research have dealt with the difficulty of maintaining a newly lowered body weight. The theory of restrained eating suggests that individuals must restrain their food intake if they do not want to regain weight.[20] Maintaining this restraint over a long period of time is difficult, however. Social pressures to consume "forbidden" foods are prevalent in Western culture, and contribute to the difficulty of maintaining dietary change.

That maintaining changes in dietary intake is difficult is supported by the literature on weight loss. Reports consistently show that people can decrease their weight but cannot maintain the initial loss. The recent consensus conference sponsored by the National Institutes of Health reported that after one year 80 to 90% of individuals who lost weight by attending weight loss programs had regained the weight, and that by five years virtually all of the individuals had regained all they had lost.[21]

The findings from the WHT feasibility studies, however, indicate that relapse can be avoided and that dietary changes can be maintained. The participants in the feasibility studies were followed for up to four years to determine the ability of women to maintain the initial changes. Two-thirds of the women in the intervention groups maintained their initial dietary changes for three to four years of follow-up.[14,22] These women did not report any detriments in social support or psychological well-being during that period; this can be taken to indicate that intensive dietary changes did not disrupt daily activities or the quality of life.

Several possible explanations exist for the differences in patterns of findings, but to our knowledge none has been tested. One explanation involves the nature of the dietary intervention, and another the intervention goal. In most weight loss programs, dietary intervention is restrictive and requires participants to deny themselves favorite foods and meals. In contrast, the WHT intervention focused on decreasing total fat intake — not reducing body weight. The WHT intervention was flexible, allowing a woman to make her own food choices. Each participant was given a daily fat consumption goal (fat grams) as the intervention goal, and the methods of reaching that goal were left up to her. Each participant learned the skills and received support to meet her daily goal. She could choose how to "spend" her allotment of fat without restricting other nonfat foods. If a participant met her goal, she could eat as much as she wanted of other foods.[14,23]

The literature has documented that dieting and weight control are problematic both physically and psychologically for women.[24] Women are more dissatisfied with their weight, diet more frequently, express dislike and shame about their body size more frequently and show patterns of disordered eating more frequently than do men.[25] In fact, wanting to be thinner is so prevalent in women that some researchers have dubbed this perspective as "a normative discontent."[20] The WHT eating plan was explicitly presented to the participants as "not a diet, but a way of eating." Replacement of energy from fat with energy from carbohydrates was encouraged, but never fully achieved.[23] Women reported to their nutritionists that for the first time in their lives, they felt able to make sense of "healthy" eating without feeling restricted or blamed. These aspects of the WHT dietary pattern may have helped these subjects to maintain changes in dietary behavior over the years.

The WHT dietary principles can be incorporated into dietary interventions. For example, exchange systems are part of every registered dietitian's repertoire. Exchanges of one food for another are particularly common in diabetic eating plans and weight loss programs. These systems involve categorizing foods into types with a daily allotment of each food category specified. Such a system is relatively rigid and regimented compared to the WHT eating plan. Alternative dietary approaches for diabetes are emerging. For example, carbohydrate counting was successfully employed in the Diabetes Control and Complications Trial.

There is evidence that women can develop coping strategies that make it easier to maintain a low-fat diet even though fat is a highly desired food for both humans and animals. Intervention participants in the WHT reported that consuming high-fat foods made them physically uncomfortable.[27] Further research[28] indicated that the explanation for this decrease in preference was due, in part, to the negative values women attached to high-fat foods based on what they had learned in the intervention study and not due to the taste of the food. Future research must explore how the psychological responses that participants developed may be used in other programs requiring maintenance of food intake changes.

III. THE ELEMENTS OF SUCCESSFUL DIETARY INTERVENTION

In the following four sections we will outline specific factors within nutrition interventions and how they might contribute to or detract from achieving dietary change. These include:

- How many elements can be changed simultaneously?
- Should all people receive the same intervention?
- Is a personalized goal best?
- Does dietary change need an "expert"?

A. SHOULD PEOPLE CHANGE ONE DIETARY ELEMENT AT A TIME OR TRY TO CHANGE ALL AT ONCE?

Current national recommendations highlight several dietary constituents that must be altered for the American diet to be considered health promoting.

Changes include reductions in total and saturated fat and in cholesterol and increased intake of complex carbohydrates, dietary fiber, and micronutrients from fruits, vegetables, and grain products. To be carried out at the population level, recommendations must also be implemented at the individual level. To do so, several changes in food intake are needed. One key question concerns the sequencing of these changes and whether one or several changes should be attempted in the intervention program.

We are aware of no published studies that directly compare a single food or nutrient goal versus one with multiple changes. We hypothesize that some changes are reciprocal and therefore can be changed in tandem. For example, reduction in fat intake in the WHT was accompanied by an increase in the fruit servings,[23] without having a specific goal for increasing fruit servings. We believe this occurred because participants substituted low fat fruit for high fat desserts and snacks. Other substitution behaviors may also lead to a decrease in fat with a concurrent increase in vegetable consumption. For example, an increase in fruit servings resulted in decreased fat intake.[29]

On the other hand, smoking cessation studies have shown that multiple intervention targets can result in focusing on one at the expense of another goal. Thus, participants in a combined smoking cessation and weight loss program focused on the weight loss portion and ignored the smoking cessation advice. The resulting smoking relapse rate among these participants was much higher than in control subjects.[30] Without prior data based on randomized comparisons of different intervention strategies intended to bring about multiple changes, caution needs to be exercised in combining multiple intervention goals. Trying to change several elements of one's eating plans simultaneously may turn out to be too complicated or confusing.

By focusing on one psychologically significant goal, such as occurred in the WHT study, secondary goals, such as higher fruit and vegetable intake, can benefit without the need to focus on these. The women in the WHT intervention increased their fruit and vegetable consumption by almost one and one-half servings per day without focusing directly on increasing fruit or vegetable consumption.[23] By making changes in dietary behaviors to meet the fat goal, women consumed more fruits and vegetables daily. Substitution of fruits and vegetables for fat-containing sweets and snacks was encouraged as part of the intervention, and adding additional fruits or vegetables to a lower-fat main dish was encouraged to prevent hunger. Given that fat and complex carbohydrate-containing foods are often reciprocally related in Western diets, focusing on fat seems to be a way to improve other nutritional elements as well.

B. SHOULD ALL PEOPLE RECEIVE THE SAME INTERVENTION?

Typical dietary change programs provide information, behavior change strategies, and necessary skills. Programs are often standardized and administered in the same way to all participants. Very little research exists whether programs should be tailored to fit the needs of the individual participants.

Current behavioral theories suggest that interventions should be adapted and tailored to the participants. The transtheoretical model of behavior change as applied to food intake[31,32] indicates that not all individuals are equally ready to change their dietary behavior. People must go through stages, from no interest in changing behavior, to considering it, to making changes, and then to maintaining them. Readiness to change can be assessed by interviewer administered questions or by self-report questionnaires. People in each stage of change require different types of interventions to move them along the change continuum. We have applied this theory to lowering dietary fat with some success[33,34] and believe that this model holds promise for understanding dietary behavior change in many types of people, including those that do not volunteer for expert-driven programs. If we are correct, it is better to provide the stage-specific intervention to achieve behavior change.

Two examples of applying the transtheoretical model to dietary change will indicate what potential the model has for nutrition intervention. The first is the 5 A Day research project in Seattle. Centers around the country are engaged in research projects to use the 5 A Day national concept in local intervention activities to increase fruit and vegetable consumption.[35] The Seattle team has chosen to deliver the 5 A Day intervention through worksites, treating each worksite rather than each individual as a unit of both intervention and analysis. We have applied the transtheoretical model to the target behavior of increasing fruit and vegetable consumption to tailor the content of the messages provided to the intervention worksites. This was done on the assumption that most people in the intervention worksites start as precontemplators. The early messages about fruits and vegetables therefore targeted precontemplators, with the intent of catching their attention and moving them along to contemplation. Six months later, contemplation-related messages were provided. One year later the messages were replaced by action messages and eventually by mainte-nance-related messages. The transtheoretical theory indicates that by hearing and considering these stage-appropriate messages, people will move to the next stage of change, i.e., from contemplating an increase in fruit and vegetable consumption, through trying it, to incorporating it into their daily intake.

Another example of the application of the transtheoretical model to dietary change involves adding staged information to written or spoken interventions. After participants or patients have been asked the staging questions and their stage determined, either by means of a brief, eight-item questionnaire, or after having been subjected to an interactive discussion at the beginning of an intervention session, participants can receive the stage-appropriate interven-tion assistance. If the intervention is written, the test can be self-scoring and the materials can refer people to separate pages for different stages. If the interven-tion is delivered in person, the interventionist can make stage-specific recom-mendations as part of the ongoing discussion. These simple-to-implement ideas can help to personalize an existing intervention or help to design a new one.

Other behavioral theories would predict that meeting the specific needs of the individual would make the intervention package more efficacious. For example, Leventhal's research on people's responses to information would indicate that a person's behavioral and emotional history, together with environmental factors, shapes the responses to health information.[36] Social Learning Theory[8] posits that behavior is influenced by the combination of the person and the environment, therefore all relevant aspects of a person's environment must be considered in intervention activities. These theories suggest that determining the needs of the person and including those needs in intervention design will promote success.

C. IS DIETARY CHANGE AN EXPERT-DRIVEN BEHAVIOR OR A COMPONENT OF SELF-CARE?

The answer to this question involves an understanding of the reasons people change the way they eat. One perspective on dietary change is that it is self-initiated, suggesting that the idea of self-care for health is highly motivating. At the opposite pole we can view health behavior change as a prescriptive change, suggesting the need for expert-initiated change with the self-care component less visible at first. For purposes of this discussion, an expert is defined as an individual health care professional or as a team of health care professionals, made up of a registered dietitian, physician, nurse, behaviorist, or allied professional. The literature on smoking cessation indicates that most smokers who quit do so on their own, without the help of a formal program or expert. There are limited longitudinal data on self-initiated change in dietary behavior. Survey data indicate that many people have already changed their dietary habits. For example, The American Dietetic Association Survey of American Dietary Habits categorized responders as already eating health-promoting foods, knowing they should, or not interested in changing eating habits.[37] Approximately one-quarter of those surveyed indicated they were already eating health-promoting foods. Over one-third of the responders believed they should make changes in the way they eat, but were not taking any actions. One-third of the responders were not interested in making changes. Two-thirds of all respondents stated that the need to maintain health generally was the reason for eating health-promoting foods.

Decades ago diets were prescribed with little or no input from patients. These dietary prescriptions were expert-driven. Readiness or willingness to change was not assessed. Patients were deemed as compliant, or more commonly, as noncompliant. Diabetic diets, a hallmark of diabetes care, were shown not to work for many reasons,[38] including:

• Not meeting patient needs
• Lack of patient understanding
• Lack of adequate teaching
• Lack of expert knowledge of diet therapy

During the past two decades, diet therapy has increasingly included behavior techniques, although success is still limited. The use of very low calorie diets (VLCDs) has been accompanied by intense expert nutrition and behavior intervention, yet success has been limited to the short-term. When the program was completed and care transferred from the expert to the patient, weight regain occurred. Weight loss from VLCDs lasts proportionally longer as behavioral support extends into the maintenance phase.[39]

We hypothesize that the need for an expert depends on an individual's readiness to change. Individuals who are in precontemplative, contemplative. or preparative stages will need time, support, and information to consider making changes, with the expert serving as facilitator and information provider. To provide information during early stages is important to dispel misconceptions that may constitute barriers to action. Individuals who are ready to change or who have already begun to make changes are likely to benefit from expert help in identifying behavioral strategies. Finally, for persons who are actively involved in change or maintenance, the expert can add skill building to the repertoire.

The role of the expert in providing information to the public is critical to bring about a change in dietary behavior. In the Survey of American Dietary Habits,[37] misconceptions were highest among persons describing themselves as already eating "healthy." For example, this group believed in the concept of good foods and bad foods. Further, 61% of all persons surveyed by the American Dietetic Association stated they are somewhat knowledgeable about public nutrition policy, yet only 7% knew that the recommended level of fat is 30% of energy. As more is learned about the relationship between dietary factors and disease, confusing messages should be reformulated so as to promote an overall eating plan for optimal disease prevention.

Taken together, the available information suggests that changing the public's dietary behaviors is more than an individual, one-on-one activity. Nutritionists should also look for opportunities to influence dietary behaviors and perceptions on a larger scale. The National Cholesterol Education Program (NCEP) is one example that public education campaigns can be successful in imparting knowledge and change.[40,41]

An example of the appropriate use of an expert is described in medical nutrition therapy, which is a model of care proposed by the American Dietetic Association. Medical nutrition therapy consists of a continuum of care provided by the registered dietitian. As such, it is expert-driven and involves both assessment and therapy. Assessment includes review of nutrition, dietary habits and medical history, along with clinical and laboratory data. Therapy is defined as including treatment and special foods. In this type of dietary intervention for medically at-risk patients, an expert is needed to influence dietary behaviors.

The success of medical nutrition therapy relies on the transfer of responsibility from the expert to the patient. Thus the patient takes on self-care or self-management under the guidance of the expert. Assessing readiness to change becomes important when moving to a self-care model. Initially, the expert could take on the role of information provider and gentle persuader, i.e., become involved at what now is defined as the precontemplative stage of change.[32] This is particularly important for persons who have been given a prescription for dietary change related to their medical condition. It is clear that if the intent is for nutritionists to act as persuader, behavior training must be joined to nutrition knowledge.

D. IS A PERSONALIZED GOAL BEST?

A hallmark of health education programs is to provide participants with personalized goals for behavior change. For example, a fat intake goal must be based on knowledge of the patient's current energy intake and a weight goal must be based on knowledge of the person's body size. Yet public health policies like the RDAs or the NCEP recommendations typically provide all people with identical goals. It is unclear which method of providing a nutritional goal is more motivating. Participants in a group or community setting with a universal goal can compare goals and have a sense of sharing difficulties. At the same time, they may wonder why all are assigned a similar calorie or body weight goal when their food intakes, family histories, and body size differ.

The complications of providing individuals with personalized goals in a public health setting argue for the simple method of assigning a common goal. The 1988 NCEP recommendations provide an example of a universal goal for all individuals.[42] Interestingly, data collected and analyzed since the 1988 NCEP guidelines have prompted the NCEP to publish revised guidelines[43] basing the clinical management on the history of heart disease and presence of risk factors. Thus, the process for the individual attaining the universal goal has become more personalized.

How the goal is stated may influence whether the goal is universal or personalized. A specific objective of losing 10 pounds represents a universal goal that also can be personalized. Yet a universal goal for all individuals to weigh 150 pounds is unrealistic and certainly not personalized. How the goal is stated also directs implementation. In the low-fat dietary interventions, such as WHT, the goal was to decrease fat intake by 50%. But this universal goal was meaningless in terms of actual food choices. It was therefore restated as a goal of obtaining 20% energy from fat, having taken into account that in the U.S. population 40% of energy was derived from fat on the average. The 20% fat goal was a universal goal, yet could be achieved because it was based on individualized energy intakes. However, it was still meaningless in terms of food choices. The next step of translating the goal into a measurable objective was to develop for each participant a personalized fat gram goal, based on height and energy intake.

IV. POTENTIAL EFFECTS OF
DIETARY INTERVENTION

Because the field of disease prevention through dietary change is relatively new, not much is known about the effects of dietary change on personal or social function. The sections to follow will summarize perspectives on effects of changing dietary behavior.

A. WILL CHANGING DIETARY PATTERNS DISRUPT ONE'S LIFE?

The concept of dietary change as being difficult, time-consuming, and ultimately hard to maintain has led to the theory that making dramatic dietary changes could be detrimental to one's quality of life. Possible effects include decreases in psychosocial well-being, in level of social support, and in the quality of interpersonal interactions. These may result from physiological factors (e.g., direct effects of nutrients or effects of deprivation), personal factors (e.g., the effort to maintain a new dietary plan), and social factors (e.g., friends and family who may be annoyed with the new eating plan and disrupt its success).

Data on how dietary behavior may change the quality of life are limited. One study found no decreases in the quality of life as a result of dietary intervention.[44] The WHT intervention did not produce any measurable disruption in social or personal interactions.[14] In fact, participation in the WHT group sessions seemed to produce improvement in several factors, e.g., social support and psychological well-being.[45]

B. DOES NUTRITION SCREENING MOTIVATE BEHAVIOR CHANGE?

Nutritional screening can be broadly defined as the measurement of nutrition-related parameters and their evaluation to the individuals on whom the measurements were taken. This occurs in hospitals and medical settings, in public health clinics, in some public places, and in research settings. The Nutrition Screening Initiative is a campaign to increase regular screening and better nutritional care for elderly people.[46] Nutritional screening is often conducted as the initial step in nutritional counseling.[47] The assumption underlying nutritional screening is that providing information about the adequacy of one's diet and nutrition-related physical parameters will cause individuals to change behavior so as to correct problems.

The traditional role for public or community screening programs has been a case-finding function, or in other words, the identification of underlying disease or malnutrition. For many years, lack of knowledge about the origins of chronic diseases barred the development of preventive strategies. New knowledge from research is steadily increasing the potential for prevention through nutritional changes. Today, the rationale for public screening also includes the educational values of these programs.[40] The guidelines developed by the National Cholesterol Education Program for public cholesterol screening[40] direct screening programs to include health information beyond the simple knowledge of a cholesterol level. As the importance of nutritional risk factors for chronic disease becomes recognized, public health nutrition screening must be expanded to include modification of nutrition-related behaviors and attack on risk factors in adolescents and adults.[48]

Little is known about the psychological effects of nutrition screening activities or about the value of combining screening and counseling approaches. Screening as an effective strategy for prevention of coronary heart disease in the community is still an issue of debate.[51] Several studies[49-54] have addressed the reduction of risk factors for coronary heart disease after community screening programs. The measurements of success reported in these studies have been confined to cholesterol levels, body mass index, body weight, and recall of recommendations including dietary recommendations. The combined results from these studies support the feasibility and efficacy of nutritional screening with brief education encounters in reducing risk factors. Despite nutrition being an important component of the education, none evaluated actual dietary, behavioral, or psychological changes that individuals participating in the screening programs may have made. One of the difficulties in screening for a particular level of fat consumption has been the inadequacy of measurement instruments that are accurate, inexpensive, and easy to use in a screening setting. Recently, a short frequency rating scale has been developed[55] that takes three to five minutes to complete and has enough accuracy to provide an individual with knowledge of a high or low risk category. Responses to this Quick Screen, composed of items selected from a larger food frequency, are entered into an algorithm which calculates an individual's percent of calories consumed as fat and can provide specific behavioral feedback about what behaviors to change.

The effects of this screening instrument have been evaluated in two social psychological laboratory studies.[56,57] The first[56] was part of a series of studies to assess the effects of perceived versus actual fat content on ice cream consumption, taste, and preference. In the relevant part of this research, subjects completed the Quick Screen. Subjects were then randomly assigned to three information groups: control subjects receiving no information, education subjects receiving general information on the link between fat consumption and disease, and feedback subjects. Feedback subjects were told: "Before we ask you to taste the ice cream, we would first like to give you some feedback on your dietary fat intake based upon the questionnaire you filled out right before coming into the taste room. In exchange for your part in our study, you will find a sheet of paper with your personal dietary fat intake. Less than 30% is generally designated by the American Dietetic Association as a healthy level. Your fat intake should be recorded on the last line of your feedback sheet. This is just for your information and is yours to keep." Feedback subjects were informed that their fat consumption was between 35 and 43% (randomly assigned), clearly higher than the recommended allowance. Then, subjects were asked to taste a dish of ice cream and rate it on taste judgment scales. In reality, the ice cream was weighed before and after the 20 minute tasting session to obtain a behavioral measure of preference. Half of the subjects were told that they were consuming a rich, creamy high fat ice cream and the other half were told that they were consuming a light, low-fat ice milk product.

The results of this study suggest that direct feedback about level of risk has strong immediate effects on overall fat and consumption. Subjects in the education group decreased consumption slightly compared to controls if they were consuming low fat ice cream, but not high fat ice cream. Subjects in the feedback group dramatically reduced their consumption of ice cream, regardless of fat content. Receiving feedback that one's level of daily fat consumption is "risky" or high resulted in immediate changes in consumption. The longevity of these behavioral changes, however, was not determined because subjects were informed of the false feedback immediately after the taste test.

A second study[57] more directly evaluated the effects of screening for fat consumption level by providing individuals with varying fat feedback and advice. In this study, 129 subjects completed the Quick Screen. Based on their actual reported fat consumption, subjects were assigned into 3 feedback groups: individuals told that they were consuming at or below the national guidelines and therefore were at low risk for cancer and cardiovascular disease; individuals told that they were consuming fat at a slightly higher level than the national guidelines and that they should reduce their fat consumption, and individuals told that their consumption was much higher than the national guidelines and that they needed to reduce fat consumption significantly. Psychological and behavioral reactions to the fat feedback were measured 15 minutes after feedback had been provided. The results of this study indicate that levels of feedback affect some, but not all, reactions. A significantly greater number of participants receiving the middle risk feedback reported intending to make changes in future fat consumption immediately after receiving the feedback, compared with either no risk or high risk category subjects. The high risk subjects recalled their correct percent fat value less frequently than did subjects in the lower two risk categories and reported more negative emotions. There were no significant differences in the frequency of subjects in each group who had tried to make changes at the one-week follow-up or who reported intentions to change in the future.

Taken together, these studies indicate that providing subjects with feedback about their level of dietary fat consumption and recommendations, even general ones, about how to reduce risk could have both positive and negative effects. The effect of feedback does not seem to be linear, in that high risk subjects are not necessarily more motivated to change than are lower risk subjects. Future studies need to address food choices, changes in fat and cholesterol intake, and the psychological effects of screening for chronic disease. Evaluation of these factors may assist in developing strategies to induce change and to enhance adoption of dietary recommendations.

V. APPLICATIONS TO THE POPULATION

A. WHAT IS PUBLIC HEALTH NUTRITION INTERVENTION?

As the field of nutrition intervention discusses and debates optimal design, it becomes necessary to transform intervention into public health programs which have a greater potential to reduce the risk of disease than dietary change made by isolated individuals. Public health nutrition intervention may be defined as follows: the intervention target must be the population as a whole, not simply volunteers; the intervention must be accessible to a broad range of people; and the intervention should be characterized by minimal or low staff intensity, i.e., the time required for contact between interventionist and participant should be relatively small. In addition, it is desirable for the intervention to be transmitted or delivered through existing channels of communication and contact, to be inexpensive, and for the desired changes to be within the abilities of the target populations. Sometimes, as in the case of changing dietary fat, people must develop new abilities and skills for food preparation.

Several national public health nutrition intervention programs have been designed and implemented in the U.S. The NCEP[40] is a national public health campaign that has demonstrated success in reducing the total blood cholesterol in American adults.[41] The NCEP recommends that dietary/physical activity therapy or pharmacological therapy be implemented based on presence of coronary heart disease or presence of coronary heart disease risk factors. The NCEP has demonstrated a reduction in total blood cholesterol in adults from 213 mg/dL in 1976–1980 to 205 mg/dL in 1988–1991.[43] The NCEP helped to achieve great public awareness about blood cholesterol, as 52% of 1000 Americans surveyed in 1991 knew that the U.S. population blood cholesterol goal is less than or equal to 200 mg/dL.[37] Nearly half of those surveyed were careful about the amount of fat they ate, and most of the people within this subset believed they were doing all they could to consume a health-promoting diet. However, only 7% of the total sample knew that the percent energy from fat should be less than or equal to 30%. These data suggest that the target for fat intake should be emphasized and translated into specific and meaningful objectives before we will see whether the US population can achieve an intake where only 30% of daily calorie intake is fat-derived.

The National 5-A-Day for Better Health Program, instituted in 1991, is another example of a national campaign to promote dietary change by getting Americans to increase their consumption of fruits and vegetables, from approximately three and one-half servings per day in 1991 to five servings per day by the year 2000.[12,35] The program includes supermarket, media, community, and research components.[35] As yet, it is too early to evaluate the impact of this program.

Project LEAN has three objectives: (1) to lower the U.S. population's fat intake to 30% of energy by teaching consumers how to identify, buy, request, or prepare low fat meals and snacks; (2) to increase the availability of low fat foods; and (3) to increase collaboration among national and community organizations. Project LEAN began in 1987 under the Henry J. Kaiser Foundation and now continues under the National Center for Nutrition and Dietetics of the American Dietetic Association. The campaign received public notice as evidenced by public service announcements reaching 50% of the U.S. television audience and the toll-free hotline receiving 300,000 calls.[58] The impact of Project LEAN on America's eating habits is unknown.

B. THE IMPORTANCE OF SMALL CHANGES IN FAT, FRUIT, VEGETABLE, AND GRAIN CONSUMPTION

Public health dietary interventions of low intensity cannot be expected to result in the dramatic changes in dietary intake often seen in intensive clinical interventions. Nevertheless, even small changes in the mean population consumption of fat, fruit, vegetables, and grain may have important and significant effects on chronic disease incidence in the population as a whole, even though the reduction in risk for any one individual may be quite small. Thus, while the diminution in risk for a given individual may not be clinically important, the impact on the population risk can be substantial, both in terms of morbidity and mortality. This is the Prevention Paradox, explained so lucidly by Sir Geoffrey Rose.[58] Rose argues for a combined approach to prevention, comprising both the public health approach and the high risk strategy, familiar to clinicians, where intensive resources are concentrated on those individuals at the extreme high end of the distribution.

The public health prevention strategy may actually lead to more significant results than may appear at first sight. For example, if the mean serum cholesterol level in the population were to be reduced by 10%, this would leave only 3% of the population with levels above the current cut-point for the top decile. The number of deaths from colon cancer that would be prevented if the entire population were, on average, to reduce its dietary fat intake by 3% (from 36% to 33% calories from fat) is considerable. The 3% reduction in fat intake corresponds to about 2,500 deaths per year saved from colon cancer alone. In turn, this represents a reduction in the colon cancer death rate of about 5%. This reduction in fat intake also corresponds to a reduction in the breast cancer death rate of about 5% and in the prostate cancer death rate of about 6%.

In our view, if nutritionists truly want to alter the incidence of disease, they must shift from a focus on individuals to one on populations. In practical terms, this means changing the question from "How can I help this person to change and maintain his/her nutrient intake?" to "How can I get more people to change their dietary habits?"

C. WHO ARE THE NECESSARY EXPERTS IN THE FIELD OF DIETARY BEHAVIOR CHANGE?

Ideally, dietary change requires a team approach. A core team should include the patient/client, a registered dietitian/nutritionist, a behaviorist, and a physician. In the past, the registered dietitian has been the only change agent, operating under a prescriptive model initiated by a physician. Early in this chapter it was proposed that nutrition and behavior science merge so as to improve the changes of dietary behavior change. Team members should therefore be cross-trained in nutrition and behavioral science to provide an effective learning environment for the patient. Ultimately the patient should become sufficiently knowledgeable so that diet management can be transferred from the health care providers to the patient. Transfer might start within days or weeks of the first intervention contact, it may also take months to become effective.

Public health nutrition intervention teams should also include an epidemiologist to assess need for intervention and to evaluate results. Classically, public health nutrition interventions, such as NCEP, have been more inclined to have a dietary change team without a behavior scientists, although the members might include physicians, nutrition scientists, and epidemiologists. Interestingly, NCEP, which starts with population screening, may later include an individual dietary consult. In this situation, the team might include a physician, nurse, registered dietitian, and perhaps a behaviorist. Thus, the necessary experts in a dietary change team might vary with the circumstances. However, current evidence suggests that a blending of nutrition and behavior skills enhances the success of dietary behavior change. At minimum, the necessary expert is a nutritionist or registered dietitian well schooled in behavior science or a behaviorist well schooled in nutrition and dietetics.

D. WHAT ARE THE ROLES OF PUBLIC HEALTH NUTRITIONISTS?

Nutritionists and policy makers must learn more about the role of nutrition in disease reduction in both developed and developing countries. The entire field of nutrition must come to understand the scope of public health nutrition and the role of a public health nutritionist. Public health nutritionists or dietitians, by counseling in government sponsored programs, e.g., Women, Infant, and Children (WIC), have brought nutrition knowledge and skills to individuals within disadvantaged populations. Others have focused on community settings attempting to influence eating behaviors. This type of public health nutrition provides minimal intervention, often in print form, to large groups of people. A third way to change the diet of the public is by increasing involvement of nutritionists in changing the food supply side. This could include changing the availability of foods (e.g., reduced-fat meats in grocery stores), supplementing critical food products (e.g., adding calcium in beverages), and making advances in food engineering (e.g., designing new foods and packaged meals to contain or reduce a certain level of a nutrient). It is unclear which of these strategies is best suited to changing dietary behaviors in the public; perhaps all are needed to achieve shifts in the public's food consumption and to provide choice to the consumers.

Nutritionists and registered dietitians are well-schooled in physiology and biochemistry. To be effective in bringing about dietary change, their training and academic curriculum must be enlarged to add behavioral science, and behavior change must become a topic within continuing education programs. In turn, behaviorists working in dietary intervention programs should have a nutrition component in their education. We must be able to assess our clients' or population's nutrition needs and readiness to change. By increasing our understanding of behavior principles we will increase our abilities to facilitate and evaluate dietary change.

VI. CONCLUDING REMARKS

Clearly, this chapter has identified more questions than answers about dietary behavior change. In many areas the field lacks solid research findings and recommendations based on empirical evidence. More collaboration among the various disciplines that make up public health nutrition will yield better research projects. These projects in turn will continue to provide us with critical findings to inform practice and policy.

REFERENCES

1. National Research Council, *What is America eating?*, National Academy Press, Washington D.C., 1986.
2. National Research Council, Diet and health: implications for reducing chronic disease risk, National Academy of Sciences, 1989.
3. U.S. Department of Agriculture, U.S. Department of Health and Human Services, Dietary Guidelines for Americans, 2nd ed., Home and Garden Bulletin No. 232, 1985.
4. U.S. Department of Agriculture, U.S. Department of Health and Human Services, Dietary Guidelines for Americans, 3rd ed., Home and Garden Bulletin Number 232, 1990.
5. U.S. Department of Agriculture, USDA's Food Guide Pyramid, Home and Garden Bulletin No. 249, 1992.
6. Snetslaar, L. G., Ed., *Nutrition Counseling Skills: Assessment, Treatment, and Evaluation,* 2nd ed., Aspen, Rockville, MD, 1988.
7. Haynes, R. B., Taylor, D. W., and Sackett, D. L., *Compliance in Health Care,* Johns Hopkins University Press, Baltimore, 1979.
8. Bandura, A., *Social Foundations of Thought and Action: A Social Cognitive Theory,* Prentice-Hall, Englewood Cliffs, N.J., 1986.
9. Kaufer, F. H. and Goldstein, A. P., *Helping People Change*, Pergamon, Elmsford, NY, 1975.
10. Mahoney, M. J. and Cagguila, A. W., Applying behavioral methods to nutritional counseling, *JADA,* 72, 1978.

11. Daily dietary fat and total food energy intakes — Third National Health and Nutrition Examination Survey, Phase 1, 1988–1991, MMWR vol. 43, 116.
12. Public Health Service, Healthy People 2000: National health promotion and disease prevention objectives, U.S. Department of Health and Human Services, Public Health Service, Washington, D.C., DHHS Publ. No. (PHS)91-50213, 1991.
13. Insull, William, Jr., Henderson, M. M., Prentice, R. L., Thompson, D. J., et al., Results of a randomized feasibility study of a low-fat diet, *Arch. Intern. Med.,* 150, 421, 1990.
14. Bowen, D. J., Henderson, M. H., Iverson, D., Burrows, E., Henry, H., and Foreyt, J., Reducing dietary fat: understanding the success of the Women's Health Trial, *Cancer Prev. Int.,* in press.
15. Caggiula, A. W., Christakis, G., Farrand, M., Hulley, S. B., Johnson, R., Lasser, N. L., Stamler, J., and Widdowson, G., The multiple risk intervention trial (MRFIT). IV. Intervention on blood lipids, *Prev. Med.,* 10(4), 443, 1981.
16. White, E., Hurlich, M., Thompson, R. S., Woods, M. N., Henderson, M. M., Urban, N., and Kristal, A., Dietary changes among husbands of participants in a low-fat dietary intervention, *Am. J. Prev. Med.,* 7, 319, 1991.
17. Bowen, D. J., Cheney, C., Kristal, A. R., Nixon, D., Sponso, R., Initiation of a volunteer program to conduct dietary intervention research for women, (Under review).
18. Marlatt, A. and Gordon, J., *Relapse Prevention,* Pergamon, New York, 1992.
19. Keesey, R. E., A set-point theory of obesity, in *Handbook of Eating Disorders: Physiology, Psychology, and Treatment of Obesity, Anorexia, and Bulimia,* Brownell, K. D. and Foreyt, J. P., Eds., Basic Books, Inc., New York, 1986.
20. Polivy, J. and Hennan, C. P., Diagnosis and treatment of normal eating, *J. Consult. Clin. Psychol.,* 55, 635, 1987.
21. U.S. Department of Health and Human Services, Consensus Conference on Weight Loss Programs, National Institutes of Health, 1993.
22. White, E., Shattuck, A. L., Kristal, A. R., Urban, N., et al., Maintenance of a low-fat diet: follow-up of the Women's Health Trial, *Cancer Epidemiol. Biomarkers Prev.,* 1, 315, 1992.
23. Bumows, E. R., Henry, J. H., Bowen, D. J., Henderson, M. M., Nutritional applications of a clinical low fat dietary intervention to public health change, *J. Nutr. Ed,* 25, 167, 1993.
24. Brownell, K. D. and Rodin, J., The dieting maelstrom: is it possble and advisable to lose weight? *Am. Psychol.,* 49(9), 781, 1994.
25. Rodin, J., Silberstein, L., and Striegel-Moore, R., Women and weight: a normative discontent, in *Nebraska Symposium on Motivations, Vol. 32, Psychology and Gender,* Sonderegger, T. B., Ed., University Press, Lincoln, 1985, p. 267.
26. Anderson, E. J., Richardson, M., Castle, G., Cercone, S., Delahanty, L., Lyon, R., Mueller, D., and Snetsellar, L., Nutrition interventions for intensive therapy in the Diabetes Control and Complications Trial, *J. Am. Dietetic Assoc.,* 93(7), 768, 1993.
27. Urban, N., White, E., Anderson, G. L., Curry, S., and Kristal, A. R., Correlates of maintenance of a low-fat diet among women in the Women's Health Trial, *Prev. Med.,* 21, 279, 1992.
28. Green, P., Bowen, D., Kestin, M., and Feng, Z., Fat preference of women on low and high fat diets, *J. Appl. Biobehavioral Res.,* in press.
29. Tinker, L. F., Schneeman, B. O., Davis, P. A., Gallaher, D. D., and Waggoner, C. R., Consumption of prunes as a source of dietary fiber in men with mild hypercholesterolemia, *Am. J. Clin. Nutr.,* 53, 1259, 1991.
30. Pirie, P. L., McBride, C. M., Hellerstedt, W., Jeffery, R. W., Hatsukami, D., Allen, S., and Lando, H., Smoking cessation in women concerned about weight, *Am. J. Public Health,* 82, 1238, 1992.
31. Prochaska, J. O., A transtheoretical model of behavior change implications for diet interventions, in *Promoting Dietary Change in Communities: Applying Existing Models of Dietary Change to Populations-Based Interventions,* Fred Hutchinson Cancer Research Center, Seattle, WA, 1992.

32. Prochaska, J. O., DiClemente, C. C., and Norcross, J. C., In search of how people change. Applications to addictive behaviors, *Am. Psychol.,* 47(9), 1102, 1992.

33. Cuny, S. J., Kristal, A. R., and Bowen, D. J., An application of the stage model of behavior change to dietary fat reduction, *Health Ed. Q.,* 7, 97, 1992.

34. Bowen, D. J., Meisehke, H., and Tomoyasu, N., Defining the processes of low-fat dietary change, *Health Ed. Res.,* 9, 172, 1994.

35. Havas, S., Heimendinger, J., Reynolds, K., Baronowski, T., Nicklas, T. A., Bishop, D., Buller, D., Sorensen, G., Beresford, S. A., Cowan, A., and Danaron, D., 5 A Day for Better Health: a new research initiative, *JADA,* 94, 32, 1994.

36. Leventhal, H. and Cameron, L., Behavioral theories and the problem of compliance, *Patient Ed. Counsel.,* 10(2), 117, 1987.

37. American Dietetic Association Survey of American Dietary Habits, the American Dietetic Association, unpublished survey, 1991.

38. West, K. M., Diet therapy of diabetes: an analysis of failure, *Ann. Int. Med.,* 79, 425, 1973.

39. National Task Force on the Prevention and Treatment of Obesity, Very low-calorie diets, *JAMA,* 270, 967, 1993.

40. National Cholesterol Education Program, Report of the Expert Panel on Population Strategies for Blood Cholesterol Reduction, U.S. Department of Health and Human Services, NIH Pub. No. 90-3046, 1990.

41. Johnson, C. L., Rifkind, B. M., Sempos, C. T., Carroll, M. D., Bachorik, P. S., Briefel, R. R., Gordon, D. J., Burt V. L., Brown, C. D., Lippel, K., and Cleeman, J. I., Declining serum total cholesterol levels among U.S. adults. The National Health and Nutrition Examination Surveys, *JAMA,* 269(23), 3002, 1993.

42. U.S. Department of Health and Human Services, Report of the Expert Panel on Detection, Evaluation, and Treatment of High Blood Cholesterol in Adults. National Heart, Lung, and Blood Institute, NIH Publ. No. 88-2925, 1988.

43. Expert Panel on Detection, Evaluation, and Treatment of High Blood Cholesterol in Adults (Adult Treatment Panel II), Summary of the Second Report of the National Cholesterol Education Program (NCEP), *JAMA,* 269(23), 3015, 1993.

44. Weidner, G., personal communication, 1993.

45. Bowen, D. J., Kestin, M., McTiernan, A., Carrell, D., and Green, P., Changes in mental health while participating in dietary intervention, *Cancer Epidemiol. Biomarkers Prev.,* in press.

46. Shoaf, L. R. and Wellman, N. S., The Nutrition Screening Initiative: responsibilities, opportunities, and challenges for dietitians, *Top. Clin. Nutr.,* 7(1), 71, 1991.

47. Aronson, V. and Fitzgerald, B., Guidebook for nutrition counselors, the Christopher Publishing House, North Quincy, MA, 1980.

48. Trowbridge, F. L., Wong, F. L., Byers, T. E., and Serdula, M. K., Methodological issues in nutrition surveillance: the CDC experience, *J. Nutr.,* 120, Suppl. 11, 1512, 1990.

49. Gans, K. M., Lasater, T. M., Linnan, L., Lapaane, K., and Carlcton, R. A., A cholesterol screening and education program: differences between older and younger adults, *J. Nutr. Educ.,* 22, 275, 1990.

50. Gill, T. P., Wahlgvist, M. L., Strauss, B. J., Dennis, P. M., and Balazs, N. D., Factors associated with successful risk reduction after a community coronary risk factor screen, *Aust. J. Public Health,* 15, 114, 1991.

52. Wiist, W. H. and Flack, J. M., A church-based cholesterol education program, *Public Health Rep.,* 105, 381, 1990.

53. Gemson, D. H., Sloan, R. P., Messeri, P., and Goldberg, I. J., A public health model for cardiovascular risk reduction: impact of cholesterol sceening with brief nonphysician counseling, *Arch. Intern. Med.,* 150, 985, 1990.

54. van Beurden, E. K., James, R., Henrikson, D., Tyler, C., and Christian, J., The North Coast Cholesterol Check Campaign. Results of the first three years of a large-scale public screening programme, *Med. J. Aust.,* 154, 385, 1991.

55. Kristal, A. R., Shattuck, A. L., Henry, H. J., and Fowler, A., Rapid assessment of dietary intake of fat, fiber, and saturated fat: validity of an instrument suitable for community intervention research and nutritional surveillance, *Am. J. Health Promotion,* 4, 288, 1990.
56. Bowen, D. J., Tomoyasu, N., Carney, M., Anderson, M., and Kristal, A., Effects of expectancies and personalized feedback on high-fat food preference, taste, and consumption, *J. Appl. Soc. Psych.,* 22, 1060, 1992.
57. Bowen, W., Fries, E., and Hopp, H., Effects of dietary fat feedback on behavioral and psychological variables, *J. Behav. Med.,* in press.
58. Samuels, S. E., Project LEAN — Lessons learned from a national social marketing campaign, *Public Health Rep.,* 108(1), 45, 1993.
59. Rose
60. Egan, M. C., Public health nutrition: a historical perspective, *J. Am. Dietetic Assoc.,* 94(3), 298, 1994.

Chapter 3

NUTRITION IN CANCER PREVENTION AND ADJUVANT THERAPY

Maryce M. Jacobs

CONTENTS

0-8493-7849-4/95/$0.00+$.50
© 1995 by CRC Press Inc.

I. INTRODUCTION

This chapter illustrates state-of-the-art research findings on nutrient and non-nutrient effects on cancer. It does not recommend specific foods that might be eaten, or others that might be avoided, in order to lower cancer risk or to diminish the spread of cancer. Many experimental studies have been carried out in an attempt to confirm the report that possibly 35% of all human cancer deaths appear to be associated with diet and nutrition.[16] Reviewing the vast literature these studies have generated on diet and cancer, one finds many studies to be contradictory. Even different conclusions have been reached by separate expert committees sponsored by the National Academy of Sciences (NAS). For example, with the abundance of data available on fat effects, neither NAS committee could recommend a precise amount, or a specific type or source, of dietary fat to consume to lower cancer risk.

The most recent dietary guidelines issued by an expert NAS committee are not highly specific, because of the inconclusiveness of the data.[55] Most recommend consuming more or less of different food groups, rather than of specific foods. Nevertheless, a variety of eating patterns might be fashioned within the guidelines that might lower risk for disease, including some cancers.

The primary guideline is to reduce fat intake to 30% or less of total calories, and to reduce saturated fatty acid intake to less than 10% of calories. Fat intake can be reduced by substituting fish, skinless poultry, lean meats, and low- or nonfat dairy products for fatty meats and whole-milk dairy products; by eating more fruits, vegetables, cereals, and legumes; and by limiting oils, fats, and fried foods. Further, the NAS committee recommends eating five or more servings of fruits and vegetables daily, maintaining moderate levels of protein intake (less than 1.6 g/kg body weight for adults); balancing food intake with exercise; maintaining adequate calcium intake (e.g., above the 800 mg/day RDA for adults); deleting or limiting alcohol consumption to one ounce per day; and limiting salt (NaCl) intake (e.g., to 6 g or less per day).[55] Research that supports the notion that these dietary recommendations might lower cancer risk, or possibly retard the spread of the disease, is illustrated in this chapter. The effects and suggested mechanisms by which nutrients and non-nutrients influence carcinogenesis and metastasis are presented. The nutrients discussed include: macronutrients that we need in large amounts (e.g., protein, fat, and carbohydrate), and micronutrients that we need in small amounts (e.g., vitamins, minerals, and trace elements). Also discussed are non-nutrient chemicals that occur naturally in foods and appear to exhibit chemopreventive potential (e.g., fiber, catechins, sulfur compounds, limonene, and isoflavones). Based on this research, the suggested dietary guidelines might lower risk for cancers of the breast, colon, or possibly other sites.

Research linking diet, nutrition, and cancer has spanned a half century and has been especially active in recent years. In a landmark study, Doll and Peto reported epidemiological data that related dietary factors to an average estimate of 35% of all cancer deaths. Their report has stimulated a large volume of contemporary research aimed at clarifying the link between diet and cancer. Studies have been carried out on both nutrient and non-nutrient food constituents. Attempts to confirm observations from human studies that suggest different foods, or food constituents, might be chemopreventive, or useful dietary adjuncts to conventional cancer therapy, have been carried out primarily in rodent models. The findings indicate that carcinogenesis can be significantly influenced by the intake of dietary fat, vitamins, minerals, lipotropes, and fiber and other non-nutrients. Further, one of the earliest, and sustained, observations has been that caloric restriction, without malnutrition, lowers the incidence of spontaneous and induced tumors, and delays their time of onset. The therapeutic potential of many dietary components has been evaluated in cell models, such as spontaneous, chemically-induced, transformed, and metastatic tumors. This chapter illustrates findings from selected studies in humans, animals, and cell models that link dietary constituents to the prevention or adjuvant therapy of cancer. Mechanisms by which several dietary components might influence carcinogenesis, tumor growth, or metastasis are indicated. Several excellent publications are recommended that exhaustively review research on diet, nutrition, and cancer.[6,7,50,55,56,59,66,67,70,78,80,82,84,97,98] These reports illustrate how our food choices might have a profound effect on our risk for cancer, as well as for our ability to enhance the beneficial attributes of conventional cancer therapy.

II. EPIDEMIOLOGY

Epidemiological studies provide the basis for many hypotheses associating dietary constituents with cancer risk. Interpretation of these epidemiological data is complex because of the wide differences in genetic, environmental, and lifestyle factors, including diet, that exist within and between populations.[6,16,17,68] Common confounding factors in interpreting human study data include inaccuracies in diet assessments, under-reporting of food intake, and lack of measurement of compliance. When assessing dietary fat effects, further complications are poor long-term adherence to diets, the combined effects of low fat, low calories, and decreased body weight, and discrepancies in adjusting energy intakes. Studies in animals, that are conducted under controlled conditions, provide opportunities to verify, or refute, prospective links between dietary components and cancer risk — observations implied from human studies. Once these links are established in experimental animals, the identification of biochemical, cellular, and molecular events specifically influenced by the nutrient, or non-nutrient constituent, in the diet can be explored. Eventually, clinical trials are undertaken to establish any preventive, or adjunct therapeutic roles, dietary constituents might have for human cancers. A large number of clinical trials involving common malignancies (e.g., breast, colon, and lung) are currently being conducted in the United States and abroad. These studies are generally of two types: double-blind placebo-controlled trials testing specific nutrients (purified, in high dose pills), and randomized dietary interventions in which the participants make a specific dietary change. This background places human studies, both epidemiological and clinical trials, in the overall scheme of identifying diet and cancer relationships. Additional references to human studies will be made in subsequent sections.

III. FAT, FIBER, AND CALORIE RESTRICTION

Dietary recommendations to prevent cancer emphasize reducing the consumption of fat and calories and increasing fiber consumption. How these recommendations might independently, or collectively, lower cancer risk, enhance conventional therapy, increase a therapeutic index, or improve the quality of life of a cancer patient is under intensive study.

A. FAT

Although the documentation of fat[7-9,14,17,32,43,60,64,65,67,97] and fiber[1,18,29,32,44,65,67,80,97] research is extensive, the distinction of independent influences of fat and fiber on cancer needs clarification. Epidemiological studies suggest that consumption of high levels of saturated fats might increase risks for breast, colon, and prostate cancer and possibly other cancers in humans. Identification of the unique effects of fat from these epidemiological data is made difficult by several factors. Some of these are the use of surrogates, such as meat for fat, the concurrent intake of high calories with high fat, the unknown impact of fats consumed in childhood on adult cancer risks, and parity and menopausal status in women.[32] Studies in which animals are provided specific types and levels of fat are helping to elucidate the effects of fat on cancers induced at specific organ sites.

In a recent conference, several presentations addressed the issue of confounding factors that influence risk for cancer.[32] Specific concerns that make it difficult to distinguish dietary fat influences from other influences on cancer were discussed. Age-adjusted epidemiological data are submitted to multiple logistic regression analyses in an effort to distinguish the influence of individual factors. In one conference presentation, these analyses of age-adjusted data indicated that former athletes had lower risks for breast and reproductive system cancers than nonathletes. To arrive at this conclusion, multiple logistic regression analyses factored out contributions of age, number of pregnancies, family history of cancer, being an athlete or nonathlete, leanness, age at menarche, ever smoked, use of oral contraceptives, and use of hormones for menopausal symptoms. The age-adjustment of the data was critical to determining the relative risk, because the population studied ranged from less than 30 to over 70 years of age. The important difference in cancer risk between former athletes and nonathletes appeared in part to be that many of the former athletes consumed low fat diets for up to five decades, while the nonathletes did not.

Based on observations in humans and animals, the NAS dietary guidelines recommend reduction of the calories derived from fat to 30% of the total caloric intake.[12,56] The current level of fat consumption in the U.S. is 37% of total calories. For prevention of cardiovascular disease, consumption of polyunsaturated vegetable fats is recommended in preference to animals fats; but for the reduction of cancer risk, the potential influence of different types of fat is still unclear. Saturated animal fats appear to be associated with increased incidences of colon, breast, and prostate cancers, although epidemiologic and experimental data both support and refute this association.[32,55] Much current research is focussed on elucidating the effects of lipids from different animal and vegetable sources on cancer risk.

Specific fats that have received considerable attention are the omega-3-fatty acids, that inhibit carcinogenesis, and the omega-6-fatty acids, that enhance carcinogenesis.[8,9,32] Several mechanisms have been proposed for their actions. Omega-3 and omega-6 fatty acids are metabolized into two different families of prostaglandins. The prostaglandins from omega-3s appear physiologically less active and counteract tumor promotion, whereas the increased prostaglandins from omega-6s appear to promote neoplasia. It has been proposed that the different families of prostaglandins may be associated with different receptor site activities in the cell membranes. Binding to different receptors might trigger a sequence of events that modulate carcinogenesis differently. Membrane alterations induced by omega-3 and omega-6 derived prostaglandins may elicit differences in cell-to-cell interactions, hence alter communication between cells, with loss of cell-to-cell communication, a fundamental characteristic of cancer cells. Another mechanism of action proposes that when omega-3 fatty acids are incorporated into a cell membrane, the permeability of the membrane is changed, this potentially increasing the sensitivity to anticancer drugs. An example is the alteration of the plasma membrane of mouse leukemia cells by omega-3 fatty acids. This alteration in turn leads to an increase in cell sensitivity to doxorubicin.[32]

B. FIBER

High level consumption of dietary fiber appears to lower colon and breast cancer risk in humans and colon and mammary carcinogenesis in animals, although observations to the contrary exist.[1,7,18,29,32,55,56,67] The differences in types of fiber that have been tested account for some of the inconsistencies among reports. The term "fiber" represents a family of compounds that express a range of chemical and physical properties. It is difficult to separate possible anticancer effects of fiber from effects due to decreased calorie and fat intake that accompanies high fiber consumption, and to decreases in weight gain that accompany high fiber consumption. High amounts of fiber in the diet may decrease intestinal transit time, decrease the time for contact of carcinogens with the colonic tissue, dilute carcinogens and bile acids (promoters of carcinogenesis) in the intestines, change the bacterial flora and fermentation capability, bind minerals (some of which inhibit carcinogenesis), and reduce the availability of vitamins (some of which inhibit carcinogenesis). All of these effects may alter carcinogensis. In addition, very high fiber in the diet may injure the mucosa of the colon and possibly enhance carcinogenesis. Researchers are exploring whether specific dimensions, physical sizes, and shapes of fibers, or specific chemical components of the fibers, are associated with enhancing or inhibiting properties.

There is evidence that certain fiber components, pentosans[12] and phytate,[20] could be the active inhibitors of carcinogenesis and metastasis. In animal models, phytate appears to inhibit colon carcinogenesis[20] and lung metastasis.[88] Phytate (inositol hexaphosphate) inhibits cell proliferation and enhances the host's defense against tumor by increasing natural killer cell activity.[88] The exact mechanisms by which phytate exerts its antitumor effects are not known. However, several mechanisms have been postulated: (1) the phytate effect is elicited by a second messenger (a less phosphorylated form of inositol such as inositol triphosphate), (2) phytate interferes with free radical generation, or (3) phytate chelates divalent cations (e.g., Fe^{++}, Zn^{++}, and Mg^{++}).[72,88] Contrary to the dogma that cell division is associated with increased calcium, the data of Shamsuddin and co-workers suggest that reduced cell growth and enhanced differentiation appear to be associated with increases in both calcium and inositol triphosphate in the presence of phytate.[72] Phytate may act as a reservoir of phosphate, and thereby has the potential to influence many cellular functions. The biological activity of a variety of macromolecules, including phosphatases, is dependent on their degree of phosphorylation. These and other chemical or physical mechanisms by which fiber acts to inhibit or enhance carcinogenesis and tumor metastasis need further clarification. Current research is focused on identifying the types of fiber, the physicochemical properties of the fiber, and the optimal levels of fiber in the diet that lower cancer risk.

C. CALORIE RESTRICTION

In 1909 Moreschi observed that "underfeeding" of mice inhibited the growth of transplanted sarcomas.[53] Since this early study, protocols have been refined in an attempt to distinguish calorie restriction from the restriction of dietary components. Calorie restriction involves reducing the level of energy in the diet. This can be accomplished by reducing the amount of fat in the diet, while maintaining constant levels of vitamins, minerals, protein, and carbohydrate. Clayson and co-workers evaluated the independent and combined effects of fat, fiber, and exercise on cell proliferation. In a series of experiments with mice, they fed diets that varied in calories, fiber, and fat content and evaluated the rate of cell proliferation in different tissues. Their studies indicated that: (1) dietary energy restriction, by itself, suppresses cell proliferation, (2) oat fiber increases proliferation of colon cells, and (3) fat from lard, Menhaden fish oil, or cod liver oil causes greater proliferation of breast and colorectal cells than fat from vegetable oils.[11] Clayson and others are now studying how these findings might be used to predict the therapeutic effects in cancer patients whose intake of calories and fat is restricted or whose fiber consumption is increased. Relevant to the issue of consuming fewer calories to lower cancer risk is the ethical question, as to whether it would be irresponsible to recommend reduced calorie consumption to cancer patients, particularly those suffering from cachexia. Tumors extract enormous amounts of energy from their cancer afflicted host for growth. This results in excessive weight loss and wasting away of muscle tissue in cancer patients.

IV. PROTEINS, AMINO ACIDS, AND CARBOHYDRATES

Restriction of either dietary protein or certain amino acids has been reported to inhibit the induction of cancer, and to suppress tumor growth and metastasis.[2,3,21,48,49,56,74,75] Assessing the direct effect of dietary protein on cancer risk is difficult, because the effects of fat and protein are not easily separated. This applies to most epidemiological studies, as well as to many animal studies. In humans, most studies address the influence of dietary protein on large bowel and breast cancers, although there are some studies on the influence of protein on pancreatic and prostate cancers. High protein may contribute to a higher incidence of these cancers. However, data suggesting this positive association are neither convincing nor have they been consistently obtained. In animals, the evidence associating protein intake with the incidence of spontaneous tumors is also inconsistent. Nevertheless, the development of transplanted and chemically-induced tumors in animals appears to be suppressed with a low (e.g., 20 to 25% total calories) protein intake level, and enhanced by high (e.g., 50% of calories) dietary protein.[56] It should be noted that tumor enhancement occurs only when amino acid intake is balanced.

In an effort to selectively retard tumor growth, while maintaining normal cell growth in the host, the independent influence of selected amino acids has been studied. For example, Meadows and co-workers have reported that restrictions in tyrosine and phenylalanine suppress growth and metastasis of melanoma and increase survival of mice that bear a tumor.[21] Tyrosine and phenylalanine may act to suppress metastasis and increase host survival by a direct effect on tumor growth, by indirectly modulating the host response, or by affecting both tumor and host and their interactions. The melanoma cells require tyrosine and phenylalanine for protein synthesis and melanoma production. Selectively restricting these amino acids not only suppresses growth and metastasis, but also increases the effectiveness of chemotherapy with levodopa. In humans, tyrosine and phenylalanine restriction modifies the immune response by increasing natural killer, T helper, and T-cytotoxic/suppressor cell activities.

Tumors are said to have unusually high requirements for selected amino acids in order to grow. If the tumor burden is large, excessive demands for these amino acids may have deleterious effects on the patient, or animal host, such as degradation of muscle protein and body weight loss. Researchers are looking for dietary regimens that will support normal cell growth, yet suppress tumor cell growth.

Chemotherapy of solid tumors has not been very successful, because many chemotherapeutic agents tend to be highly toxic to both host and tumor cells. Some cancer cells have metabolic defects that can be exploited to selectively kill them. Methionine dependence is one such defect that occurs in several tumor cell lines. This defect has been the basis for studies on the preferential inhibition of tumor growth.[75] Studies show that when methionine is replaced with its precursor, homocysteine, the following result: (1) methionine-dependent tumor cells are locked into late S and G2 phases of the cell growth cycle, (2) the therapeutic index is improved, and (3) the percentage of tumor cells that are sensitive to chemotherapy is increased.[75]

Considerable research based on another metabolic defect has led to human clinical trials. L-asparaginase has been reported to inhibit tumor growth preferentially. It induces complete remissions in up to 80% of patients with acute lymphoblastic leukemia.[74] The mechanisms of L-asparaginase action, still under investigation, in part involve transamination reactions and alterations in the glutamine and asparagine pools. Normal cells do not require asparagine from an outside source, because they possess the enzyme asparagine synthetase which permits them to synthesize asparagine from glutamine and aspartic acid. Certain leukemia and lymphoma cells lack this enzyme and depend on an outside source for asparagine. If large doses of L-asparaginase are administered to treat the leukemia, the amino group is removed from asparagine and the circulating blood levels of asparagine are depleted. This causes the leukemia cells to become depleted of this amino acid and to die. Normal cells of the host survive because they continue to synthesize their own asparagine, hence leukemia patients can go into remission. However, L-asparaginase therapy is effective for only a limited period of time, because the tumor cells eventually adapt by inducing asparagine synthetase and manufacturing their own asparagine. Consequently, L-asparaginase must be combined with other chemotherapeutic agents in the sustained treatment of children with leukemia.

Many tumors avidly consume glutamine. Consequently, with progressive tumor growth, the host is depleted of glutamine. Animal and human studies utilizing glutamine-supplemented diets have indicated that this supplement may be beneficial[74] because supplementation keeps the host from developing the glutamine deficiency that would otherwise result from the increased demand for glutamine by the tumor cells.

Some research has addressed a possible link between cancer and carbohydrate, and in particular glucose, and its metabolism. Cancer patients may appear diabetic, yet have normal to high levels of insulin.[77] They exhibit insulin resistance, that is, an impaired response to insulin stimulation of glucose uptake and metabolism, of lipid synthesis, and many other anabolic processes. Initially, more insulin is produced by the pancreas in response, but as the demand for greater pancreatic insulin secretion continues, a "pancreatic exhaustion" results in reduced insulin secretion, along with elevated blood glucose levels, and an increase in lactate production. This can be simulated by subjecting rats to acute food restriction or high fat diets, or by inducing diabetes experimentally. In obese humans, the adipocytes overproduce lactate. Because these responses in animals and humans parallel those observed in cancer patients, they constitute good models for investigating the mechanisms that bring about high levels of lactate and insulin resistance in human cancers. If these studies were to lead to strategies for dietary modifications, the ability of patients to tolerate full courses of conventional therapy might be enhanced.

A discussion of nutrient effects would not be complete without some attention to the problem of malnutrition or cachexia, a common problem in the cancer patient. This condition may arise because of unbalanced diets, or malabsorption and defective utilization of nutrients.[45] It develops in about 75% of the cancer patients and therefore, constitutes a major concern, yet a basic understanding of the etiology, progression, and treatment of cachexia is still lacking.[54] Many cancer patients suffer anorexia (loss of appetite), severe losses in muscle tissue and in body weight as a whole. Cancer cachexia adversely affects the quality of life of patients and reduces their ability to withstand optimal courses of conventional therapy. The nutritional problems that arise from cancer cachexia, anorexia, malabsorption, physical and psychological problems, and conventional treatment are complex. The challenge to physicians is to select dietary regimens that alleviate rather that aggravate these nutritional problems.

Much of the research to understand the etiology of cachexia has focussed on cachectin, or tumor necrosis factor. This is produced by macrophages and can alter gene expression. It stimulates fibroblast growth, bone resorption and collagenase release, promotes angiogenesis, induces growth factors, and other activities. Cachectin appears to function by different mechanisms. It suppresses the expression of lipoprotein lipase and other adipose specific enzymes and prevents normal uptake and storage of exogenous triglycerides, causing a net loss of triglycerides from fat.[23,45,54,86] Investigations currently underway deal with nutritional modifications that might block cachectin associated activities and restore normal metabolism, and normal storage of fat and other nutrients. Other studies deal with the impact of changes in gene expression, in hormone and enzyme activities, and in fat, protein, carbohydrate, vitamin, and mineral metabolism on the development and progression of malnutrition.

Many of the numerous nutrient and non-nutrient components of foods that have been identified for their chemopreventive properties are now being evaluated for their potential value as adjuncts to cancer therapy. Diet and cancer research has addressed issues that include the use of: (1) dietary and endogenous factors to prevent or reverse cancer anorexia and cachexia, (2) nutritional factors to reduce toxicity or improve the efficacy of conventional cancer therapy, and (3) nutritional components to selectively arrest tumor cell growth and metastasis.

V. MICRONUTRIENTS

A large number of micronutrients express antitumorigenic and anticarcino-genic activities.[6,13,15,22,24,27,28,31,40-42,46,47,51,52,58,61,62,73,83,87,93,94,102,104] Although re-search has emphasized chemopreventive properties, it has also addressed the therapeutic potential of several nutrients. In this section, chemoprevention and modes of action are illustrated for several micronutrients.

A. VITAMINS

Epidemiological studies have associated low dietary consumption of sev-eral vitamins with increased incidence of human cancers at different sites. Adequate or greater intakes of vitamin A, retinoids, and carotenoids, have been associated with decreased human cancers of the bladder, breast, cervix, colorectum, esophagus, gastrointestinal tract, larynx, lung, oral cavity, pan-creas, prostate, skin, and stomach; vitamin C with human cancers of the breast, cervix, colorectum, esophagus, larynx, lung, oral cavity, prostate, and stomach; and vitamin E with human cancers of the bladder, breast, colorectum, lung and stomach. Experimental animal studies and *in vitro* models have validated these associations and have implicated specific mechanisms by which various vitamins, and their metabolites, appear to protect against carcinogenesis.[31,40-42,46,47,51,52,58,61,62,66,73,83,87,93,94,98,102,104]

Retinoids, beta-carotene, and vitamins C, D, and E, and their active metabo-lites, have been reported to influence the growth of cancer cells by several mechanisms.[7,31,51,66] Selected receptor-mediated antiproliferative activities are shared by vitamins A, D, and E. The genomic actions of these vitamins involve the binding of the vitamins to their cytosolic receptors and translocation to the nucleus for eventual mediation of gene expression. Pyridoxal phosphate, the biologically active form of vitamin B_6, can interfere with glucocorticoid recep-tor binding to DNA with subsequent modulation of gene expression.[47]

Vitamins C and E are perhaps best known for the activity they express at the level of carcinogen activation; however, as noted below, vitamin E also influ-ences the immune response and other cellular processes. Nitrosation reactions, the conversion of nitrites and amines to nitrosamines, can be inhibited by vitamin C in aqueous environments, and by vitamin E in lipid environments.[51,93] Nitrosamines are potent carcinogens that are frequently used in experimental models to induce cancers of the esophagus, stomach, and urinary bladder. They are also associated with cancers of the esophagus and stomach in humans. It is important that their formation be prevented and that their mechanism(s) of action be elucidated.

1. Vitamin C

Water soluble vitamin C has been widely reported to inhibit nitrosation reactions and hence prevent chemical induction of cancers of the esophagus and stomach.[51] In the United States, processed foods that are high in nitrates or nitrites, such as sausage and bacon, are supplemented with ascorbic acid in order to prevent the formation of carcinogenic nitrosamines.

2. Vitamin E

Lipid soluble vitamin E, alpha-tocopherol, can also inhibit nitrosation reactions. In experimental animals, vitamin E has the capacity to inhibit a broad range of chemical carcinogens. Vitamin E inhibits 7,12-dimethylbenz(a)anthracene-induced mammary carcinogenesis and 1,2-dimethylhydrazine-induced colon carcinogenesis in addition to the nitrosation reactions.[51] Research indicates that vitamin E influences a variety of cell functions. Alpha-tocopherol is best known for its ability to scavenge free radicals, and thus prevent oxidative damage that can lead to cell death.[22] It also reduces the expression of c-myc and H-ras oncogenes, and induces differentiation and growth of tumor cells. In addition to its chemopreventive properties, vitamin E also has therapeutic potential. As an antiproliferative factor, vitamin E binds to its cytosolic receptor and is translocated to the nucleus where DNA binding domains on the receptor mediate gene regulation. Retrovirus-induced tumorigenesis involves transformation of normal cells into tumor cells. These cells undergo uncontrolled proliferation and express immune dysfunction. There is evidence that vitamin E might ameliorate this immune dysfunction by interacting with macrophages and/or T lymphocytes. This can result in the down-regulation of prostaglandin E2, a potent inhibitor of the immune response, or the up-regulation and enhanced production of interleukin-2.[40-42]

3. Vitamin D

Gene amplification is the mechanism by which transformed cells make multiple copies of discrete regions of their genomes. Some episomes, or circular DNA molecules, carry amplified genes that cause resistance to antineoplastic drugs. These or other episomes carry amplified oncogenes that cause tumor progression *in vivo*. Detection of these episomes, and therefore of their gene amplifications, has been of prognostic significance in some malignancies. Elimination of these episomes might provide a potential means for decreasing tumor progression, or decreasing resistance of a patient's tumor to chemotherapy. Vitamin D_3 has been reported to inhibit incorporation of extra chromosomally located c-myc into a chromosomal site. This may lead to a strategy that would make this episome more susceptible to elimination.[87]

Recent work suggests a possible use of 1,25-dihydroxyvitamin D_3 and retinoic acid in the adjuvant therapy of retinoblastoma, a childhood tumor. The binding of retinoic acid and 1,25-dihydroxyvitamin D_3 to their receptors sets off a cascade of events. The bound receptor is translocated to the nucleus where there is regulation of the retinoblastoma gene and regulation of selected oncogene expressions as mediators in the control of cell proliferation and differentiation.[102]

4. Vitamin A

Retinoids and carotinoids have been implicated in preventive and therapeutic roles with cancer. Green and yellow vegetables contain large amounts of beta-carotene, which is the precursor of vitamin A. The retinoids are synthetic analogues and retinoic acids are probably the most extensively studied vitamins. Both retinoids and carotenoids inhibit neoplastic transformation, and current data suggest they share similar mechanisms of action. Both compounds act to up-regulate gap junctional communication between cells.[6] In humans, 13-*cis*-retinoic acid prevents secondary tumors in patients treated for squamous cell carcinoma of the head and neck[27] and all-*trans*-retinoic acid produces a high percentage of remissions in acute promyelocytic leukemia patients.[28] Side-effects of all-*trans*-retinoic acid include dry lips and skin, headache, nausea, vomiting, liver toxicity, and bone pain. In an effort to reduce these toxic side effects, *in vitro* studies have been performed in which granulocyte colony-stimulating factor has been observed to enhance the ability of retinoic acid to induce terminal differentiation in several leukemia cell lines.[46] In studies with keratinocytes in culture, retinoids have been found to be potent modulators of growth and differentiation and can reverse the effects of cervical human papilloma virus (HPV) infection. Retinoic acid suppresses HPV mediated transformation associated with cervical cancer and inhibits the expression of HPV16 oncogenes.[61] In other reports on the mode of action of retinoic acid, this form of the vitamin prevents growth stimulation by promoters in that it controls the activity of protein kinase C.[58] Although this activity has been observed only in melanoma cells in culture, it suggests that retinoic acid might be used therapeutically to induce differentiation and prevent the growth of melanoma *in vivo*.

In a comparison of the modes of action of retinoids and carotenoids, both types of agents have been found to up-regulate gap junctional communication between cells.[6] Gap junctions serve as conduits for growth regulatory signals. Cancer cells have low levels of communication, because of diminished gap junctions. Addition of retinoids can reestablish the conduits and can enhance communication between cells, thereby ultimately slowing the rate of proliferation and tumor growth.

5. Vitamin B$_6$

The B vitamins, pyridoxal phosphate and folic acid, have been extensively evaluated for their therapeutic potential. Pyridoxal phosphate, the biologically active form of vitamin B$_6$, interferes with the binding of its glucocorticoid receptor to DNA. Specific lysine residues on zinc fingers of the DNA binding domain of the receptor are the apparent targets of pyridoxylation. The data indicate that pyridoxal killing of human and mouse melanoma cells involves inhibition of glucocorticoid receptor translocation to the nucleus.[47]

6. Folic Acid

In humans, a folate deficiency has been associated with dysplasia or carcinoma of the gastrointestinal tract, uterine cervix, respiratory tract, and bone marrow. Dietary folate deficiency, or abnormal absorption and metabolism of folate, appear to contribute to the serum folate deficiency and associated cancer.[70] The potential risks and benefits of folate administration to cancer patients have been debated for decades. Low serum folic acid levels are observed in cancer patients, yet replacement therapy has been reported to promote tumor growth. Research to develop folate antagonists as chemotherapeutic agents has grown out of attempts to overcome the folate dilemma in cancer patients.

7. Lipotropes

Lipotropes (choline, methionine, folic acid and vitamin B_{12}) have been associated with human cancers of the bone marrow, cervix, esophagus, gastrointestinal tract, liver and respiratory tract. Methyl groups are supplied in the diet primarily by methionine and choline, and normal methyl metabolism requires, in addition, the nutrients, folate and vitamin B_{12}. Many researchers have reported that lipotrope deficient diets increase susceptibility to chemically-induced carcinogenesis.[31,69,70,89] The relationship between the dietary methyl supply and cancer was first observed in studies designed to induce fatty liver and cirrhosis in rats that served as models for liver disease in human alcoholics. In these studies, rats were fed diets deficient in choline, methionine, or folate. The animals were noted to have a propensity for developing liver tumors, hepatocellular carcinomas.[69,70,89] Folate deficiency-induced biochemical and morphological changes have been reported in human cancer patients, as well as in animal and cell culture systems. Normal and cancer cells share many similar pathways for the transfer of methyl groups in the metabolism of macromolecules. Associated with dietary methyl deficiency are alterations in xenobiotic metabolism, nucleic acid methylation, purine and pyrimidine synthesis, membrane phospholipids, cell adhesive properties, signal transduction pathways, chromosome anomalies (e.g., gaps, breaks, and condensations), and increased cell division.[26,100] Many current investigations are focused on the induction by dietary methyl deficiency of hypomethylation of specific oncogenes during early and late stages of hepatocarcinogenesis.[31,70,89]

B. MINERALS

Epidemiological studies and laboratory animal investigations have suggested that a number of minerals and trace elements (especially selenium) might reduce the risk for some cancers in humans and inhibit carcinogenesis in animals.[10,30,31,33-36,38,57,71,76,85,93,99] The modulation of chemical carcinogenesis by minerals has been recently reviewed in detail.[36] Research on the therapeutic attributes of minerals began when platinum coordination complexes and selenium compounds were found to be effective in cancer therapy.[38,95] Inhibition of chemical carcinogenesis in a variety of animal models has helped elucidate the mechanism(s) of action of minerals. Among minerals reported to have chemopreventive properties are different organic and inorganic forms of copper, zinc, magnesium, calcium, lead, iron, potassium, sodium, arsenic, iodine, and germanium.[36] Modulation of carcinogenesis with dietary selenium has been the focus of a large number of studies. An interesting paradox is that on one hand minerals can inhibit chemical induction of carcinogenesis, and, on the other hand, some of the same minerals can also enhance the growth of established tumors. These contrasting activities are expressed by different redox states, different organic and inorganic forms, and different doses. For some minerals there are sufficient data to suggest that the response elicited is dose-dependent. Moreover, it is not uncommon for deficiencies in some minerals to increase neoplasia. The various organic and inorganic forms of chromium, copper, and other metals appear to be the basis for the contrasting risks and benefits. The anion or ligand can determine its physico-chemical properties, and these affect the solubility, absorption, and distribution of the mineral to different sites, and thus relate to the anticarcinogenic, or toxic, effects reported for that mineral.

1. Selenium

In humans, low serum selenium levels have been observed in gastrointestinal cancer patients.[71] In rodents, dietary supplements of selenium have been shown to inhibit colon, mammary gland, liver, skin, pancreatic, and stomach carcinogenesis.[10,33-35,57,71,76,85,99] Mechanisms of action proposed for selenium are for it to: (1) inhibit carcinogen activation, (2) enhance glutathione peroxidase activity to prevent lipid peroxidation and damage to cell membranes, (3) enhance glutathione *S*-transferase activity for detoxification of carcinogenic electrophiles, especially alkylating agents, (4) induce DNA repair, and (5) induce the immune response by affecting T and B lymphocytes and natural killer cells. Some data suggest that the potential protective effects of selenium might be nullified with antioxidants, or high fat diets.[33] Since inorganic selenium compounds can be toxic at high concentrations, studies are needed to identify the dietary concentrations, especially in humans, that will protect against carcinogenesis, afford therapeutic potential against established tumors, and not be highly toxic to the host.

Research on other minerals indicates chemopreventive effects of zinc, copper, and potassium. In humans, low blood and diseased tissue levels of zinc have been observed in esophageal, prostatic, and bronchial cancer patients, while in laboratory animals a zinc deficiency appears to enhance carcinogenesis.[34,36,57,62,76] In experimental animals, organic and inorganic forms of copper have been noted to inhibit hepatocarcinogenesis and colon carcinogenesis. In the last few years, several reports have documented chemopreventive effects for potassium. In humans, experimental animals, and cell culture systems, increased potassium levels have been associated with decreased tumor cell growth and inhibition of carcinogenesis.[30,37]

Serum iron, transferrin, and ferritin influence cancer risk and cancer cell growth.[79] Epidemiological studies show cancers of lung, colon, bladder, and esophagus have a high correlation with increased serum iron and increased transferrin saturation. In contrast, many cancer patients develop low serum iron and serum transferrin levels. Since many tumor cells require iron for growth, it has been postulated that the increased accumulation of iron by the tumor depresses the serum iron level in cancer patients. In mice with subcutaneous tumor implants, a low iron diet reportedly results in less rapid tumor growth, in support of this hypothesis. The mechanisms by which iron influences tumor growth are under investigation. In humans with acute leukemia, ten times higher levels of serum ferritin are observed than is normal. In addition, in people with cancers of the liver, pancreas, kidney, breast, or stomach, the serum ferritin is reported to be markedly elevated. Much of the research to explain these observations deals with the relationship of the ratio of bound to free iron to the rate of tumor cell growth. The prognostic use of serum ferritin levels to predict the extent of disease, or tumor burden, is being investigated.

VI. NON-NUTRIENTS

Non-nutrient chemicals with cancer preventive potential have been identified in many natural products. Among these are catechins, sulfur compounds, limonene, and isoflavins found in tea, broccoli, garlic, citrus fruit, and soybean. The mechanisms of action of the active compounds from these plants are being intensely studied. There is interest in developing hybrids, and bioengineered designer foods that are fortified with the active compounds, in the event that these new foods might offer increased protection against cancer or other diseases.

A. CATECHINS

With the large consumption of tea around the world, there has been considerable interest in investigations into the purported anticarcinogenic properties of green and black teas. It has been shown that green tea extracts contain catechins and black tea extracts contain the catechin fermentation products, theaflavins and thearubigins.[39,90,91] These compounds inhibit the chemical induction of lung, esophageal, skin, and forestomach tumors in rodents. Their activities include inhibition of promotion, protection against oxidative damage from lipid peroxidation and DNA strand breaks, inhibition of carcinogen activation, and trapping of ultimate carcinogens. Many of the non-nutrient compounds, including polyphenol extracts from green and black teas, enhance antioxidant enzymes and induce phase II enzymes.[39]

B. SULFUR COMPOUNDS

Sulfur compounds from several commonly eaten foods have been found to possess chemopreventive properties. Much attention has been directed to the compound, sulforaphane, from broccoli. This compound increases the phase II enzymes that detoxify chemical carcinogens.[103] Garlic and related allium vegetables contain the organosulfur compounds, diallylsulfide and *S*-allyl-cysteine, that can induce cytochrome P450 enzymes. These enzymes can inhibit carcinogen activation and selectively prevent cancers of the colon, esophagus, lung, liver, nasal cavity, and other tissues.[92,101] Organosulfur compounds also afford protection against chemical carcinogenesis by depressing demethylase activity and stimulating glutathione peroxidase activity. Although there is a large body of literature on the chemopreventive properties of garlic, it is unclear whether the organosulfur compounds are the only active ingredients.

C. LIMONENE

Limonene is a major monoterpene, found in citrus fruits, that has been extensively studied for its chemopreventive properties. This compound has the ability to prevent isoprenylation and oncogene expression. There is some evidence suggestive of a possible therapeutic potential whereby limonene causes regression of DMBA-induced mammary tumors.[19]

D. ISOFLAVONES

Breast and prostate cancers share the common feature of being sex-hormone dependent.[4] Patients with these cancers are often treated with estrogen-like drugs. For breast cancer, the antiestrogen drug, tamoxifen, is used to prevent the metastatic growth of estrogen-dependent primary tumors. One mechanism suggested for its action is for tamoxifen to recognize and bind to the estrogen receptor, thereby interfering with estrogen binding and eliciting the subsequent events associated with the stimulation of tumor growth. Tamoxifen might also be an antipromoter, and is currently being tested in a chemoprevention trial in women at high risk for breast cancer. For prostate cancer, the nonsteroidal synthetic estrogen drug, diethylstilbestrol, is used to reduce the synthesis of testosterone.

Soybeans contain the isoflavones, genistein and daidzein. These phyto-estrogens are weak estrogen agonists and can interfere with the promotive effects of both estrogens and androgens in tumors. Dietary soybean inhibition of the chemical induction of mammary tumors has been attributed to crude soybean extracts and purified forms of the isoflavones.[4] Both genistein and daidzein slow the growth of human breast carcinoma cell lines. They were effective in two cell lines, MDA-468, which is estrogen receptor negative, and MCF-7, which is estrogen receptor positive.[63] Inhibition of carcinogenesis by soybean has been attributed not only to its constituent isoflavones, but also to soybean trypsin inhibitor and to other protease inhibitors in soybeans.[81]

VII. NUTRIENT INTERACTIONS

Most experimental and clinical research has focussed on the independent effect of specific macronutrient, micronutrient, or non-nutrient food constituents. In our diets, however, a large number of these active nutrient and non-nutrient compounds are intermingled. They have the potential to interact and to modify each other's actions. Changes in the intake of one dietary component may alter the balance and intake of other components. The requirement for one nutritional component may be raised or lowered in the presence of an excess or deficiency of another. For example, even in a cancer-free state, the requirement that rats have for selenium is decreased when vitamin E is at an adequate nutritional level.[25] One can speculate that new or enhanced interactions might arise in cancer patients. Changes in nutrient requirements that occur in cancer patients may evolve from nutrient interactions, as well as from the well documented effects of tumor growth and metastasis and conventional therapies of radiation, chemotherapy, and surgery.

VIII. CONCLUSION

Clearly there are numerous nutrient and non-nutrient constituents in foods in our diet that have the potential to confer chemopreventive properties or enhance conventional therapy. Preventive effects of low dietary fat against the major cancers (e.g., breast) is perhaps best documented. There is evidence that vegetables and fruits, rich sources of fiber and antioxidant vitamins C, E, and beta-carotene might protect against cancers at several sites. Although more conclusive data are still being sought to establish the cancer preventive activity of many foods and their active components, the general advice to lower cancer risk is to consume less fat, and to consume more fruits, vegetables, cereals and legumes. Even if this recommendation were not effective in lowering cancer risk, at the least, people would benefit because this change in diet protects against cardiovascular disease. The current consensus is that reducing calorie consumption and eating a variety of foods in moderation is perhaps the best recipe for lowering cancer risk.

REFERENCES

1. American Dietetic Association, Position of the American Dietetic Association: health implications of dietary fiber, Technical Support Paper, *J. Am. Dietetic Assoc.*, 88(2), 217, 1988.
2. Appleton, B. S. and Campbell, T. C., Dietary protein intervention during the post-dosing phase of aflatoxin B1-induced hepatic preneoplastic lesion development, *J. Natl. Cancer. Inst.*, 70, 547, 1983.
3. Asselin, B. L., Ryan, D., Frantz, C. N., Bernal, S. D., Leavitt, P., Sallan, S. E., and Cohen, H. J., In vitro and in vivo killing of acute lymphoblastic leukemia cells by L-asparaginase, *Cancer Res.*, 49, 4363, 1989.
4. Barnes, S., Grubbs, C., Setchell, K. D. R., and Carlson, J., Soybeans inhibit mammary tumors in models of breast cancer, in: *Mutagens and Carcinogens in the Diet*, Pariza, M., Ed., Alan R. Liss, New York, 1990.
5. Bertram, J. S., Cancer chemoprevention by retinoids and carotenoids: proposed role of gap junctional communication, in *Vitamins and Minerals in the Prevention and Treatment of Cancer*, Jacobs, M. M., Ed., CRC Press, Boca Raton, 1991, chap. 3.

6. Bertram, J. S., Kolonel, L. N., and Meyskens, F. L. Jr., Rationale and strategies for chemoprevention of cancer in humans, *Cancer Res.,* 47, 3012, 1987.
7. Boutwell, R. K., An overview of the role of diet and nutrition in carcinogenesis, in *Nutrition, Growth, and Cancer,* Alan R. Liss, Inc., New York, 1988.
8. Broitman, S. A., Vitale, J. J., Vavrousek-Jakuba, E., and Gottlieb, L. S., Polyunsaturated fat, cholesterol and large bowel tumorigenesis, *Cancer (Phila.),* 40, 2455, 1977.
9. Carroll, K. K., Braden, L. M., Bell, J. A., and Kalamegham, R., Fat and cancer, *Cancer,* 58, 1818, 1986.
10. Clark, L. C., The epidemiology of selenium and cancer, *Fed. Proc.,* 44(9), 2584, 1985.
11. Clayson, D. B., Lok, E., Scott, F., Mongeau, R., Ratnayake, W. M. N., Nera, E. A., and Jee, P., Calories, fat, fibers, and cellular proliferation in Swiss Webster mice, in *Exercise, Calories, Fat, and Cancer,* in: *Advances in Experimental Medicine and Biology,* Vol. 322, Plenum Press, New York, 1992, chap. 8.
12. Cohen, L. A., Diet and cancer, *Sci. Am.,* 257(56), 42, 1987.
13. Colditz, G. A., Stampfer, M. J., and Willett, W. C., Diet and lung cancer: a review of the epidemiologic evidence in humans, *Arch. Intern. Med.,* 147, 157, 1987.
14. Craven, P. A., DeRubertis, F. R., and Fox, J. W., Fatty acid-dependent benzo(a)pyrene oxidation in the colonic mucosal microsomes: evidence for a distinct metabolic pathway, *Cancer Res.,* 43, 35, 1983.
15. Davis, D. L., Natural anticarcinogens, carcinogens, and changing patterns in cancer: some speculation, *Exp. Res.,* 50, 322, 1989.
16. Doll, R. and Peto, R., The causes of cancer: quantitative estimates of avoidable risks of cancer in the United States, today, *J. Natl. Cancer. Inst.,* 66(6), 1193, 1981.
17. Dwyer, J. T., Dietary fat and breast cancer: testing interventions to reduce risks, in *Exercise, Calories, Fat, and Cancer,* Jacobs, M. M., Ed., *Advances in Experimental Medicine and Biology,* Vol. 322, Plenum Press, New York, 1992, chap. 14.
18. Eastwood, M., Dietary fiber and the risk for cancer, *Nutr. Rev.,* 45, 193, 1987.
19. Elegbede, J. A., Elson, C. E., Qureshi, A., Tanner, M. A., and Gould, M. N., Inhibition of DMBA-induced mammary cancer by monoterpene *d*-limonene, *Carcinogenesis,* 5, 661, 1984.
20. Elsayed, A., Chakravarthy, A., and Shamsuddin, A., Inositol hexaphosphate from corn decreased the frequency of colorectal cancer in azomethane-treated rats, *Lab. Invest.,* 56, 21, 1987.
21. Elstad, C. A., Meadows, G. G., Aslakson, C. J., and Starkey, J. R., Evidence for nutrient modulation of tumor phenotype: impact of tyrosine and phenylalanine restricition, in *Diet and Cancer: Markers, Prevention, and Treatment,* Jacobs, M. M., Ed., *Advances in Experimental Medicine and Biology,* Vol. 354, Plenum Press, New York, 1994, chap. 13.
22. Fariss, W., Oxygen toxicity: unique cytoprotective properties of vitamin E succinate in hepatocytes, *Free Rad. B.,* 9, 333, 1990.
23. Harvey, K. B., Bothe, A., and Blackburn, G. L., Nutritional assessment during oncological therapy, *Cancer,* 42, 2065, 1979.
24. Hennekens, C. H., Mayrent, S. L., and Willett, W., Vitamin A, carotenoids, and retinoids, *Cancer,* 58, 1837, 1986.
25. Hoekstra, W. G., Biochemical function of selenium and its relation to vitamin E. *Fed. Proc. Fed. Am. Soc. Exp. Biol.,* 43, 2083, 1975.
26. Hoffman, R. M., Altered methionine metabolism, DNA methylation and oncogene expression in carcinogenesis, *Biochim. Biophys. Acta,* 738, 49, 1984.
27. Hong, W. K., Lipman, S. M., Itri, L. M., Karp, D. D., Lee, J. S., Byers, R. M., Shantz, S. P., Kramer, A. M., Lotan, R., Peters, L. J., Dimery, I. W., Brown, B. W., and Goepfert, H., Prevention of second primary tumors with isotretinoin in squamous-cell carcinoma of the head and neck, *N. Engl. J. Med.,* 323, 796, 1990.
28. Huang, M., Ye, Y., Chen, S., Chai, J., Lu, J. X., Zhoa, L., Gu, L., and Wang, Z., Use of all-trans retinoic acid in the treatment of acute promyelocytic leukemia, *Blood,* 72, 567, 1988.

29. Jacobs, L. R., Dietary fiber and cancer, *J. Nutr.*, 117, 1319, 1987.
30. Jacobs, M. M., Potassium inhibition of DMH-induced small intestinal tumors in rats, *Nutr. Cancer*, 14, 95, 1990.
31. Jacobs, M. M., Ed., *Vitamins and Minerals in the Prevention and Treatment of Cancer*, CRC Press, Boca Raton, FL, 1991.
32. Jacobs, M. M., Ed., Exercise, Calories, Fat, and Cancer, in *Advances in Experimental Medicine and Biology*, Vol 322, Plenum Press, New York, 1992.
33. Jacobs, M. M. and Griffin, A. C., Effects of selenium on chemical carcinogenesis: comparative effects on antioxidants, *Biol. Trace Ele. Res.*, 1, 1, 1979.
34. Jacobs, M. M. and Griffin, A. C., Trace elements and metals as anticarcinogens, in *Inhibition of Tumor Induction and Development*, Zedeck, M. S. and Lipkin, M., Eds., Plenum Press, New York, 1981.
35. Jacobs, M. M., Jansson, B., and Griffin, A. C., Inhibitory effects of selenium on 1,2-dimethylhydrazine and methylazoxymethanol acetate induction of colon tumors, *Cancer Lett.*, 2, 133, 1977.
36. Jacobs, M. M. and Pienta, R. J., Modulation by minerals, in *Chemical Induction of Cancer: Modulation and Combination Effects*, J. C. Arcos, M.F. Argus, and Y-T. Woo, Eds., Lewis Press, New York, in press.
37. Jacobs, M. M. and Pienta, R. J., Relationships between potassium and cancer, in *Vitamins and Minerals in the Prevention and Treatment of Cancer*, Jacobs, M. M., Ed., CRC Press, Boca Raton, 1991, chap. 16.
38. Kazantzis, G., Role of cobalt, iron, lead, manganese, mercury, platinum, selenium, and titanium in carcinogenesis, *Environ. Health Persp.*, 40, 143, 1981.
39. Khan, S. G., Kartiyar, S. K., Agarwal, R., and Mukhtar, H., Enhancement of antioxidant and phase II enzymes by oral feeding of green tea polyphenols in drinking water to SKH-1 hairless mice: possible role in cancer prevention, *Cancer Res.*, 52, 4050, 1992.
40. Kline, K., Cochran, G. S., and Sanders, B. G., Growth inhibitory effects of vitamin E succinate on retrovirus-transformed tumor cells in vitro, *Nutr. Cancer*, 14, 27, 1990.
41. Kline, K., Rao, A., Romach, E. H., Kidao, S., Morgan, T. J., and Sanders, B. G., Vitamin E effects on retrovirus-induced immune dysfunctions, *Ann. N.Y. Acad. Sci.*, 587, 294, 1990.
42. Kline, K. and Sanders, B. G., Modulation of immune suppression and enhanced tumorigenesis in retrovirus tumor challenged chickens treated with vitamin E, *In Vivo*, 3, 161, 1989.
43. Kritchevsky, D. Fat, calories and cancer, *Front. Gastrointest. Res.*, 14, 188, 1988.
44. Kritchevsky, D., Webber, M. M., and Klurfield, D. M., Dietary fat versus caloric content in initiation and promotion of 7,12-dimethylbenz(a)anthracene-induced mammary tumorigenesis in rats, *Cancer Res.*, 44, 3174, 1984.
45. Lawson, D. H., Richmond, A., Nixon, D. W., and Rudman, D., Metabolic approaches to cancer cachexia, *Ann. Rev. Nutr.*, 2, 277, 1982.
46. Li, J. and Sartorelli, A. C., Synergistic induction of the differentiation of WEH1-3B D+ Myelomonocytic leukemia cells by retinoic acid and granulocyte colony-stimulating factor, *Leukemia Res.*, 16, 571, 1992.
47. Litwack, G., Robertson, N. M., Maksymowych, A. B., and Celiker, M., Vitamin B_6 and other inhibitors of glucocorticoid receptor function and cell death of B_{16} melanoma cells, in *Vitamins and Minerals in the Prevention and Treatment of Cancer*, Jacobs, M. M., Ed., CRC Press, Boca Raton, FL, 1991, chap. 2.
48. Meadows, G. G. and Oeser, D. E., Response by B16 Melanoma-bearing mice to varying levels of phenylalanine and tyrosine, *Nutr. Rep. Int.*, 28, 1073, 1983.
49. Meadows, G. G., Pierson, H. F., Abdallah, R. M., and Desai, P. R., Dietary influence of tyrosine and phenylalanine on the response of B16 Melanoma to carbidopalevodopa methyl ester chemotherapy, *Cancer Res.*, 42, 3056, 1982.
50. Meyskens, F. L., Jr., Strategies for prevention of cancer in humans, *Oncology (Huntingt)*, 6(2), 15, 1992.

51. Mirvish, S. S., Effects of vitamins C and E on N-nitroso compound formation, carcinogenesis, and cancer, *Cancer*, 58, 1842, 1986.
52. Moon, R. C. and Mehta, R. G., Anticarcinogenic effects of retinoids in animals, in *Essential Nutrients in Carcinogenesis*, Poirier, L. A., Newberne, P. M., and Pariza, M. W., Eds., Plenum Press, New York, 1986.
53. Moreschi, C., Beziehungen Zwischen Ernahrung und Tmorwachstum, *Z. Immunitatsforsch*, 2, 651, 1909.
54. Morrison, S. D., Control of food intake in cancer cachexia: a challenge and a tool, *Physiol. Behav.*, 17, 705, 1976.
55. National Academy of Sciences, *Diet and Health: Implications for Reducing Chronic Disease Risk*, National Academy Press, Washington, DC, 1989.
56. National Academy of Sciences, *Diet, Nutrition and Cancer*, National Academy Press, Washington, DC, 1982.
57. Nielsen, F. H., Effect of trace minerals and vitamins on tumor formation, *Food Technol.*, March, 1983.
58. Niles, R. M. and Loewy, B. P., Induction of protein kinase C in mouse melanoma cells by retinoic acid, *Cancer Res.*, 49, 4483, 1989.
59. Nutrition and health promotion, *Cancer Res.*, Suppl., 52, 2019s, 1992.
60. Pariza, M. W., Dietary fat, calorie restriction, ad libitum feeding, and cancer risk, *Nutr. Rev.*, 45(1), 1, 1987.
61. Pirisi, L., Batova, A., Jenkins, G. R., Hodam, J. R., and Creek, K. E., Increased sensitivity of human keratinocytes immortalized by human papillomavirus type 16 DNA to growth control by retinoids, *Cancer Res.*, 52, 187, 1992.
62. Petering, H. G., Diet, nutrition and cancer, in *Advances in Experimental Medicine and Biology*, Plenum Press, New York, 1978.
63. Peterson, G. and Barnes, S., Genistein inhibition of the growth of human breast cancer cells: independence from estrogen receptors and multi-drug resistance gene, *Biochem. Biophys. Res. Commun.*, 179, 661, 1991.
64. Prentice, R. L., Kakar, K., Hursting, S., Sheppard, L., Klein, R., and Kushi, L. H., Aspects of the rationale for the women's health trial, *J. Natl. Cancer. Inst.*, 80, 802, 1988.
65. Reddy, B. S., Dietary fat, calories, and fiber in colon cancer, *Prev. Med.*, 22(5), 738, 1993.
66. Reddy, B. S. and Cohen, L. A. Eds., Macronutrients and cancer, in *Diet, Nutrition, and Cancer: A Critical Evaluation* Vol. I, CRC Press, Boca Raton, FL, 1986.
67. Reddy, B. S. and Cohen, L. A., Eds., Micronutrients, nonnutritive dietary factors, and cancer, in *Diet, Nutrition, and Cancer: A Critical Evaluation*, Vol. II, CRC Press, Boca Raton, FL, 1986.
68. Ritenbaugh, C., Dietary supplementation: the case for placebo-controlled trials, *Prev. Med.*, 22(5), 667, 1993.
69. Rogers, A. E., Zeisel, S. H., and Akhtar, R., Choline, methionine, folate and chemical carcinogenesis, in *Vitamins and Minerals in the Prevention and Treatment of Cancer*, Jacobs, M. M., Ed., CRC Press, Boca Raton, FL, 1991, chap. 10.
70. Rogers, A. E., Zeisel, S. H., and Groopman, J., Diet and carcinogenesis, *Carcinogenesis*, 14(11), 2205, 1993.
71. Shamberger, R. J., Rukovena, E., Longfield, A. K., Tytco, S. A., Deodhar, S., and Willis, C. E., Antioxidants and cancer. I. Selenium in the blood of normals and cancer patients, *J. Natl. Cancer Inst.*, 50, 867, 1973.
72. Shamsuddin, A. M., Baten, A., and Lalwani, D., Effects of inositol hexaphosphate on growth and differentiation in K-562 erythroleukemia cell line, *Cancer Lett.*, 64, 195, 1992.
73. Shubik, P., Progression and promotion, *J. Natl. Cancer. Inst.*, 73(5), 1005, 1984.
74. Souba, W. W., Glutamine and cancer, *Ann. Surg.*, 218(6), 715, 1993.
75. Stern, P. H. and Hoffman, R. M., Enhanced in vitro toxicity of chemotherapeutic agents for human cancer cells based on a metabolic defect, *J. Natl. Cancer Inst.*, 76, 629, 1986.

76. Stout, M. G. and Rawson, R. W., Minerals, trace elements and cancer, in *Nutrition and Cancer: Etiology and Treatment*, Newell, G. R. and Ellison, N. M., Eds., Raven Press, New York, 1981.
77. Thacker, S. V., Nickel, M., and DiGirolamo, M., Effects of food restriction on lactate production from glucose by rat adipocytes, *Am. J. Physiol.*, 253, E336, 1987.
78. Thorling, E. B., Dietary non-nutritive cancer protective factors, *Eur. J. Cancer. Prev.*, 2(2), 95, 1993.
79. Torti, F. M. and Torti, S. V., Cytokines, iron homeostasis and cancer, in *Diet, and Cancer: Markers, Prevention, and Treatment*, Jacobs, M. M., Ed., *Advances in Experimental Medicine and Biology*, Vol. 354, Plenum Press, New York, 1994.
80. Trock, B., Lanza, E. and Greenwald, P., Dietary fiber, vegetables, and colon cancer: Critical review and meta-analysis of the epidemiologic evidence, *J. Natl. Cancer. Inst.*, 82(8), 650, 1990.
81. Troll, W., Frenkel, K., and Wiesner, R., Protease inhibitors as anticarcinogens, *J. Natl. Cancer Inst.*, 73, 1245, 1984.
82. U.S. Department of Health and Human Services, *The Surgeon General's Report on Nutrition and Health*, Public Health Service DHHS (PHS) Publication No. 88-50210, 1988.
83. Van Poppel, G., Carotenoids and cancer: an update with emphasis on human intervention studies, *Eur. J. Cancer*, 29A(9), 1335, 1993.
84. Vecchia, C. L., Harris, R. E., and Wynder, E. L., Comparative epidemiology of cancer between the United States and Italy, *Cancer Res..*, 48, 7285, 1988.
85. Vernie, L. N., Selenium in carcinogenesis, *Biochim. Biophys, Acta*, 738, 203, 1984.
86. Vlassara, H., Brownlee, M., Monague, K. R., Dinarello, C. A., and Pasagian, A., Cachectin/TNF and IL-1 induced by glucose-modified proteins: role of normal tissue remodeling, *Science*, 240, 1546, 1988.
87. Von Hoff, D. D. and Van Devanter, D. R., Optimal detection of the effect of vitamin D3 on extrachromosomal oncogene sequences, in *Vitamins and Minerals in the Prevention and Treatment of Cancer*, Jacobs, M. M., Ed., CRC Press, Boca Raton, FL, 1991, chap. 13.
88. Vucenik, I., Tomazic, V. J., Fabian, D., and Shamsuddin, A. M., Antitumor activity of phytic acid (inositol hexaphosphate) in murine transplanted and metastatic fibrosarcoma, a pilot study, *Cancer Lett.*, 65, 9, 1992.
89. Wainfan, E., Kilkenny, M., and Dizik, M., Comparison of methyltransferase activities of pair-fed rats given adequate or methyl-deficient diets, *Carcinogenesis*, 9(5), 861, 1988.
90. Wang, Z. Y., Agarwal, R., Khan, W. A., and Mukhtar, H., Protection against benzo(a)pyrene and N-nitrosodiethylamine-induced lung and forestomach tumorigenesis in A/J mice by water extracts of green tea and licorice, *Carcinogenesis*, 13, 1491, 1992.
91. Wang, Z. Y., Hong, J.-Y., Huang, M.-T., Reuhl, K., Conney, A. H., and Yang, C. S., Inhibition of N-nitrosodiethylamine and 4-(methylnitrosamino)-1-(3-pyridyl)-1-butanone-induced tumorigenesis in A/J mice by green tea and black tea, *Cancer Res.*, 52, 1943, 1992.
92. Wargovich, M. J., Sumiyoshi, H., Baer, A., and Imada, O., Chemoprevention of gastrointestinal cancer in animals by naturally occuring organosulfur compounds in allium vegetables, in *Vitamins and Minerals in the Prevention and Treatment of Cancer*, Jacobs, M. M., Ed., CRC Press, Boca Raton, FL, 1991, chap. 6.
93. Watson, R. R. and Leonard, T. K., Selenium and vitamins A, E, and C: nutrients with cancer prevention properties, *Perspectives in Practice*, 86, 505, 1986.
94. Wattenberg, L. W., Inhibition of carcinogenesis by minor dietary constituents, *Cancer Res.*, 52, 2085s, 1992.
95. Weisburger, A. S. and Suhrland, L. G., Studies on analogues of L-cysteine and L-cystine. III. The effect of selenium cystine on leukemia, *Blood*, 10, 19, 1955.
96. Weisburger, J. H., Role of fat, fiber, nitrate, and food additives in carcinogenesis: A critical evaluation and recommendations, *Nutr. Cancer*, 8, 47, 1986.

97. Weisburger, J. H., Carcinogens in our food and cancer prevention, in *Nutritional and Toxicological Consequences of Food Processing*, Friedman, M., Ed., Plenum Press, New York, 1991.

98. Weisburger, J. H., Nutritional approach to cancer prevention with emphasis on vitamins, antioxidants, and carotenoids, *Am. J. Clin. Nutr.*, 53, 226S, 1991.

99. Whanger, P. D., Selenium in the treatment of heavy metal poisoning and chemical carcinogenesis, *J. Trace Elem. Electrolytes Health Dis.*, 6(4), 209, 1992.

100. Wilson, M. J., Shivapurkar, N., and Poirier, L. A., Hypomethylation of hepatic nuclear DNA in rats fed with a carcinogenic methyl-deficient diet, *Biochem. J.*, 218, 987, 1984.

101. Yang, C. S., Wang, Z.-Y., and Hong, J. Y., Inhibition of tumorigenesis by chemicals from garlic and tea, in *Diet and Cancer: Markers, Prevention, and Treatment*, Jacobs, M. M., Ed., *Advances in Experimental Medicine and Biology*, Vol. 354, Plenum Press, New York, 1994, chap. 8.

102. Yen, A., Chandler, S., Forbes, M. E., Fung, Y.-K., T'Ang, A., and Pearson, R., Coupled down-regulation of the RB retinoblastoma and c-myc genes antecedes cell differentiation: possible role of RB as a "status quo" gene, *Europ. J. Cell. Biol.*, 57, 210, 1992.

103. Zhang, Y., Talalay, P, Cho, C.-G., and Posner, G. H., A major inducer of anticarcinogenic protective enzymes from broccoli: isolation and elucidation of structure, *Proc. Natl. Acad. Sci. U.S.A.*, 89, 2310, 1992.

104. Ziegler, R. G., Subar, A. F., Craft, N. E., Ursin, G., Patterson, B. H., and Graubard, B. I., Does beta-carotene explain why reduced cancer risk is associated with vegetable and fruit intake?, *Cancer Res.*, 52, 2060s, 1992.

Chapter 4

CHOLESTEROL AND CARDIOVASCULAR DISEASE: HOW CAN NUTRITION HELP?

David Kritchevsky

CONTENTS

I. INTRODUCTION

Cardiovascular disease is conceded to be a disease of multiple etiology. In the absence of an unequivocal diagnosis for the impending coronary we have developed a number of surrogate statistical diagnoses which we call risk factors. A risk factor, then, is a statistical rather than a medical indication of susceptibility. Since risk factors essentially represent the odds of a coronary event, we cannot expect them to be infallible, but they will be right more often than not. Conversely, in many cases the risk factors are identified as the disease which is the wrong way to regard them.

Hopkins and Williams[57] identified 246 risk factors for coronary disease. Not all were of equal importance but the number indicates how diverse the field of study is. The major risk factors are male gender, hypercholesterolemia, hypertension, cigarette smoking and obesity. Family history of coronary disease is also important, but it and gender are beyond medical control. Hypertriglyceridemia was once generally considered to be a risk factor, then was relegated to non-risk factor, and is now being rehabilitated into risk factor status. Havel[46] has reviewed newer aspects of the role of triglyceride rich lipoproteins in atherosclerosis.

In 1950 Gofman and his co-workers[38] demonstrated the possibility of separating plasma lipoproteins into classes based on their hydrated density. Their work led to a huge refinement in risk classification over the previous one of simply measuring total serum or plasma cholesterol. Originally they classified the lipoproteins by S_f units (S_f = Svedberg units of flotation). More familiarly these classes are now identified as chylomicrons (large in size, low in density, and consisting mainly of triglycerides); VLDL or very low density lipoproteins which are rich in triglycerides; low density lipoproteins (LDL) which are rich in cholesterol and are considered to be a risk factor when elevated; and high density lipoproteins (HDL) which are protein-rich and offer a negative risk for coronary disease. In the popular press LDL is said to carry the "bad" cholesterol and HDL to carry the "good" cholesterol. It was shown several decades ago by Rothblat et al.,[128] that cholesterol entered cells in culture when they were suspended in medium containing a lipid-protein mix resembling LDL and that cholesterol was removed from cells suspended in HDL-like medium.

The definition of lipoprotein classes by their physical characteristics (hydrated density) means that their chemical composition, as presented in Table 1, is approximate. And indeed, we are now discovering that LDL may consist of large or small particles and that the size of the particle and its composition may be crucial to the metabolic behavior of that particle. Small LDL particles may enter cells more readily than large ones. Stender and Zilversmit[139] showed that molecular size was a determinant of lipoprotein influx into aortas of cholesterol-fed rabbits. More recent studies[121] involving isolation of LDL from cholesterol-fed normal and diabetic rabbits and injection of the iodine labeled lipoproteins back into the rabbits, show that relative arterial initial clearance of

TABLE 1
Properties of the Plasma Lipoproteins

	Class					
	CM	VLDL	IDL	LDL	HDL2	HDL3
Density (g/ml)	<0.95	<1.006	1.006–1.019	1.019–1.063	1.063–1.125	1.125–1.21
Mean diameter (nm)	10^2–10^3	43	27	22	9.5	6.6
Protein (%)	1–2	10	18	25	40	55
Lipid (%)	98–9	90	82	75	60	45
Total Cholesterol (%)	3	17	41	59	43	38
(%Ester)	(46)	(57)	(66)	(70)	(74)	(81)
Triglycerides	88	56	32	7	6	7
Phospholipid	9	19	27	28	42	41

Note: CM = chylomicrons; VLDL = very low density lipoprotein; IDL = intermediate density lipoprotein; LDL = low density lipoprotein; HDL = high densitylipoprotein.

From Thompson, G. R., *A Handbook of Hyperlipidemia,* Current Science, London, 1989.

the lipoproteins is inversely related to their relative molecular weight. Marzetta and Rudel[105] suggested that differences in severity of diet-induced atherosclerosis between cynomolgus and African green monkeys might be due to size and composition of their LDL. Babiak and Rudel[10] have reviewed data which indicate that small, cholesterol ester-depleted LDL is associated with coronary heart disease.

Austin et al.[9] analyzed subclasses of LDL by gradient gel electrophoresis. The LDL were obtained from plasma of 109 cases with confirmed myocardial infarction and 121 controls. The LDL subclass pattern characterized by increased levels of small, dense LDL particles was associated with a threefold increased risk of myocardial infarction. The correlation was independent of age, sex, and relative weight. While total plasma cholesterol levels of cases and controls were not significantly different (226 ± 47 vs. 215 ± 40), triglyceride levels were (214 ± 104 vs. 157 ± 68) ($p < 0.01$).

The interest in the proteins which accompany the lipids (apolipoproteins) has expanded the breadth of research in this field and offers the opportunity for genetic characterization. Thus apolipoprotein B (apo B), which is the sole apoprotein of LDL, presents another basis for risk assessment and diagnosis. The polymorphism of apo E[150,164] presents a way to classify subjects by apo E phenotype and thus obtain a more accurate diagnosis of susceptibility and greater insight as to mode of treatment. Jenkins et al.[66] have reported on the effects of dietary fiber on serum lipids in a cohort of 43 men and 24 women. Apo E phenotype and genotype were determined for each proband. Reductions in LDL cholesterol levels were significantly different (p = 0.048) depending on apo E allele. The level of LDL cholesterol reduction in apo E2 carriers was greater than for apo E3 homozygotes or apo E4 carriers. Thompson[143] has written a very useful monograph covering hyperlipidemia.

Cholesterol is a very important component of the biological economy.[74,116] It is a component of every cell and a precursor of essential compounds such as corticosteroids, bile acids and sex hormones. In general cholesterol comprises about 0.2% of body weight with most of the body's cholesterol being present in muscle and nervous tissue. Cholesterol is synthesized endogenously by the liver and other tissues and in most cases we synthesize more cholesterol than we ingest. Cholesterol feeding inhibits hepatic cholesterol synthesis. How did this essential chemical achieve the status of a major nutritional and physiological villain?

The focus of cholesterol as a factor in atherogenesis arose from the experiments by Anitschkow and Chalatow[8] and Wacker and Hueck[153] in which they produced aortic lesions in rabbits fed cholesterol for several months. Their experiments stimulated untold numbers of studies carried out in many species. The level of cholesterol in the blood did not always correlate with the severity of aortic lesions but since cholesterol feeding elevated plasma cholesterol it was natural to hypothesize that high blood cholesterol was related to aortic deposition. Today we are admonished to be aware of our serum cholesterol

TABLE 2
Seasonal Variation of Plasma Total and
HDL-Cholesterol in Israeli Men

		Cholesterol (mg/dl)		
Month	Subjects	Total	HDL	%HDL
1	208	201	43.1	21.4
2	156	203	41.6	20.0
3	191	202	42.3	20.9
4	125	199	41.2	20.7
5	315	197	40.4	20.5
6	338	194	39.5	20.4
7	288	195	39.3	20.2
8	273	199	40.9	20.6
9	138	199	40.2	20.2
10	77	210	41.0	19.5
11	170	202	41.3	20.4
12	180	205	42.7	20.8

From Harlap, S., Kark, J. D., Baras, M., Eisenberg, S., and Stein, Y., *Isr. J. Med. Sci.,* 18, 1158, 1982.

level and to keep it within a desirable range by means of diet (low cholesterol, low fat) and if that fails to consider pharmacologic intervention.

To deal intelligently with serum cholesterol levels we must be aware that in most people cholesterol levels fluctuate over the course of the year. In 1924 Currie[23] studied serum cholesterol levels in cancer patients and controls and found seasonal variations in both groups. Several years later Schube[132] studied the cholesterol levels of 10 men over a 16-week period. While the weekly group average was relatively constant individual levels varied by as much as 31%. Thomas et al.[141] carried out monthly cholesterol determinations in 16 young prisoners over a year. In eight subjects with cholesterol levels below 225 mg/dl the mean cholesterol value over the year was 202 ± 2; the range of average values was 168 to 242. In four subjects whose cholesterol ranged from 225 to 274 mg/dl, the year average and range were 244 ± 7 and 214–295 mg/dl respectively and for four individuals whose cholesterol levels were above 275 mg/dl the year average was 301 ± 3 mg/dl and the range was 240 to 376 mg/dl. Harlap et al.[45] found seasonal variations in 2459 men and 2787 women studied in the Jerusalem Lipid Research Clinic (Table 2). They concluded, "...clinicians should take season into account when diagnosing hyperlipidemia and when evaluating success or failure of its treatment." Groover et al.[43] studied 177 army officers in the Pentagon over a five-year period during which they obtained at least six cholesterol determinations yearly for each individual. For the entire cohort the variation averaged about 25% with variations of plasma cholesterol of less than 20 or more than 50% being observed in 20 and 21% of the probands, respectively. Gordon et al.[39] analyzed seasonal variations in plasma lipids and lipoproteins in 1446 hypercholesterolemic men who comprised the placebo group in the Lipid Research Clinics Coronary Primary Prevention Trial. They found highly significant ($p < 0.001$) seasonal cycles for total, LDL, and HDL cholesterol. Total and LDL-cholesterol variations were inversely and significantly correlated with hours of daylight and HDL-cholesterol variations were significantly and positively correlated with ambient temperature. There was no correlation between seasonal fluctuations and body mass index or seasonal intake of total calories, fat, or cholesterol. They concluded, "While the etiologic mechanisms of seasonal plasma lipid and lipoprotein cycles remain uncertain there can no longer be any doubt that these cycles exist." Robinson et al.[127] have shown these variations in a cohort of over 200,000 Britons and Japanese. The subject has been reviewed recently.[53,77,79] Thus we must consider cholesterol levels and their relation to risk in light of our knowledge concerning this cyclical phenomenon.

What nutrient is the principal contributor to cholesterolemia? The first instinct is to indict cholesterol itself. However, most studies show that cholesterol plays a relatively minor role in cholesterolemia. In 1950 Gertler et al.[36] studied two cohorts of 40 men each separated into four ten-man subgroups according to high or low serum cholesterol or low or high cholesterol intake. The 40-man groups were composed of men who did or did not have coronary disease. As Table 3 shows, in every subgroup the men with coronary disease had significantly higher cholesterol levels but there was no correlation with

TABLE 3

Dietary and Serum Cholesterol in Control Subjects and those with Coronary Disease (10 Men in each Subgroup)

	Serum Cholesterol		
	Control	**CHD**	***p<***
Lowest serum cholesterol			
Serum cholesterol, mg/dl	162 ± 2	196 ± 5	0.001
Dietary cholesterol, g/wk	3.8 ± 0.3	3.3 ± 0.5	NS
Highest serum cholesterol			
Serum cholesterol, mg/dl	313 ± 3	416 ± 7	0.001
Dietary cholesterol, g/wk	4.3 ± 0.4	4.1 ± 0.6	NS
Lowest cholesterol intake			
Serum cholesterol, mg/dl	222 ± 16	271 ± 14	0.05
Dietary cholesterol, g/wk	1.4 ± 0.1	1.3 ± 0.1	NS
Highest cholesterol intake			
Serum cholesterol, mg/dl	213 ± 11	288 ± 22	0.01
Dietary cholesterol, g/wk	7.0 ± 0.3	5.7 ± 0.2	0.01

From Gertler, M. M., Garn, S. M., and White, P. D., *Circulation*, 2, 696, 1950.

TABLE 4
Daily Nutrient Intake and Coronary Heart Disease (CHD)
in Three Trial Locations

	Framingham		Puerto Rico		Hawaii	
	No CHD	CHD	No CHD	CHD	No CHD	CHD
No. subjects	780	79	1932	286	7008	264
Total Calories	2622	2488	2395	2289	2319	2210*
Protein (g)	101	99	86	85	95	95
Carbohydrate (g)	252	248	280	262*	264	249*
Sugar (g)	72	78	52	50	46	45
Starch (g)	117	118	180	167*	165	155*
Other (g)	61	52*	48	45	52	48
Fat (g)	114	111	95	94	87	86
P/S	0.39	0.41	0.45	0.49	0.54	0.57
Cholesterol(mg)	529	534	417	419	555	549
Alcohol (g)	25	12*	12	8	14	8*

* Significantly different from No CHD.

From Gordon, T., Kagan, A., Garcia-Palmieri, M., Kannel, W. B., Zukel, W. J., Tillotson, J., Sorbie, P., and Hjortland, M., *Circulation,* 63, 500, 1981.

level of cholesterol intake. Dawber et al.[26] found no connection between cholesterol intake and serum cholesterol levels in the Framingham study. Earlier studies of other free-living populations have found no relation between dietary cholesterol intake and serum or plasma cholesterol levels.[125,136] Flynn et al.[31] fed a group of 47 men and 29 women diets which supplied daily 5 oz of beef (70 mg cholesterol per 100 g) or of poultry (75 mg cholesterol per 100 g) or fish (50 mg cholesterol per 100 g). Each dietary period was of three months' duration. After a wash-out period all subjects were fed 5 oz of pork (65 mg cholesterol per 100 g) daily. Otherwise, the diets were self-selected but also contained one egg per day. There were no differences in serum cholesterol levels between the dietary periods. A similar study[32] was repeated in a cohort of 74 men and 55 women and again there were no differences in any serum lipids among the men, but the women showed significant elevations in triglyceride levels when eating poultry and fish. Scott et al.[133] have reported recently that lean beef and chicken had similar results on plasma lipids and lipoproteins when added to a Step 1 Diet. The diets were fed for 5 weeks and contained 85 g of either cooked beef or cooked chicken A study of heart disease and diet among subjects in three large prospective studies of coronary disease[40] found no significant differences between intakes of fat and cholesterol and coronary disease (Table 4). McNamara[108] analyzed data from 68 studies involving 1490 subjects and concluded that the average effect of dietary cholesterol on blood cholesterol is about 2.3 ± 0.2 mg/dl per 100 mg of dietary cholesterol.

Mention should be made of current interest in the effects of low plasma cholesterol levels on noncoronary death. There have been reviews of data from a number of primary prevention trials[20,55,115] discussing possible causes of noncoronary mortality in these trials. A report from the Lipid Research Clinics program[19] found increased risk of colon cancer in men whose plasma cholesterol level is below 187 mg/dl. Review of a large number of trials (yielding 68,406 deaths) found that plasma cholesterol levels below 160 mg/dl were not advantageous[65] and prompted an editorial[61] suggesting rethinking of our health policy regarding blood cholesterol. The review[65] found that men whose cholesterol levels were below 160 mg/dl had 20% more cancer deaths, 40% more noncardiovascular, noncancer deaths, 35% more deaths from injury, and 50% more digestive system deaths. A review[101] of low cholesterol levels and risk of cancer found the risk surfaced in the course of the cholesterol lowering trials and not afterward, suggesting that metabolic abnormalities which occurred during the cholesterol lowering regimen could determine the observed outcomes. The foregoing do not lead one to question the role of elevated cholesterol as a risk factor; based on current knowledge and medical theory elevated cholesterol levels should be reduced but as a recent meta-analysis has shown cholesterol reduction is beneficial primarily in cases of severe hypercholesterolemia.[25]

II. FAT

The type of fat present in the diet is the principal determinant of the plasma cholesterol level. Saturated fat is much more atherogenic for rabbits than unsaturated fat regardless of the cholesterol content of the diet.[87,88,95] Ahrens[2] demonstrated that serum cholesterol levels of subjects given formula diets containing 40% fat were generally related to the level of unsaturation of the particular fat. There are exceptions, however. Fats rich in stearic acid, such as cocoa butter are less atherogenic than might be adduced from their level of saturation.[90,92] Keys et al.[70] and Hegsted et al.[52] formulated equations for predicting changes in cholesterol level as a function of the levels of saturated and unsaturated fatty acids present in the diet. In both cases stearic acid was regarded as neutral. The Keys and Hegsted formulas have proved useful adjuncts to research.

The original Keys formula[70] was:

$$\Delta C = 1.35 \ (2\Delta S - \Delta P) + 1.5 \ \Delta Z$$

where ΔC represents the change in cholesterol level, S and P represent saturated and unsaturated fatty acids, respectively, and Z represents the square root of mg of dietary cholesterol per 1000 kcal.

The Hegsted formula[52] is:

$$\Delta C = 2.16 \ \Delta S - 1.65 \ \Delta P + 0.168 \ \Delta C \ (mg/1000 \ kcal) + 85$$

Recently other investigators have developed other regression equations to predict the effects of fat on cholesterol levels. Hayes and his co-workers[48,49,72] have been studying the effects of mixed fats on cholesterolemia in monkeys, hamsters, and man in order to delineate effects of specific fatty acids. In preparing the fats used in his studies Hayes blended various amounts of naturally available oils so that the fatty acid spectra of the blends provided the proper test material, but all the fatty acids were in their normal distribution within each triglyceride. They conclude that linoleic acid is hypocholesterolemic until it reaches the level of about 4% of dietary calories and then has no further effect. Myristic acid is thought to be hypercholesterolemic at any level and palmitic acid is cholesterolemic only under specific conditions such as high cholesterol (>400 mg/day) diet. Hayes[47] has developed a predictive formula useful for persons on cholesterol free diets:

$$\text{Cholesterol} = 229 + 8E_{14:0} - 3.6 \ E_{18:2}$$

where E represents the energy contribution of the specific fatty acids.

Derr et al.[29] have devised a formula which addresses specific fatty acids, namely:

$$\Delta C = 2.3 \ \Delta \ 14:0 + 3.0 \ \Delta \ 16:0 - 0.8 \ \Delta \ 18:0 - 1.0 \ \text{PUFA}$$

where PUFA represents polyunsaturated fatty acids.

Cobb and Teitlebaum[18] have studied responsiveness of plasma cholesterol to diet and have determined that age plays a role. Their formulas for predicting changes in total, LDL- and HDL-cholesterol are:

$$\Delta \ \text{Total Cholesterol (mg/L)} = 0.79 \ (\text{age in years}) + 1.03 \ (\% \ \Delta SFA)$$

where SFA represents saturated fatty acids.

$$\Delta \ \text{LDL-C (mg/L)} = 0.71 \ (\text{age, years}) + 1.03 \ (\% \Delta SFA)$$
$$+ 0.22 \ \text{baseline LDL,(mg/L)} - 28.41$$

and

$$\Delta \ \text{HDL - C (mg/L)} = 0.31 \ (\% \ \Delta SFA) - 0.40 \ (\% \ \Delta PUFA)$$
$$+ 0.13 \ \text{baseline HDL-C (mg/L)}$$

Flynn et al.[33] followed 144 men over a 20-year period and found no significant change in serum cholesterol with age.

TABLE 5
Plasma Lipids (mg/dl) in Subjects Fed Saturated (SFA) or Unsaturated (PUFA) fat and High or Low Levels of Cholesterol

Dietary Cholesterol	Plasma Lipids[a]	
	Total Cholesterol (mg/dl)	LDL/HDL
PUFA (39 subjects)		
Low Cholesterol	218 ± 49	3.12
High Cholesterol	224 ± 46	3.14
SFA (36 subjects)		
Low Cholesterol	243 ± 50	3.20
High Cholesterol	248 ± 51	3.26

Note: PUFA = P/S about 1.5; SFA = P/S about 0.3; Low cholesterol about 250 mg/d; High cholesterol about 800 mg/d.

[a] The difference between cholesterol levels of subjects on PUFA-low cholesterol or PUFA-high cholesterol was 2.8%; that between the two groups on SFA was 2.1%. Difference between PUFA-high cholesterol and SFA — high cholesterol was 10.7% and between PUFA and SFA low cholesterol was 11.5%.

From McNamara, D. J., Kolb, R., Parker, T. S., Batwin, H., Samuel, P., Brown, C. D., and Ahrens, E. H., Jr., *J. Clin. Invest.*, 79, 1729, 1987.

Thus, in a general sense, saturated fatty acids are more cholesterolemic and possibly more atherogenic than unsaturated fats. There are anomalies, however. Peanut oil, a relatively unsaturated fat, is surprisingly atherogenic for rats,[42] rabbits,[98] and monkeys.[84,152] Autointeresterification (randomization) of peanut oil alters the structure of its component triglycerides and reduces significantly its atherogenicity.[92,96] Fats containing predominate levels of specific fatty acids prepared by interesterifying specific triglycerides (trilaurin, tripalmitin, etc.) with commercially available plant oils do not reflect the hypercholesterolemic properties imputed to naturally occurring oils containing those fatty acids.[91,106] The reason for the difference may lie in the randomization.

The relative effects of saturated and unsaturated fats on human cholesterolemia are shown clearly in a study by McNamara et al.[109] in which volunteers were fed diets high or low in cholesterol and containing saturated or unsaturated fat (Table 5). The effect of fat saturation far overrode the effects of cholesterol level. They also found that about two-thirds of their subjects compensated for increased dietary cholesterol by reducing endogenous synthesis.

After reviewing 420 dietary observations from 141 groups of subjects, Hegsted et al.[51] concluded that saturated fatty acids are the principal determinants of serum cholesterol levels, polyunsaturated fatty acids lower serum cholesterol, monounsaturated fats have no independent effect, and dietary cholesterol raises serum cholesterol levels.

A recent concern has involved the effects of fats containing trans-unsaturated double bonds. The term "trans fat" refers to fats containing unsaturated fatty acids containing double bonds in the transconfiguration. The effects of trans fats were reviewed a few years ago,[78] but a few new questions have arisen. Trans fats occur in nature — in plants and in animal tissues — but the principal source of trans fat in the human diet is hydrogenated fat.

Trans fatty acids are generally metabolized like their cis counterparts. Carboxyl labeled oleic and eladic acids are decarboxylated at the same rate.[122] Uniformly labeled (with ^{14}C) oleic and elaidic were catabolized to $^{14}CO_2$ at rates of 70 and 65% respectively.[7] Rats fed partially hydrogenated soybean oil show presence of cis and trans fatty acids in triglycerides and phospholipids of all tissues.[162] Rats[114] or monkeys[84] fed trans fat accumulate trans unsaturated fatty acids in liver and blood but these acids disappear soon after the dietary stimulus has been removed. The concern about TFA is not new. McMillan's group fed cholesterol and TFA-rich fats to rabbits more than 30 years ago. They found the diets to be more cholesterolemic but not more atherogenic than the control diets.[107,155] When rabbits were fed semi-purified, cholesterol-free diets containing 3.2 or 6.0% TFA, cholesterol levels were increased but the severity of their atherosclerosis was like that of the control; the diets had no effect on the activities of a number of hepatic enzymes.[129] Houtsmuller[58] concluded that TFA should be regarded as quasi-saturated fatty acid. Some experiments suggest that dietary TFA lead to increase of 10% or more in human cholesterol levels,[3,28,113] whereas others find more modest increases.[160,110,117] One current concern is that TFA may reduce HDL-cholesterol levels and increase the level of lipoprotein (a), Lp(a), a particularly dangerous lipoprotein.[12,59] However, other studies do not find an elevation of Lp(a).[103,161] The effect of TFA on Lp(a) may reflect the action of a specific trans-unsaturated fatty acid.

Hydrogenation leads to double bond shifts in fatty acids with the result that margarines may contain double bonds (both cis and trans) anywhere between carbon atoms 4 and 16 of an 18-carbon atom fatty acid.[30] More definitive work is required in this area. Two studies have shown that the trans fatty acid content of the tissues of subjects who died of coronary disease was the same as that of control.[50,142] There has been muted public concern about the long standing advice to substitute margarine for butter.

The data show that fat saturation is the principal determinant of plasma cholesterol levels. However, it is becoming apparent that specific fatty acids have unique effects which may be further influenced by dietary cholesterol. Until all the variables have been clearly identified the best general advice vis-a-vis cholesterolemia is moderation in fat intake.

III. PROTEIN

Ignatowski[63,64] conducted the first studies devoted purely to diet and atherosclerosis. Previous work had included other aspects, such as mechanical injury, stress, or administration of noxious agents. Ignatowski found that adult rabbits developed nephritis, cirrhosis and atherosclerosis when fed meat and that weanling rabbits given milk and egg yolk developed atherosclerosis, anemia, renal disorders and cirrhosis. Other investigators of that era also observed that diets containing animal protein tended to be atherogenic for rabbits.[104,131,138,140] Knack[73] showed that a normal rabbit diet plus 500 to 4500 mg of cholesterol was less atherogenic than one containing milk and one egg which provided 300 mg cholesterol. Research on protein effects in atherosclerosis was dealt a setback in 1913 when Anitschkow and Chalatow[8] demonstrated the atherogenic potential of pure cholesterol. For decades thereafter atherosclerosis research entailed aspects of cholesterol feeding with little attention being paid to the influence of other components of the diet.

In the course of studies of Bright's disease, Newburgh[118] found that rabbits developed atherosclerosis when fed 15 to 30 g of casein daily. Newburgh and Squier[120] showed that rabbits fed casein or beef exhibited atherosclerosis with the severity being dependent upon the duration of feeding. Newburgh and Clarkson[119] confirmed that severity of atherosclerosis depended on protein level and duration of feeding. The diets they used provided between 28 and 36 mg per day of cholesterol, which is not enough to be atherogenic per se. To establish this point Clarkson and Newburgh[17] fed rabbits varying doses of cholesterol for different time periods and showed that, under their conditions, 253 mg of cholesterol daily did not become atherogenic until fed more than three months.

Meeker and Kesten[111,112] were the first investigators to compare directly proteins of animal or plant origin. They maintained rabbits on a diet providing 15% protein. They compared this control diet with diets high (38%) in animal protein (casein) or high (39%) in plant protein. In some experiments they added cholesterol to the diets. On the cholesterol-free diets, average plasma cholesterol levels (mg/ml) were approximately 55 (basal), 65 (soy) or 145 (casein). Carroll and Hamilton[16] found a wide range of cholesterolemic effects of animal or plant protein with the former being more cholesterolemic (Table 6).

We proposed the possibility that the lysine/arginine ratio might play a role in atherogenesis.[75] The reasoning was based, in part, on the known antagonism between lysine and arginine in chicks[67] and rats.[68] Using a semipurified, cholesterol-free diet as the vehicle, we examined the effects of casein, soy protein, casein plus enough arginine to provide the lysine/arginine ratio found in soy protein, and soy plus sufficient lysine to provide the ratio of lysine to arginine found in casein.[24,76] Soy protein was significantly less cholesterolemic and atherogenic than casein. Addition of arginine to casein did not affect lipidemia but reduced atherosclerosis by 25%. Addition of lysine to soy protein increased serum cholesterol levels by about 50% and atherosclerosis by 60%. The differences in atherogenicity were reflected in levels of IDL (intermediate density lipoprotein). Beef protein or casein is more cholesterolemic and atherogenic for rabbits than is textured soy protein (TVP), but a 1:1 mixture of TVP and beef protein is no more atherogenic and only slightly more

TABLE 6
Influence of Protein Source on Serum Cholesterol Levels in Rabbits

Animal Protein	Serum Cholesterol (mg/dl)	Plant Proteins	Serum Cholesterol (mg/dl)
Egg yolk	260	Wheat Gluten	80
Skim Milk	230	Peanut	80
Turkey	217	Oat	77
Lactalbumen	210	Cottonseed	73
Casein	200	Sesame seed	70
Whole egg	183	Alfalfa	67
Fish	167	Soy isolate	67
Beef	153	Sunflower Seed	53
Chicken	147	Pea	40
Pork	107	Fava Bean	30
Egg White	100		

Note: Rabbits fed 30% defatted protein, 1% corn oil for 1 month.

From Carroll, K. K. and Hamilton, R. M. G., *Food Sci.*, 40, 118, 1975.

cholesterolemic than TVP alone.[93] Rabbits fed casein exhibit larger body pools of cholesterol and slower cholesterol turnover and excretion than those fed soy protein.[35,80]

In a review of the literature conducted in 1957, Yerushalmy and Hilleboe[163] concluded that the intake of animal protein was better correlated than fat intake with risk of atherosclerosis. Hodges et al.[54] fed six volunteers diets containing a variety of combinations of fat and carbohydrate mixtures in a series of four-week studies. To avoid another variable, the subjects were switched from their habitual mixed protein diet to one containing only plant protein. The consequent reduction in plasma cholesterol was greater than that seen on any of the test diets (Table 7). Sirtori et al.[134,135] have shown that soy protein significantly lowers cholesterol levels in a number of hypercholesterolemic subjects. Not all studies in man have shown soy protein to be hypocholesterolemic.[56]

The reason why protein of animal origin is relatively cholesterolemic is not clear. It may be due to the fat associated with animal protein and it may be due to its amino acid composition. Protein of animal origin is a good source of trace minerals such as zinc and iron and provides B vitamins as well. More work is needed in this area especially since most experiments involve substitution of all of one protein for another rather than mixing proteins in the proportions normally ingested. The animal studies[93] suggest that a diet balanced in protein is most advantageous.

IV. CARBOHYDRATE

Elevated triglyceride levels are associated with lipoprotein abnormalities which are considered to be atherogenic, namely, high LDL and low HDL.[60]

High carbohydrate diets elevate triglycerides levels[13] and substitution of sucrose or fructose for starch results in hypertriglyceridemia.[102]

Sucrose is more cholesterolemic and atherogenic than glucose for cholesterol-fed rabbits[41] or chickens,[86] and lactose is very atherogenic when fed with cholesterol.[156] When fed as part of an atherogenic semi-purified, cholesterol-free diet sucrose and fructose are more atherogenic than either glucose or lactose.[89,96]

Truswell[146] has discussed the effects of carbohydrates on plasma lipids and has reviewed the reasons for the triglyceridemic effects of fructose and sucrose. Fructose is almost totally taken up by the liver, phosphorylated to fructose-2-phosphate and rapidly converted to trioses whereas part of the glucose intake goes to muscle. During fructose infusion there is less oxidation of fatty acids and increased fatty acid esterification with more synthesis of triglycerides.

When fed to Vervet monkeys as part of a semi-purified, cholesterol-free diet, sucrose and fructose were more cholesterolemic than glucose and fructose was much more sudanophilic than either sucrose or glucose.[82] Sudanophilia is a measure of lipid deposition in arterial tissue. The tissue is exposed to a red dye (Sudan IV) which is taken up by the lipid which has been deposited in the vessel wall. Baboons that were fed similar diets (containing glucose, fructose, sucrose or starch) exhibited cholesterol levels that were similar in all four groups (155 ± 3 mg/dl), but triglycerides were highest in animals fed fructose or sucrose.[83] Inclusion of lactose in the diet did not influence lipemia or cholesterolemia, However, when 0.1% cholesterol was also added, lactose proved to be significantly more cholesterolemic and sudanophilic than fructose, glucose, sucrose or starch.[81]

TABLE 7
Serum Lipids in 6 Subjects Fed Various Fats,
Carbohydrates and Protein

Protein	CHO[a]	%Fat (en%)	Lipids, (mg/dl)	
			Cholesterol	Triglyceride
Mixed (12)	23/20	45	217 ± 13	159 ± 22
Plant (15)	8/32	45	194 ± 17	$122 + 8$
Plant (18)	13/54	15	202 ± 11	109 ± 21
Plant (13)	58/14	15	$189 + 10$	161 ± 29
Plant (18)	13/54	15	203 ± 10	119 ± 115
Plant (13)	58/14	15	$173 + 7$	203 ± 31
Plant (12)	34/9	45	199 ± 10	135 ± 21
Mixed (12)	23/20	45	267 ± 11	159 ± 11

Note: Each diet fed for 4 weeks.

[a] Ratio of simple/complex carbohydrate.

From Hodges, R. E., Krehl, W. A., Stone, D. B., and Lopez, A., *Am. J. Clin. Nutr.,* 20, 198, 1967.

Epidemiologically,[146] high carbohydrate intake is associated with low plasma cholesterol levels and variability in plasma triglyceride concentrations. Type IV hyperlipoproteinemia (hypertriglyceridemia) is not the most common type of lipidemia but should be treated where it occurs. As more data emerge on triglyceride levels as a risk factor for coronary disease the effects of high carbohydrate diets will certainly come under more care scrutiny.

V. FIBER

The fiber hypothesis suggests that populations ingesting diets high in fiber are relatively free of Western diseases.[14,145] Fiber is defined as plant material which is impervious to our digestive secretions; it is a generic term covering a variety of materials of unique chemical structure and specific physiological effects. The fiber hypothesis is based on observation of populations which ingest a high fiber diet. The fiber in that diet exists in its indigenous form and is accompanied by a number of other substances such as plant sterols and phytoestrogens which may also influence lipidemia. In 1954 Walker and Arvidsson[154] proposed that the absence of coronary disease in African black populations was due to the high levels of fiber in their diets. Vegetarians also have low levels of plasma cholesterol and triglycerides.[130] An early study of Seventh Day Adventists showed that the vegans in this group had a higher fiber intake and lower cholesterol levels than the lacto-ovo vegetarians or omnivores in that group.[44] A later study[94] confirmed the earlier findings and found that the major difference in fiber intake among the various sub groups was that the vegans ingested considerably more pectin-rich foods (Table 8).

TABLE 8
Serum Lipids and Fiber Intake of Seventh Day Adventists

	Group			
	VEG (18)	**LOV (25)**	**NV(25)**	**GP(22)**
Serum Lipids (mg/dl)				
Total Cholesterol	149 ± 8	192 ± 7	207 ± 7	214 ± 7
% HDL-C	24.4 ± 20	24.3 ± 1.6	21.8 ± 1.6	25.7 ± 1.8
Triglycerides	174 ± 17	142 ± 14	138 ± 14	97 ± 15
Fiber Intake (g/kcal/d)				
Cellulose	2.5 ± 0.3	2.0 ± 0.2	1.5 ± 0.1	2.0 ± 0.2
Hemicellulose	11.0 ± 2.5	11.5 ± 1.0	11.0 ± 1.0	10.4 ± 1.0
Pectin	7.5 ± 1.0	4.5 ± 0.3	4.0 ± 0.2	4.0 ± 0.2
Lignin	0.8 ± 0.2	0.7 ± 0.2	0.5 ± 0.1	0.4 ± 0.1

Note: VEG, vegan; LOV, lacto-ovo vegetarian; NV, non-vegetarian; GP, general population. Number of subjects.

From Kritchevsky, D., Tepper, S. A., and Goodman, G., *Am. J. Clin. Nutr.,* 40, 921, 1984.

Fiber may also be extracted from food in essentially the same form in which it exists in the food. One example of this type of fiber is wheat bran, which has virtually no effect on plasma cholesterol. Recently Truswell and Beynen[174] reviewed data from 35 studies in which wheat bran had been fed to human subjects for varying lengths of time. No effect was seen in 26 of the studies, 7 showed cholesterol decreases and 2 showed increases.

Fiber may be extracted from food and fed in a purified concentrated form which does not resemble its natural state. The soluble fibers, pectin, guar gum, and psyllium, are fed in this form and all show hypocholesterolemic properties. The first report on the hypolipidemic effect of pectin was by Keys et al.[71] who fed 24 subjects 15 g/d of citrus pectin (in biscuits) and observed a significant (4.7%) reduction in cholesterol levels. Most subsequent studies have used citrus pectin but apple pectin appears to be as effective. Ginter et al.[37] found ascorbic acid to enhance the hypocholesterolemic effect of pectin. Eighteen studies of pectin fed 15 ± 2 g/day for 10 ± 4 weeks with an average cholesterol lowering of $27.5 \pm 1.6\%$. There appears to be little difference in efficacy between low and high methoxyl preparations.[69]

The effects of guar gum have been studied extensively, especially in diabetic patients since guar gum may also lower plasma glucose levels. In eleven studies carried out in nondiabetic subjects, an average of 19 subjects were fed 15 ± 1 g/day of guar gum for 11 ± 4 weeks. The average reduction in plasma cholesterol was $11 \pm 1.4\%$. Seventeen studies in which the subjects were diabetic contained an average of 20 probands who were fed 14.4 ± 1.4 g/day of guar gum for 9.7 ± 1.1 weeks. The average reduction in plasma cholesterol was $14 \pm 2\%$.[147]

Another fiber source that has been tested to a great extent is oat bran or oat meal. Thirty years ago de Groot et al.[27] fed rolled oats (140 g/day) in bread to 21 male volunteers for 3 weeks and observed an 11% drop in plasma cholesterol levels. Anderson et al.[4,5] carried out studies under metabolic ward conditions in which men were fed 100 g/day of oat bran and recorded cholesterol reductions of about 20% in each experiment. In 8 other studies in which oat bran or oat cereal was used there was an average of 29 probands who were fed 53 ± 11 g/day of fiber for 5 ± 1 weeks and recorded cholesterol reduction of $6.5 \pm 1.2\%$.[147]

Psyllium is a fiber that has attracted recent attention. Abraham and Mehta[1] fed 21 g of psyllium daily to seven men for three weeks and achieved a significant reduction in total and LDL cholesterol. Anderson et al.[6] observed a 15% reduction in total cholesterol and a 20% reduction in LDL cholesterol in 15 men fed fiber 8 g/day of psyllium (as a commercial preparation) over a 10-week period. Bell et al.[11] saw a 6% reduction in total and LDL cholesterol in men given a psyllium-enriched cereal. Flaxseed is a rich source of linoleic acid as well as a soluble fiber. Relatively high doses of flaxseed oil have been shown to lower serum cholesterol in man.[15,22,123] Ten volunteers (five male, five female) were fed 50 g of flaxseed daily in the form of muffins. After four weeks, their plasma total cholesterol levels and the ratio of LDL/HDL cholesterol had both fallen by 6%.[21]

The original observations leading to the fiber hypothesis were made in populations eating high fiber diets. The studies cited involving pectin, guar gum, and psyllium were essentially pharmacologic studies. Oat bran and oat meal may be regarded as indigenous fiber. Truswell and Beynen[147] cite several studies in which legumes (beans, peas, lentils, etc.) exerted significant hypocholesterolemic effects.

The foregoing discussion has dwelt on the effects of specific dietary components and many of the studies, especially those using animals have total replacement of one nutrient with another (corn oil vs. coconut oil for instance). Such studies provide easily interpretable data but they do not reflect how people eat. Difficult as it may be, we must do more work in which interactions of dietary ingredients are examined. The experiment showing effects of an equal mixture of animal and plant protein has already been cited.[93] The influence of dietary protein on experimental atherosclerosis is also influenced by the type of fiber present in the diet. Thus soy protein is less cholesterolemic than casein when the dietary fiber is cellulose, but the two are equivalent when the fiber is alfalfa.[100] Mixtures of animal and plant proteins and fats and carbohydrates were made up to resemble the American diets of 1909 and 1972.

The diets were made up to resemble the ratios of animal to plant protein (1.07 in 1909 and 2.16 in 1972); sucrose to starch (0.47 in 1909 and 1.11 in 1972); animal to vegetable fat (4.77 in 1909 and 1.61 in 1972); and the 1909 diet contained more fiber. The contributions of protein, carbohydrate and fat to total calories were 11.6%, 56.1%, and 32.2% in 1909, and 12.1%, 45.5%, and 42.2% in 1972. When fed to rats or rabbits their effects on cholesterol metabolism or atherosclerosis were identical.[93] In rabbits, serum cholesterol levels were higher on the 1972 diet, but the average severity of atherosclerosis was 27% lower (possibly due to the increased levels of corn oil). In rats there were no differences in serum or liver lipids and cholesterol synthesis, degradation and absorption were the same in animals on both diets.

Despite the many demonstrations of short term effects of dietary fibers on human lipidemia the important question involves long-term dietary effects on coronary heart disease. Humble et al.[62] have assessed the effect of dietary fiber on coronary heart disease in hypercholesterolemic middle-aged men. Their data were obtained from 1801 men in the placebo arm of the Lipid Research Clinic Coronary Primary Prevention Trial. Over a 9.6-year follow-up period there were 249 suspect or definite coronary events.

Mechanism(s) by which fiber may lower blood cholesterol have been propounded by a number of authors but to date none have been generally adopted or proved satisfactorily. Vahouny[151] discussed possible mechanisms of fiber action and suggested that there were direct effects including enhanced gastric emptying, altered transit time, interference with bulk phase diffusion and sequestration of micellar components including bile acids. Among possible indirect effects were influence on bile acid pool size in which increased steroid excretion and bile acid synthesis both played a role, influence on gut hormones and structural changes in intestinal tissue. Every one of these possibilities has been investigated but none provides a totally satisfactory explanation.

One other aspect of nutrition which has a profound influence on many of the risk factors for coronary disease is obesity. As an excellent recent review shows, obesity carries a number of adverse health consequences including effects on blood pressure, lipidemia, coronary heart disease and diabetes.[124]

Despite the general agreements of the effects of diet on risk of heart disease, there are a few disquieting data: In a review of coronary artery disease in Japan, Toshima[144] showed that the traditional Japanese diet had changed; currently Japanese ingest 25% of calories from fat, 60% from carbohydrate and 15% from protein. Their salt intake is about 12 g/day. Despite these changes there has been reduced incidence of stroke and no increase in coronary heart disease. Another study[148] found that between 1950 and 1985 cardiovascular mortality in Japanese men and women aged 30 to 69 had decreased by over 38%.

The "French Paradox" is well publicized. The French eat more red meat than any other Europeans[149] and their consumption of dairy fat is seventh highest in Europe,[126] still their incidence of heart disease is among the lowest in Europe. It has been suggested that the antioxidants present in red wine may play a role in the paradox.[34] St. Leger et al.[137] noted an inverse correlation between per capita wine consumption and coronary heart disease in Europe.

In summary, many aspects of diet may influence factors which are prominent in the etiology of heart disease. The dietary guidelines for health begin by telling us to eat a variety of foods and to maintain desirable weight. The guide to healthy nutrition for most people is moderation, variety and balance. There is still much to learn about diet and coronary disease. Based on what we already know we should be prudent but with so much left to learn we shouldn't succumb to panic.

ACKNOWLEDGEMENT

Supported, in part, by a Research Career Award (HL00734) from the National Institutes of Health.

REFERENCES

1. Abraham, Z. D. and Mehta, T., Three week psyllium-husk supplementation: effect on plasma cholesterol concentrations, fecal steroid excretion and carbohydrate absorption in men, *Am. J. Clin. Nutr.*, 47, 67, 1988.
2. Ahrens, E. H., Jr., Nutritional factors and serum lipid levels, *Am. J. Med.*, 23, 928, 1957.
3. Anderson, J. T., Grande, F., and Keys, A., Hydrogenated fats in the diet and lipids in the serum of man, *J. Nutr.*, 75, 388, 1961.

4. Anderson, J. W., Spencer, D. B. M., Hamilton, C. C., Smith, S. F., Tietyen, J. M., Bryant, C. A., and Oeltgen, P., Oat bran cereal lowers serum total and LDL cholesterol in hypercholesterolemic men, *Am. J. Clin. Nutr.,* 52, 495, 1990.
5. Anderson, J. W., Story L., Sieling, B., Chen, W. J. L., Petro, M. S., and Story, J., Hypercholesterolemic effects of oat bran or bean intake for hypercholesterolemic men, *Am. J. Clin Nutr.,* 40, 1146, 1984.
6. Anderson, J. W., Zettwoch, N., Feldman, T., Tietyen-Clark, J., Oeltgen, P., and Biship, C. W., Cholesterol-lowering effects of psyllium hydrophilic mucilloid for hypercholesterolemic men, *Arch. Int. Med.,* 148, 292, 1988.
7. Anderson, R. L. and Coots, R. H., The metabolism of geometric isomers of uniformly ^{14}C-labeled Δ9 octadecenoic acid and uniformly ^{14}C labeled Δ9, 12-octadecadienoic acid by the fasting rat, *Biochem. Biophys. Acta,* 144, 525, 1967.
8. Anitschkow, N. and Chalatow, S., Uber experimentelle Cholesterinsteatose und ihre Bedeutung fur die Entstchung einiger pathologischer Prozesse, *Z. Allg. Pathol Anat.,* 24, 1, 1913.
9. Austin, M. A., Breslow, J. L., Hennekens, C. H., Buring, J. E., Willett, W. C., and Krauss, R. M., Low-density lipoprotein subclass patterns and risk of myocardial infarction, *J. Am. Med. Assoc.,* 260, 1917, 1988.
10. Babiak, J. and Rudel, L. L., Lipoproteins and Atherosclerosis, *Baillieres' Clin. Endocrinol. Metab.,* 1, 515, 1987.
11. Bell, L. P., Hectorne, K., Reynolds, H., Balm, T. K., and Hunninghake, D. B., Cholesterol-lowering effects of psyllium hydrophilic mucilloid: adjunct therapy to a prudent diet for patients with mild to moderate hypercholesterolemia, *J. Am. Med. Assoc.,* 261, 3419, 1989.
12. Berg, K., A new serum type system in man-the Lp system, *Acta. Pathol.,* 59, 369, 1963.
13. Bierman, E. L. and Porte, D., Jr., Carbohydrate intolerance and lipemia, *Ann. Int. Med.,* 68, 926, 1968.
14. Burkitt, D. P., Walker, A. R. P., and Painter, N. S., Dietary Fiber and Disease, *J. Am. Med. Assoc.,* 229, 1068, 1974.
15. Carlson, L. A. and Walldius, G., Association beteen a low adipose tissue content of polyunsaturated fatty acids and both glucose intolerance and hypertriglyceridemia in apparently healthy men, *Acta Med. Acad.,* 197, 295, 1975.
16. Carroll, K. K. and Hamilton, R. M. G., Effects of dietary protein and carbohydrate on plasma cholesterol levels in relation to atherosclerosis, *Food Sci.,* 40, 118, 1975.
17. Clarkson, S. and Newburgh, L. H., The relation between atherosclerosis and ingested cholesterol in the rabbit, *J. Exp. Med.,* 43, 595, 1926.
18. Cobb, M. M. and Teitlebaum, H., Determinants of plasma cholesterol responsiveness to diet, *Br. J. Nutr.,* 71, 271, 1994.
19. Cowan, L. D., O'Connell, D. I., Criqui, M. H., Barrett-Conner, E., Bush, T. L., and Wallace, R. B., Cancer mortality and lipid and lipoprotein levels. The Lipid Research Clinics Program Mortality Follow-up Study, *Am. J. Epidemiol.,* 131, 468, 1990.
20. Criqui, M. H., Cholesterol, primary and secondary prevention and all-cause mortality, *Ann Int. Med.,* 115, 973, 1991.
21. Cunnane, S. C., et al., *Am. J. Clin. Nutr.,* in press.
22. Cunnane, S. C., Ganguli, S., Menard, C., Liede, A. C., Hamadeh, M. J., Chen, Z. Y., Wolever, T. M. S., and Jenkins, D. J. A., High alpha-linoleic acid flaxseed (Linum usitatissimum): some nutritional properties in humans, *Br. J. Nutr.,* 69, 443, 1993.
23. Currie, A. N., The cholesterol of blood in malignant disease, *Br. J. Exp. Path.,* 5, 293, 1924.
24. Czarnecki, S. K., Effects of dietary proteins on lipoprotein metabolism and atherosclerosis in rabbits. Ph.D. dissertation, University of Pennsylvania, Philadelphia, PA, 1982.
25. Davey Smith, G., Song, F. and Sheldon T. A., Cholesterol lowering and mortality: the importance of considering initial level of risk, *Br. Med. J.,* 306, 1367, 1993.
26. Dawber, T. R., Nickerson, R. J., Brand, F. N. and Pool, J., Eggs vs. serum cholesterol and coronary heart disease, *Am. J. Clin Nutr.,* 36, 617, 1982.

27. de Groot, A. P., Luyken, R. and Pikaar, N. A., Cholesterol lowering effect of rolled oats, *Lancet,* 2, 303, 1963.

28. de Jongh, H., Beerthius, K. R., den Hartog, C., Dalderup, L. M. and Van der Speck., Influence of some dietary fats on serum lipids in man, *Bibl. Nutr. Dieta.,* 7, 137, 1965.

29. Derr, J., Kris-Etherton, P. M., Pearson, T. A. and Seligson, F. H., The role of fatty acid saturations on plasma lipids, lipoproteins, and apolipoproteins. II. The plasma total and ow-density lipoprotein cholesterol response to individual fatty acids, *Metabolism,* 42, 130, 1993.

30. Dutton, H. J., Hydrogenation of fats and its significance, in *Geometric and Positional Fatty Acid Isomers.* Emken, E. A. and Dutton, H. J. Eds., American Oil Chemists Society, Champaign, IL, 1979.

31. Flynn, M. A., Herne, B., Nolph, G. B., Naumann, H. D., Parisi, E., Ball, D., Krause, G., Ellersieck, M., and Ward, S. S., Serum lipids in humans fed diets containing beef or fish and poultry, *Am. J. Clin. Nutr.,* 34, 2734, 1981.

32. Flynn, M. A., Naumann, H. D., Nolph, G. B., Krause, G., and Ellersieck, M., Dietary "meats" and serum lipids, *Am. J. Clin. Nutr.,* 35, 935, 1982.

33. Flynn, M. A., Nolph, G. B., Baker, S., and Krause, G., Aging in Humans: a continuous 20 year study of physiologic and dietary parameters, *J. Am. Coll. Nutr.,* 11, 660, 1992.

34. Frankel, E. N., Kanner, J., German, J. B., Parks, E., and Kinsella, J. E., Inhibition of oxidation of human low density lipoprotein by phenolic substances in red wine, *Lancet,* 341, 454, 1993.

35. Fumagalli, R., Paoletti, R., and Howard A. N., Hypocholesterolaemic effect of soy, *Life Sci.,* 22, 947, 1978.

36. Gertler, M. M., Garn, S. M., and White, P. D., Serum cholesterol and coronary artery disease, *Circulation,* 2, 696, 1950.

37. Ginter, E., Kubec, F. J., Vozar, J., and Bobeck, P., Natural hypercholesterolemic agent: pectin plus ascorbic acid, *Int. J. Vitam. Nutr. Res.,* 49, 406, 1979.

38. Gofman, J. W., Lindgren, F., Elliott, H., Mantz, W., Hewitt, J., Strisower, B., Herring, V., and Lyon, T. P., The role of lipids and lipoproteins in atherosclerosis, *Science,* 111, 166, 1950.

39. Gordon, D. J., Hyde, J., Trost, D. C., Whaley, F. S., Hannan, P. J., Jacobs, D. R., and Ekelund, L. G., Cyclic seasonal variation in plasma lipid and lipoprotein levels: the lipid research clinics coronary primary prevention trial placebo group, *J. Clin. Epidemiol.,* 41, 679, 1988.

40. Gordon, T., Kagan, A., Garcia-Palmieri, M., Kannel, W. B., Zukel, W. J., Tillotson, J., Sorlie, P., and Hjortland, M., Diet and its relation to coronary heart disease and death in three populations, *Circulation,* 63, 500, 1981.

41. Grant, W. C. and Fahrenbach, M. J., Effect of dietary sucrose and glucose on plasma cholesterol in chicks and rabbits, *Proc. Soc. Exp. Biol. Med.,* 100, 250, 1959.

42. Gresham, G. A. and Howard, A. N., The independent production of atherosclerosis and thrombosis in the rat, *Br. J. Exp. Pathol.,* 41, 395, 1960.

43. Groover, M. E., Jr., Jernigan, J. A., and Martin, C. D., Variations in serum lipid concentration and clinical coronary artery disease, *Am. J. Med. Sci.,* 239, 133, 1960.

44. Hardinge, M. G., Chambers, A. C., Crooks, H., and Stare, F. J., Nutritional studies of vegetarians. III. Dietary level of fiber, *Am. J. Clin Nutr.,* 6, 523, 1958.

45. Harlap, S., Kark, J. D., Baras, M., Eisenberg, S., and Stein, Y., Seasonal changes in plasma lipid and lipoprotein levels in Jerusalem, *Isr. J. Med. Sci.,* 18, 1158, 1982.

46. Havel, R., McCollum Award lecture 1993: Triglyceride-rich lipoproteins and atherosclerosis — new perspectives, *Am. J. Clin Nutr.,* 59, 795, 1994.

47. Hayes, K. C., Personal communication, 1994.

48. Hayes, K. C. and Khosla, P., Dietary fatty acid thresholds and cholesterolemia, *FASEB J.,* 6, 2600, 1992.

49. Hayes, K. C., Pronczuk, A., Lindsey, S., and Diersen-Schade, D., Dietary saturated fatty acids (12:0, 14:0, 16:0) differ in thier impact on plasma cholesterol and lipoproteins in nonhuman primates, *Am. J. Clin. Nutr.,* 53, 491, 1991.

50. Heckers, H., Korner, M., Tusihen, T. W. L., and Melcher, F. W., Occurrence of individual trans isomeric fatty acids in human myocardium, jejunum, and aorta in relation to different degrees of atherosclerosis, *Atherosclerosis,* 28, 389, 1977.

51. Hegsted, D. M., Ausman, L. M., Johnson, J. A., and Dallal, G. E., Dietary fat and serum lipids: an evaluation of the experimental data, *Am. J. Clin. Nutr.,* 57, 875, 1993.

52. Hegsted, D. M., McGandy, R. B., Myers, M. L., and Stare, F. J., Quantitative effects of dietary fat on serum cholesterol in man, *Am. J. Clin Nutr.,* 17, 281, 1965.

53. Hegsted, D. M. and Nicolosi, R. J., Individual variation in serum cholesterol levels, *Proc. Natl. Acad. Sci. U.S.A.,* 84, 6259, 1987.

54. Hodges, R. E., Krehl, W. A., Stone, D. B., and Lopez, A., Dietary carbohydrates and low cholesterol diets: effects on serum lipids of man, *Am. J. Clin. Nutr.,* 20, 198, 1967.

55. Holme, J., An analysis of randomized trials evaluating the effect of cholesterol reduction on total mortality and CHD incidence, *Circulation,* 82, 1916, 1990.

56. Holmes, W. L., Rubel, G. B., and Hood, S. S., Comparison of the effect of dietary meat versus dietary soybean protein on plasma lipids of hyperlipidemic individuals, *Atherosclerosis,* 36, 379, 1980.

57. Hopkins, P. N. and Williams, R. R., A survey of 246 suggested coronary risk factors, *Atherosclerosis.,* 40, 1, 1981.

58. Houtsmuller, U. M. T., Biochemical aspects of fatty acids with trans double bonds, *Fette, Seifen, Anstrichm.,* 80, 162, 1978.

59. Howard, G. C. and Pizzo, S. V., Biology of Disease. Lipoprotein (a) and its role in atherothrombotic disease, *Lab Invest.,* 69, 373, 1993.

60. Hulley, S. B., Rosenman, R. H., Bawol, R. D., and Brand, R. J., Epidemiology as a guide to clinical decisions. The association between triglycerides and coronary heart disease, *N. Engl. J. Med.,* 302, 1383, 1980.

61. Hulley, S. B., Walsh, J. M. B., and Newman, T. B., Health Policy on Blood Cholesterol. Time to change directions, *Circulation,* 86, 1026, 1992.

62. Humble, C. G., Malarcher, A. M., and Tryoler, H. A., Dietary fiber and coronary heart disease in middle-aged hypercholesterolemic men, *Am. J. Prev. Med.,* 9, 197, 1993.

63. Ignatowski, A., Influence de la nourriture animale sur l'organisme des lapins, *Arch. Med. Exp. Anat. Path.,* 20, 1, 1908.

64. Ignatowski, A., Uber die Wirkung des tiereschen eiweisses auf die aorta und die parenchymatosen organe der kaninchen,*Virchows Arch. Pathol. Anat. Physiol. Klin. Med.,* 198, 248, 1909.

65. Jacobs, D., Blackburn, H., Higgins, M., Reed, D., Iso, H., McMillan, G., Neaton, J., Nelson, J., Potter, F., Rifkind, B., Rossouw, J., Shekelle, R., and Yusuf, S., Report of the conference on low blood cholesterol: mortality associations, *Circulation,* 86, 1046, 1992.

66. Jenkins, D. J. A., Hegele, R. A., Jenkins, A. L., Connelly, P. W., Hollak, K., Bracci, P., Kashtan, H., Corey, P., Pintilia, M., Stern, H., and Bruce, R., The apolipoprotein E gene and the serum low-density lipoprotein cholesterol response to dietary fiber, *Metabolism,* 42, 585, 1993.

67. Jones, J. D., Lysine-arginine antagonism in the chick, *J. Nutr.,* 84, 313, 1964.

68. Jones, J. D., Wolters, R., and Burnett, P. C., Lysine-arginine electrolyte relationships in the rat, *J. Nutr.,* 89, 171, 1966.

69. Judd, P. A. and Truswell, A. S., Comparison of the effect of high and low methoxyl pectins on blood and faecal lipids in men, *Br. J. Nutr.,* 48, 451, 1982.

70. Keys, A., Anderson, J. T., and Grande, F., Serum cholesterol response to changes in the diet. IV. Particular saturated fatty acids in the diet, *Metabolism,* 14, 776, 1965.

71. Keys, A., Grande, F., and Anderson, J. T., Fiber and pectin in the diet and serum cholesterol concentrations in man, *Proc. Soc. Exp. Biol. Med.,* 106, 555, 1961.

72. Khosla, P. and Hayes, K. C., Comparison between the effects of dietary saturated (16:0) monounsaturated (18:0) and polyunsaturated (18:2) fatty acids on plasma lipoprotein metabolism in cebus and rhesus monkeys fed cholesterol free diets, *Am. J. Clin. Nutr.,* 55, 51, 1992.

73. Knack, A. V., Uber cholesterinsklerose, *Virchows Arch. Pathol. Anat. Physiol. Klin. Med.,* 220, 36, 1915.
74. Kritchevsky, D., *Cholesterol,* John Wiley and Sons, New York, 1958.
75. Kritchevsky, D., Vegetable protein and atherosclerosis, *J. Am. Oil Chem. Soc.,* 56, 135, 1979.
76. Kritchevsky, D., Dietary protein and atherosclerosis, in *Diet and Drugs in Atherosclerosis,* G. Noseda, Lewis, B., and Paoletti, R., Eds., Raven Press, New York, 1980, 9.
77. Kritchevsky, D., Variation in serum cholesterol levels, in *Nutrition Update, Vol. 2,* Weiniger, J. and G. M., Briggs, Eds., John Wiley & Sons, Inc., New York, 1985, 91.
78. Kritchevsky, D., Trans unsaturated fat in nutrition and health, in *Edible Fats and Oils Processing: Basic Principles and Modern Practice,* Erikson, D., Ed., AOCS Press, Champaign, IL, 1990, 158.
79. Kritchevsky, D., Variation in plasma cholesterol levels, *Nutrition Today,* 27(5), 21, 1992.
80. Kritchevsky, D., Dietary protein and experimental atherosclerosis, *Ann. N.Y. Acad. Sci.,* 676, 180, 1993.
81. Kritchevsky, D., Davidson, L. M., Kim, H. K., Krendel, D. A., Malhotra, S., Mendelsohn, D., van der Watt, J. J., du Plessis, J. P., and Winter, P. A. D., Influence of type of carbohydrates on atherosclerosis in baboons fed semi-purified diets plus 0.1% cholesterol, *Am. J. Clin. Nutr.,* 33, 1869, 1980.
82. Kritchevsky, D., Davidson, L. M., Kim, H. K., Krendel, D. A., Malhotra, S., van der Watt, J. J., du Plessis, J. P., Winter, P. A. D., Ipp, T., Mendelsohn, D., and Bersohn, I., Influences of semipurified diets on atherosclerosis in African green monkeys, *Exp. Mol. Pathol.,* 26, 28, 1977.
83. Kritchevsky, D., Davidson. L. M., Shapiro, I. L., Kim, H. K., Kitagawa, M., Malhotra, S., Nair, P. P, Clarkson, T. B., Bersohn, I., and Winter, P. A. D., Lipid metabolism and experimental atherosclerosis in baboons: influence of cholesterol-free semi-synthetic diets, *Am. J. Clin. Nutr.,* 27, 29, 1974.
84. Kritchevsky, D., Davidson, L. M., Weight, M., Kreik, N. P. J., and du Plessis, J., Influence of native and randomized peanut oil on lipid metabolism and aortic sudanophilia in the vervet monkey, *Atherosclerosis,* 42, 53, 1982.
85. Kritchevsky, D., Davidson, L. M., Weight, M., Kriek, N. P. J., and duPlessis, J., Effect of trans-unsaturated fats on experimental atherosclerosis in Vervet monkeys, *Atherosclerosis,* 51, 123, 1984.
86. Kritchevsky, D., Grant, W. C., Fahrenbach, M. J., Riccardi, B. A., and McCandless, R. F. J., Effect of dietary carbohydrate on the metabolism of cholesterol-4-C^{14} in chickens, *Arch. Biochem. Biophys.,* 75, 142, 1958.
87. Kritchevsky, D., Moyer, A. W., Tesar, W. G., Logan, J. B., Brown, R. A., Davies, M. C., and Cox, H. R., Effect of cholesterol vehicle in experimental atherosclerosis, *Am. J. Physiol.,* 178, 30, 1954.
88. Kritchevsky, D., Moyer, A. W., Tesar, W. C., McCandless, R. E. J., Logan, J. B., Brown, R. A., and Englert, M., Cholesterol vehicle in experimental atherosclerosis. II. Effect of unsaturation, *Am. J. Physiol.,* 185, 279, 1956.
89. Kritchevsky, D., Sallata, P., and Tepper, S. A., Experimental atherosclerosis in rabbits fed cholesterol-free diets. 2. Influence of various carbohydrates, *J. Atheroscler. Res.,* 8, 697, 1968.
90. Kritchevsky, D. and Tepper, S. A., Cholesterol vehicle in experimental atherosclerosis. 7. Influence of naturally occurring saturated fats, *Med. Pharmacol. Exp.,* 12, 315, 1965.
91. Kritchevsky, D. and Tepper, S. A., Cholesterol vehicle in experimental atherosclerosis X. Influence of specific saturated fatty acids, *Exp. Mol. Pathol.,* 6, 394, 1967.
92. Kritchevsky, D., Tepper, S. A., Bises, G., and Klurfeld, D. M., Experimental atherosclerosis in rabbits fed cholesterol-free diets. 10. Cocoa butter and palm oil, *Atherosclerosis,* 41, 279, 1982.
93. Kritchevsky, D., Tepper, S. A., Czarnecki, S. K., Klurfeld, D. M., and Story, J. A., Experimental atherosclerosis in rabbits fed cholesterol free diets. 9. Beef protein and textured vegetable protein, *Atherosclerosis,* 39, 169, 1981.

94. Kritchevsky, D., Tepper, S. A., and Goodman, G., Diet, nutrition intake and metabolism in populations at high and low risk for colon cancer: relationship of diet to serum lipids, *Am. J. Clin. Nutr.,* 40, 921, 1984.

95. Kritchevsky, D., Tepper, S. A., Kim, H. K., Story, J. A., Vesselinovitch, D., and Wissler, R. W., Experimental atherosclerosis in rabbits fed cholesterol-free diets. 5. Comparisons of peanut, corn, butter and coconut oils, *Exp. Mol. Pathol.,* 24, 375, 1976.

96. Kritchevsky, D., Tepper, S. A., and Kitagawa, M., Experimental atherosclerosis in rabbits fed cholesterol-free diets. 3. Comparison of fructose with other carbohydrates, *Nutr. Rep. Int.,* 7, 193, 1973.

97. Kritchevksy, D., Tepper, S. A., Morrissey, R. B., Klurfeld, D. M., and Story, J. A., Comparison of diets approximating American intake of 1909 and 1972: effect on lipid metabolism in rabbits and rats, *Nutr. Rep. Int.,* 28, 1, 1983.

98. Kritchevsky, D., Tepper, S. A., Vesselinovitch, D. and Wissler, R. W., Cholesterol vehicle in experimental atherosclerosis. 11. Peanut oil, *Atherosclerosis,* 14, 53, 1971.

99. Kritchevsky, D., Tepper, S. A., Vesselinovitch, D., and Wissler, R. W., Cholesterol vehicle in experimental atherosclerosis. 13. Randomized peanut oil, *Atherosclerosis,* 17, 225, 1973.

100. Kritchevsky, D., Tepper, S. A., Williams, D. E., and Story, J. A., Experimental atherosclerosis in rabbits fed cholesterol-free diets. 7. Interaction of animal or vegetable protein with fiber, *Atherosclerosis,* 26, 397, 1977.

101. Kritchevsky, S. B. and Kritchevsky, D., Serum cholesterol and cancer risk. An epidemiological perspective, *Ann. Rev. Nutr.,* 12, 391, 1992.

102. Kuo, P. T., Dietary sugar in the production of hypertriglyceridemia in patients with hyperlipemia and atherosclerosis, *Trans. Assoc. Am. Physicians.,* 78, 97, 1965.

103. Lichtenstein, A. H., Ausman L. M., Carrasco, W., Jenner, J. L., Ordovas, J. M., and Schaefer, E. J., Hydrogenation impairs the hypolipidemic effect of corn oil in humans. Hydrogenation, trans fatty acids and plasma lipids, *Arteriosclerosis Thrombosis,* 123, 154, 1993.

104. Lubarsch, O., Zur pathogenese der atherosclerose der arteien, *Munch. med. Wochenschr.,* 56, 1819, 1909.

105. Marzetta, C. A. and Rudel, L. L., A species comparison of low density lipoprotein heterogeneity in non-human primates fed atherogenic diets, *J. Lipid Res.,* 27, 753, 1986.

106. McGandy, R. B., Hegsted, D. M., and Meyers, M. L., Use of semi-synthetic fats in determining effects of specific dietary fatty acids on serum lipids in man, *Am. J. Clin. Nutr.,* 23, 1288, 1970.

107. McMillan, G. C., Silver, M. D., and Weigensberg, B. I., Elaidinized olive oil and cholesterol atherosclerosis, *Arch. Pathol.,* 76, 105, 1963.

108. McNamara, D. J., Relationship between blood and dietary cholesterol, in *Meat and Health. Adv. Meat Res.,* Vol. 6, Pearson, A. M. and T. R. Dutson, Eds., Elsevier Applied Science, London, 1990, 63.

109. McNamara, D. J., Kolb, R., Parker, T. S., Batwin, H., Samuel, P., Brown, C. D., and Ahrens, E. H., Jr., Hetrogeneity of cholesterol homeostasis in man. Response to changes in dietary fat quality and cholesterol quantity, *J. Clin. Invest.,* 79, 1729, 1987.

110. McOsker, D. E., Mattson, F. H., Sweringen, B., and Kligman, A. M., The influence of partially hydrogenated dietary fats on serum cholesterol levels, *J. Am. Med. Assoc.,* 180, 380, 1962.

111. Meeker, D. R. and Kesten, H. D., Experimental atherosclerosis and high protein diets, *Proc. Soc. Exp. Biol. Med.,* 45, 543, 1940.

112. Meeker, D. R. and Kesten, H. D., Effect of high protein diets on experimental atherosclerosis of rabbits, *Arch. Pathol.,* 31, 147, 1941.

113. Mensink, R. P. and Katan, M. B., Effect of dietary trans fatty acids on high-density and low density lipoprotein cholesterol levels in healthy subjects, *N. Eng. J. Med.,* 323, 439, 1990.

114. Moore, C. E., Alfin-Slater, R. B., and Aftergood, L., Incorporation and disappearance of trans fatty acids in rat tissues, *Am. J. Clin Nutr.,* 33, 2318, 1980.

115. Muldoon, M., Manuck, S., and Matthews, K., Lowering cholesterol concentrations and mortality: a quantitative review of primary prevention trials, *Br. Med. J.,* 301, 309, 1990.
116. Myant, N. B., *The Biology of Cholesterol and Related Sterols,* W. Heinemann Medical Books, Ltd., London, 1981.
117. Nestel, P., Noakes, M., Belling, B., McArthur, R., Clifton, P., Janus, E., and Abbey, M., Plasma lipoprotein lipid and Lp(a) changes with substitution of elaidic acid for oleic acid in the diet, *J. Lipid Res.,* 33, 1029, 1992.
118. Newbergh, L. H., The production of Bright's disease by feeding high protein diets, *Arch Intern. Med.,* 24, 359, 1919.
119. Newburgh, L. H. and Clarkson, S., Production of atherosclerosis in rabbits by diets rich in animal protein, *J. Am. Med. Assoc.,* 79, 1106, 1922.
120. Newburgh, L. H. and Squier, T. L., High protein diets and atherosclerosis in rabbits. A preliminary report, *Arch. Intern. Med.,* 26, 38, 1920.
121. Nordestgaard, B. G. and Zilversmit, D. B., Comparison of arterial intimal clearances of LDL from diabetic and nondiabetic cholesterol-fed rabbits. Differences in intimal clearance explained by size difference, *Arteriosclerosis,* 9, 176, 1989.
122. Ono, K. and Frederickson, D. S., The metabolism of ^{14}C-labeled cis and trans isomers of octadecadienoic acids, *J. Biol. Chem.,* 239, 2482, 1964.
123. Owren, P. A., Hellem, A. J., and Odegaard, A., Linoleic acid or the prevention of thrombosis and myocardial infarction, *Lancet,* 2, 975, 1964.
124. Pi-Sunyer, F. X., Medical hazards of obesity, *Ann. Intern Med.,* 119, 655, 1993.
125. Porter, M. W., Yamanaka, W., Carlson, S. D., and Flynn, M. A., Effect of dietary egg on serum cholesterol and triglyceride of human males, *Am. J. Clin. Nutr.,* 30, 490, 1977.
126. Renaud, S. and De Lorgeril, M., Wine, alcohol, platelet and the French Paradox for coronary heart disease, *Lancet.,* 339, 1523, 1992.
127. Robinson, D., Bevan, E. A., Hinohara, S., and Takabashi, T., Seasonal variation in serum cholesterol levels-evidence from the UK and Japan, *Atherosclerosis,* 95, 15, 1992.
128. Rothblat, G. H., Buchko, M. K., and Kritchevsky, D., Cholesterol uptake by L-5178Y tissue culture cells: studies with delipidized serum, *Biochem Biophys. Acta,* 164, 327, 1968.
129. Ruttenberg, H., Davidson, L. M., Little, N. A., Klurfeld, D. M., and Kritchevsky, D., Influence of trans unsaturated fats on experimental atherosclerosis in rabbits, *J. Nutr.,* 113, 835, 1983.
130. Sacks, F. M., Castelli, W. P., Donner, A., and Kass, E. H., Plasma lipids and lipoproteins in vegetarians and controls, *N. Eng. J. Med.,* 292, 1148, 1975.
131. Saltykow, S., Experimentelle atherosclerose, *Beitr. Patholog. Anat. Allg. Pathol.,* 57, 415, 1913.
132. Schube, P. G., Variations in the blood cholesterol of man over a period of time, *J. Lab. Clin. Med.,* 22, 280, 1936.
133. Scott, L. W., Dunn, J. K., Pownall, H. J., Branchi, D. J., McMann, M. C., Herd, J. A., Harris, K. B., Savell, J. W., Cross, H. R., and Gotto, A. M., Jr., Effects of beef and chicken consumption on plasma lipid levles in hypercholesterolemic men, *Arch. Int. Med.,* 154, 1261, 1994.
134. Sirtori, C. R., Agradi, E., Conti, F., Mantero, O., and Gatti, E., Soybean protein in the treatment of type II hyperlipoproteinaemia, *Lancet,* 1, 275, 1977.
135. Sirtori C., R., Gatti, E., Mantero, O., Conti, F., Agradi, E., Tremoli, E., Sirtori, M., Fraterrigo, L., Tavazzi, I., and Kritchevsky, D., Clncial experience with the soybean protein diet in the treatment of hypercholesterolemia, *Am. J. Clin Nutr.,* 32, 1645, 1979.
136. Slater, G., Mead, J., Dhopeshwarkar, G. M. Robinson, S., and Alfin-Slater, R. B., Plasma cholesterol and triglycerides in men with added eggs in the diet, *Nutr. Rep. Int.,* 14, 249, 1976.
137. St. Leger, A. S., Cochrane, A. L., and Moore, F., Factors associated with cardiac mortality in developed countries with particular reference to the consumptions of wine, *Lancet,* 1, 1017, 1979.
138. Steinbiss, W., Uber experimentelle alimentare atherosklerose, *Virchows Arch. Pathol. Anat. Physiol. Klin. Med.,* 212, 152, 1913.

139. Stender, D. and Zilversmit, D. B., Transfer of plasma lipoprotein components and of plasma proteins into aortas of cholesterol-fed rabbits. Molecular size as a determinant of plasma lipoprotein influx, *Arteriosclerosis*, 1, 38, 1981.

140. Stuckey, N, W., Uber die veranderungen der kaninchen aorta bei der futterung mit verschiedenen fettsorten, *Z. Allg. Pathol. Patholog. Anat.*, 23, 910, 1912.

141. Thomas, C. B., Holljes, H. W. D., and Eisenberg, F. A., Observations on seasonal variations in total serum cholesterol level among healthy young prisoners, *Ann. Int. Med.*, 54, 413, 1961.

142. Thomas, C. B., Jones, P. R., Winter, J. A., and Smith, H., Hydrogenated oils and fats: the presence of chemically modified fatty acids in human adipose tissue, *Am. J. Clin. Nutr.*, 34, 877, 1981.

143. Thompson, G. R., *A Handbook of Hyperlipidemia*, Current Science, London, 1989.

144. Toshima, H., Coronary Artery Disease in Japan, *Jap. Circulation J.*, 58, 166, 1994.

145. Trowell, H., Ischemic heart disease and dietary fiber, *Am. J. Clin Nutr.*, 25, 926, 1972.

146. Truswell, A. S., Food carbohydrates and plasma lipids — an update, *Am. J. Clin. Nutr.*, 59, 710S, 1994.

147. Truswell, A. S. and Beynen, A. C., Dietary fibre and plasma lipids: potential for prevention and treatment of hyperlipidaemias, in *Dietary Fibre A Component of Food*, Schweizer, T. F. and Edwards, C. A., Eds., Springer Verlag, London, 1992, 295.

148. Uemura, K. and Pisa, Z., Trends in cardiovascular disease mortality in industrialized countries since 1950, *World Health Stat. Quart.*, 41, 155, 1988.

149. Ulbricht, T. L. V. and Southgate, D. A. T., Coronary heart disease: seven dietary factors, *Lancet*, 338, 985, 1991.

150. Utermann, G., Hees, M., and Steinmetz, A., Polymorphism of apolipoprotein E and occurrence of dysbetalipoproteinemia in man, *Nature*, 269, 604, 1977.

151. Vahouny, G. V., Dietary fibers and intestinal absorption of lipids, in *Dietary Fiber in Health and Disease*, Vahouny, G. V. and Kritchevsky, E., Eds., Plenum Press, New York, 1982, 203.

152. Vesselinovitch, D., Getz, G. S., Hughes, R. H., and Wissler, R. W., Atherosclerosis in the rhesus monkey fed three food fats, *Atherosclerosis*, 20, 303, 1974.

153. Wacker, L. and Hueck, W., Uber experimentelle Atherosklerose und Cholesterinamie, *Munch. Med. Wochenschr.*, 60, 2097, 1913.

154. Walker, A. R. P. and Arvidsson, U. B., Fat intake serum cholesterol concentration and atherosclerosis in the South African Bantu. I. Low fat intake and age trend of serum cholesterol concentration in the South African Bantu, *J. Clin Invest.*, 33, 1358, 1954.

155. Weigensberg, B. I., McMillan, G. C., and Ritchie, A. C., Elaidic acid: effect on experimental atherosclerosis, *Arch. Pathol.*, 72, 126, 1961.

156. Wells, W. W. and Anderson, S. C., The increased severity of atherosclerosis in rabbits on a lactose-containing diet, *J. Nutr.* 68, 541, 1959.

157. Wood, R., Kubena, K., O'Brien, B., Tseng, S., and Martin, G., Effects of butter, mono- and poly-unsaturated fatty acid-enriched butter, trans fatty acid margarine and zero trans fatty acid margarine on serum lipids and lipoproteins in healthy men, *J. Lipid Res.*, 34, 1, 1993.

158. Wood, R., Incorporation of dietary cis and trans octadecenoate isomers in the lipid classes of various rat tissues, *Lipids*, 14, 975, 1979.

159. Yerushalmy, J. and Hilleboe, H. E., Fat in the diet and mortality from heart disease: a methodologic note, *N.Y. State J. Med.*, 57, 2343, 1957.

160. Zannis, V. I. and Breslow, J. L., Human very low density lipoprotein apolipoprotein E isoprotein polymorphism is explained by genetic variation and post-translational modification, *Biochemistry*, 20, 1033, 1981.

161. Zock, P. L. and Katan, M. B., Hydrogenation alternatives: effects of trans fatty acids and stearic acid versus linoleic acid on serum lipids and lipoproteins in humans, *J. Lipid Res.*, 33, 399, 1992.

Chapter 5

CALCIUM NUTRITION AND OSTEOPOROSIS

Felix Bronner and Wilfred D. Stein

CONTENTS

> *"...and your bones shall flourish like young grass..."*
>
> (Isaiah 66:14)

With the aging of the American population, osteoporosis, defined as a thinning of bone structure that leads to great susceptibility to bone fracture

0-8493-7849-4/95/$0.00+$.50
© 1995 by CRC Press Inc.

(Figure 1), has become a significant public health problem.[7] This chapter will review what is known about calcium metabolism and nutrition, inasmuch as calcium is the major mineral component of bone, and relate this to the epidemiology of osteoporosis, and to the biology of the skeleton and of the cells that construct this largely extracellular structure.

I. THE ROLE OF CALCIUM

Over 99% of the calcium content of the human body, typically 1 to 1.5 kg, is found in the skeleton.[15] In the first two decades of life, skeletal growth and calcium accumulation in bones tend to go in parallel. By the end of the third decade of life, with skeletal growth having come to an end some 10 to 12 years earlier, there occurs a reversal in the relationship between bone calcium deposition and removal. Whereas the bone calcium deposition rate exceeds the bone removal rate, leading to a positive calcium balance during the period of skeletal growth, deposition and resorption after the age of 30 begin to decline, with deposition decreasing faster than resorption. As a result, the mass of bone

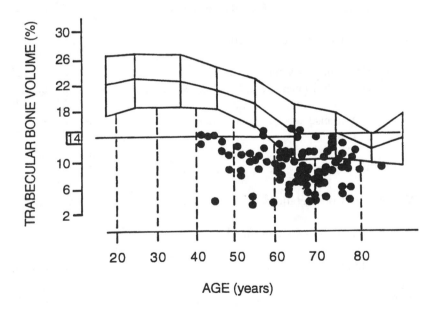

FIGURE 1.   Trabecular bone volume in women as a function of age. The boxes represent mean values (± SEM) for normal women. The individual data points are from 106 women with primary vertebral osteoporosis, aged 65.6 ± 9.9 years, with a mean trabecular volume of 10.0 ± 28%. A value of 14 is considered the vertebral fracture threshold (vft) in women with osteoporosis. *Note:* The term "fracture threshold" represents a statistical concept, not an absolute value only below which fractures might occur. Indeed, actual fracture risk is continuous and progressive over a fairly wide range of bone mineral density. (From Meunier, P. J., *Molecular and Cellular Regulation of Calcium and Phosphate Metabolism,* Wiley-Liss, New York, 1990. With permission).

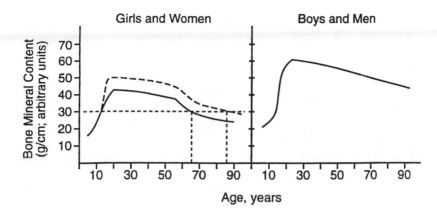

FIGURE 2. Bone mineral content as a function of age, determined by photon absorptiometry. The dashed line indicates a theoretical fracture limit. Accordingly, the bone of women 65 years or older would be subject to ready fracture. If, however, bone mineral content of the females had increased as indicated by the stippled curve, the likelihood of ready fracture would be delayed to the age of 86 and beyond. (From unpublished data kindly provided by C. Christiansen, Denmark.)

calcium begins to decrease (Figure 2). This decrease is quite gradual, almost imperceptible, until the age of 50. Thereafter, it accelerates. In women, at the menopause, the loss of bone calcium is sudden and rapid and does not begin to slow until the seventh decade of life (Figure 2). It is obvious that the greater the rate of bone calcium loss, the greater must be the difference in the rates of bone calcium deposition and resorption. Moreover, although both of these rates decline with age (Figure 3), their rates of decline must differ, thereby giving rise to bone calcium loss.

What is the effect of changes in calcium intake? How does a high or low calcium intake affect bone mass and skeletal height?

Body conformation is, as animal breeders have known for a long time, the result of the interaction between genetic endowment and the environment. Breeders have therefore searched for animal specimens that most closely represent the sought-for characteristics and brought up the offspring under optimum conditions. A number of experiments in nature are known regarding body height and skeletal mass in people.

Spain, following the Napoleonic wars in the early 19th century, suffered economic deprivation, hunger and poverty. Costumes and clothing worn by the Spanish population in that period reflect the very small body height of many (5 ft [155 cm] and under), yet contemporary Spaniards are as tall as other Europeans.

The Japanese who, before World War II, had, compared with other comparable societies, among the lowest calcium intake (10 mmol/d)[14] were also the shortest. Changes in protein and calcium intake that occurred as a result of the American occupation and the subsequent marked development of the Japanese

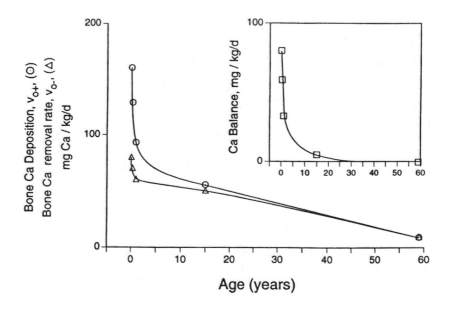

FIGURE 3. Bone calcium deposition (v_{o+}) and resorption (v_{o-}) rates as a function of age. Data based on estimates from the literature (references 1–3, 25, 61), refer to both sexes in the babies (1 year old and under), but only to females in the 13 year and 59 year old individuals. The bone balance is the difference between v_{o+} and v_{o-}.

economy have led to significant increases in body height of contemporary Japanese.

In a controlled study, Matkovic and associates[58] analyzed the incidence of bone fractures in two Yugoslav villages, with a presumably comparable genetic background, which differed in their habitual calcium intake. One village was accustomed to a low calcium intake, the other, to a moderately high calcium intake. Most fractures occurred earlier and tended to be more severe in the village population accustomed to a low calcium intake.

Subsequent studies, in which bone density was measured directly,[44,57] have confirmed the association between calcium intake during the growth phase and subsequent skeletal height and bone strength.

A. CALCIUM ABSORPTION

Intestinal absorption of calcium proceeds by two routes:[20,22] a saturable, transcellular pathway, regulated almost exclusively by vitamin D, and a nonsaturable, paracellular pathway that is not subject to acute regulation.

The saturable pathway, located principally in the duodenum, becomes expressed slowly after birth and reaches maximum expression in the rat of about six to seven weeks of age, i.e., at a time that coincides approximately with maximum growth.[72] There are no comparable data for humans, but there is general information that calcium absorption is higher in childhood and youth.

Since the nonsaturable component of calcium absorption does not appear to vary significantly with age,[72] it seems reasonable to infer that active absorption in people is high in the years of growth and is downregulated in adulthood. Since, moreover, bone calcium is lost on a steady basis in maturity, it is likely that the active, regulatable component of intestinal calcium transport remains downregulated in older people as well.

The proportion of absorbed calcium that is transported actively varies with age, vitamin D status, and total calcium intake. In growing and vitamin D-replete rats on a low calcium intake, as much as half of the absorbed calcium may be absorbed by the active route.[22] In contrast, in mature, i.e., non-growing rats on a high calcium intake, virtually all calcium is absorbed paracellularly, i.e., by the nonsaturable route.[73] Raising calcium intake in a normal animal will result in down regulation of the active transport route, but will increase the amount transported by the nonsaturable, paracellular route. Thus, the saturable transport route appears to constitute the mechanism by which the body can minimize the effects of low calcium intake. This ability is totally dependent on vitamin D, as the biosynthesis of the calcium-binding protein, calbindin D_{9k} ($M_r \approx$ 9kDa), the molecule primarily involved in assuring active calcium transport,[22] requires vitamin D.[75]

The mechanism by which calbindin D_{9k} assures active calcium transport across the duodenal cell is not yet fully established. The most likely mechanism involves a calcium ferrying function, not unlike the manner by which hemoglobin binds and transfers oxygen.[96] The rate at which calcium can self-diffuse through an intestinal cell devoid of calbindin D_{9k} is only about 1/70 of the rate at which calcium is in fact transported.[22] Vitamin D, in its biologically active form of 1,25-dihydroxyvitamin D_3, induces in the duodenal cell the genomically mediated biosynthesis of calbindin D_{9k}.[75] The amount of calbindin D_{9k} a cell contains under conditions of maximum calcium transport is just sufficient to enhance the otherwise low self-diffusion rate by a factor of about 70.[22] In addition, the amount of calbindin D_{9k} is directly and linearly proportional to the experimental maximum transport rate, V_m.[22]

The V_m of active transport varies inversely with calcium intake,[22] goes up in the period between birth and maximum growth[72] and goes up in pregnancy.[26] As bone matures, active calcium transport is down regulated.[16] Consequently, in adults with a mature skeleton, active calcium absorption contributes relatively little to the total absorbed, with the bulk of calcium being transported by the nonsaturable, paracellular route. The major factor that determines the amount of calcium that is absorbed is the quantity ingested. This is particularly true when paracellular transport dominates, as when calcium intake is high or when the skeleton is mature.[73]

B. CALCIUM EXCRETION

Calcium is lost from the body by two routes: renal and intestinal. Somewhere between 20 and 25% of the cardiac output goes to the kidney, where the inorganic and ionized plasma calcium is filtered through the glomerulus.

Bound calcium will only enter the lumen of the nephron, along with ionized calcium, if the binding molecule can be filtered. For all practical purposes, the calcium concentration of the glomerular filtrate is equal to half that of the plasma. About two-thirds of the calcium in the ultrafiltrate is reabsorbed in the proximal nephron. That movement is largely passive and paracellular. Additional calcium is reabsorbed in the thick ascending limb of the loop of Henle and the connecting and collecting duct portions of the nephron, again by a passive, paracellular transport mechanism. Active calcium reabsorption occurs in the distal convoluted tubule and probably utilizes the same general transcellular mechanism as in the intestine: passive entry, down an electro-chemical gradient, probably via calcium channels, intracellular diffusion significantly enhanced by the cytosolic vitamin D-dependent calbindin D_{28K}, extrusion via the CaATPase. The renal calbindin is a different gene product than the intestinal calbindin; its molecular weight is about 28 kDa and it has four calcium-binding sites. Its cytosolic concentration is probably similar to that of the intestinal calbindin;[17] it probably also amplifies calcium transport by about the same factor as the intestinal calbindin, i.e., about 70 times.[23]

The amount of calcium lost in the urine varies with age and maturity. Children excrete only a few percent of their net calcium absorption,[97] whereas in postmenopausal women this can constitute 25%.[15,45] Urinary calcium excretion of adults ranges typically between 2.5 and 7.5 mmol/d.

Reports in the literature indicate that high protein intakes lead to increased urinary calcium output.[56] It has been suggested that this increased loss may play a role in causing osteoporosis.

As will be discussed in greater detail below, skeletal mass decreases with age regardless of the level of prior calcium intake, but, as shown in the Matkovic et al. study,[58] lower calcium intakes lead to fractures at an earlier age (Figure 3). Thus, if the protein-induced calciuria were to be maintained for a long period, it would be more correct to say fractures might occur sooner than in the absence of such hypercalciuria. On the other hand, the very existence of this condition has been questioned.[87]

Calcium is lost from the body in the feces, via endogenous calcium that finds its way into the intestinal lumen by way of intestinal secretions like bile, loss of intestinal lining cells and some serosal-to-mucosal leakage.[15] Some of that endogenous calcium is reabsorbed, but some is lost from the body. It seems unlikely that the loss of endogenous calcium in the feces represents a significant clearance process subject to regulation.[15] In humans the amount of endogenous calcium lost in the feces approximately equals in amount the urinary calcium output. The quantity lost appears to increase with increased calcium intake, but diseases or conditions of markedly changed output are rare.[45] Calcium in the stool thus stems from two sources — unabsorbed food calcium and endogenous calcium that failed to be reabsorbed as it mixed with the luminal contents and moved distally in the intestine toward the colon.

C. CALCIUM IN BONE

Calcium, along with phosphate, constitutes the principal structural substance that gives vertebrates their internal support and allows people to stand erect. The skeleton constitutes about 16% of an adult's body weight. 47% of the skeletal weight is dry, fat-free bone and 26% of the latter is calcium.[21]

At least 90% of the crystalline calcium phosphate in bone is hydroxyapatite $[C_{10}(PO_4)_6(OH)_2]$; other calcium phosphates include whitlockite, octacalcium phosphate and brushite, as well as an amorphous calcium phosphate with variable phosphate content.[85]

The precise order in which calcium is precipitated and the path it follows as calcium salts mature and become increasingly less soluble is not yet known. The initial calcium phosphate is deposited on or inside collagen fibrils that have formed extracellularly from collagen molecules that had been extruded by osteoblasts, the bone-forming cells. Additional calcium phosphate is deposited by accretion so that the calcium salt is arranged in a very orderly fashion. The resulting crystals are plate-like, with the surface layers of the bone crystals constituting 50% of the newly formed crystals, but ultimately, in the fully mature crystal, the surface layers constitute only about 25% of the fully mature crystal volume.[85]

Calcium exists in bone in two forms: in a liquid state, as part of the fluid that surrounds and exists in bone, termed "bone calcium pool," and in a solid state, as the bone salts described above. The bone calcium pool contains five to six times more calcium than found in the extracellular fluid, but constitutes only a small fraction of the total body calcium. For example, in a 200 g male rat, the extracellular calcium amounts to 0.67 mmol Ca, the bone calcium pool contains about 3.45 mmol Ca, whereas the total skeletal calcium amounts to about 120 mmol Ca.[82]

The bone calcium pool serves two functions: as the source of calcium that becomes deposited as bone salt, and as the source of exchangeable calcium, i.e., the calcium that leaves and reenters blood, with the concentration of blood plasma calcium determined by the average calcium binding capacity of the bone salt.[24]

The fraction of calcium entering the bone calcium pool that then undergoes a phase transformation to become bone salt diminishes with age. Bone calcium resorption, i.e., the phase transformation of solid to liquid and the return of that calcium into the circulation, also decreases with age, but somewhat less rapidly than does the bone calcium deposition rate. As a result, the individual goes into negative bone calcium balance, i.e., the bone mass decreases. This is illustrated in Figure 3.

II. THE BIOLOGY OF BONE

As indicated above, bone is a largely extracellular structure. It is made up of a collagen network impregnated with calcium phosphate salts. The collagen network together with a large variety of proteins, which includes osteonectin (a protein that binds calcium, hydroxyapatite, and collagen), at least four cell attachment proteins (fibronectin, thrombospondin, osteopontin, and bone sialoprotein), and two proteoglycans,[91] is termed the extracellular matrix and is synthesized by the osteoblasts. Bone formation is the process that results from synthesis of the extracellular matrix and its subsequent calcification. Bone growth takes place by a complex cell-directed process, with bone formation coupled to bone destruction in many, but not all situations, such that the macroscopic overall form of bone is preserved. Bone destruction, termed bone resorption, is accomplished by specialized multinucleated cells, the osteoclasts, which release protons and lysosomal enzymes that solubilize bone salt and lyse the matrix.

It is convenient to divide bone into trabecular and cortical bone, with trabecular bone, also termed cancellous bone, a lattice of large plates and rods known as trabeculae, comprising the spongy interior of many bones. In long bones, the metaphyses, the regions that are most amply supplied with blood vessels and that provide the major portals of entry, are trabecular in nature, whereas shin bones are largely cortical. The hip bone and vertebrae are largely trabecular; the bones of the skull are cortical in nature.

Cortical bone is a dense mass, perforated by microscopic channels, which makes up the exterior bones. Mature bone is constantly undergoing remodelling, i.e., it is destroyed and formed by, respectively, osteoclasts and osteoblasts, acting in concert as a bone remodelling unit. In adults, trabecular bone has a mean turnover time of about 4 years and cortical bone one of about 20 years.

A. THE EFFECTS OF AGING ON THE SKELETON

Figures 4A and 4B are representative of the available information on how the mineral mass of the skeleton changes with age in women and men. In women (Figure 4A), a very modest decline in bone mineral mass between the ages of 20 and menopause is followed by a sharp, exponential decline for the next decade, with a farther, more modest, apparently linear decline thereafter. The rapid loss of bone mineral mass that occurs in women in the decade after menopause accounts for some 13% of the total body bone density at menopause and largely affects trabecular bone. In men (Figure 4B), on the other hand, bone mineral mass declines linearly, with a rate of approximately 0.2% per year from a peak mass reached in the third decade of life. The Framingham cross-sectional population study showed that elderly men and women well past the menopause have a bone mass that decreases with age in both groups in a linear and equivalent fashion.[46]

Loss of trabecular bone volume may involve the loss of whole trabecular plates,[74] rather than their mere thinning, as is the case for cortical bone. As a result, "...the mainly continuous trabecular network characteristic of a young person [is transformed] into the mainly discontinuous network characteristic of the elderly..."[74] Compressive strength of trabecular bone depends importantly on the connections between these structural elements. Once lost, a trabecular

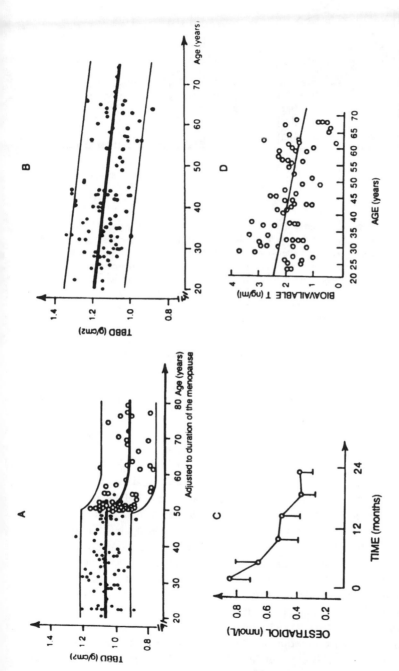

FIGURE 4. Total body bone density (TBBD) as a function of age in women (A) and men (B). Plasma oestradiol concentration (C) in 31 women, 47–54 years old, with irregular menses during a two-year period. Bioavailable testosterone levels in plasma of men (D). TBBD was obtained by measuring total bone mineral content of the body by gadolinium 153 scanning, normalized to skeletal surface area. (Figures A and B taken from Gotfredsen, A., Hadberg, A., Nilas, L., and Christiansen, C., *J. Lab. Clin. Med.,* 110, 362, 1987. Figure C taken from Nilas, L. and Christiansen, C., *Brit. J. Obstet. Gynecol.,* 96, 580, 1989. Figure D taken from Nahoul, K. and Roger, M., *J. Steroid. Biochem.,* 35, 293, 1990. All reproduced with permission.)

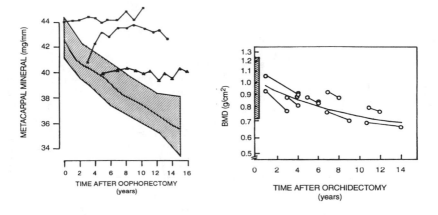

FIGURE 5.   The effect of gonadectomy on bone. A. In Women. Hatched area is mean ± SD. Single lines represent mean bone loss values in three groups of women given estrogen treatment at 0 (■), 3 (●), and 6 (▲) years after oophorectomy. B. In men. In 8 of the 12 patients, the measurement was repeated after 1 to 3 years. The line is a second order regression. The hatched bar indicates the range of bone mineral density (BMD) in 20 men matched for age. (Figure A from Aitken, J. M., Hart, D. M., Anderson, J. B., Lindsay, R., and Smith, D. A., *Brit. Med. J.*, 1, 325, 1973. Figure B from Stepan, J. J., Lachman, M., Zverina, J., Pacovsky, V., and Baylink, D. J., *J. Clin. End. Metab.*, 69, 523, 1989. With permission).

plate cannot be restored. Hence a major aim of therapy must be prevention of loss of the trabecular elements, as well as slowing the thinning of cortical bone.

B. GONADAL HORMONES AS MAJOR REGULATORS OF BONE CELL FUNCTION

It was Albright[5] who first related osteoporosis in women to the menopause. The incisiveness of this insight is illustrated in Figure 4 which shows how the abruptness of loss in gonadal hormone function in women (Figure 4C) parallels the abruptness with which their skeleton weakens (Figure 4A). The figure also shows how the gradual loss of bone mass in males (Figure 4B) is paralleled by a comparably gradual loss in functional testosterone levels (Figure 4D). What is more, gonadectomy in both females (Figure 5A) and males (Figure 5B) is followed by a rapid drop in bone mass, the rate of which is comparable to that in Figure 4B. For example, the bone mineral density of men castrated by orchidectomy (whose testosterone levels were at least an order of magnitude lower than those of controls) fell exponentially to stabilize at some 70% of the initial density.[89] This value and the rate of fall ($t_{1/2} \approx 3y$) are comparable to those that can be calculated from Figure 4A for the rapid phase of bone loss that follows the menopause in women. The exponential rate of bone loss of castrates (Figure 5B) is 100 times greater than normal (Figure 4B). Swartz and Young[90] have reported that in 62 male geriatric patients, mean age 69 years, fractures involving limbs, hips, and ribs occurred twice as frequently in men whose morning levels of serum testosterone were at or below 1040 nmol/L than in those whose testosterone levels were higher. They also report that two or more separate incidents of fracture occurred five times more frequently in hypogonadal than eugonadal men.[90] Recently Murphy et al.[64] were able to demonstrate that, in the hip of healthy men, there was a consistently positive relationship between bone mineral density and the logarithm of the ratio of testosterone to serum hormone binding globulin. This ratio is an index of free testosterone levels.

The effects of gonadectomy on bone metabolism are rapid and dramatic. Thus, in oophorectomized women, losses in urine of hydroxyproline and calcium increased within three weeks[71] and estrogen treatment of only one week was associated with a clear reversal of the effects of oophorectomy.[71] Figure 5A shows how promptly metacarpal bone mineral levels stopped dropping when oophorectomized women were treated with estradiol. Similar responses have been reported in men.[8,37] In situations where puberty is delayed due to gonadal hormone deficiency, in boys,[39] or in young women with anorexia nervosa,[12] normal peak bone density is not reached. Similarly, men who suffer from hypogonadism due to a deficiency of the hypothalamic gonadotropin releasing factor, GnRH, evince a marked decrease in bone density. This can be raised by gonadal hormone replacement,[46] the treatment being more effective in younger men, with a less mature bone structure. These effects of gonadal hormone deficiencies and replacements in both males and females show that osteoporosis is not a disease confined to women, associated only with the loss of circulating estrogens. Rather, its cause must be searched for in how both male and female hormones modulate bone cell metabolism.

C. CELLULAR EFFECTS OF GONADAL HORMONES

Osteoblast-like cells possess receptors for both androgens and estrogens[29,32,34] and for the insulin-like growth factor (somatomedin C).[33] Moreover, these bone cells, whether isolated from men or women, bind male and female hormones.

Osteoclasts also seem to possess gonadal hormone receptors, though the evidence is somewhat less direct. Avian osteoclasts in culture have been shown to diminish their osteolytic activity in a dose-dependent fashion in response to the addition of estrogens.[69] Cells from human giant cell tumors (an osteoclastoma) contain estrogen and respond in vitro to 17β-estradiol.[70] Those reports thus provide functional evidence for the existence of estrogen receptors in osteoclasts.

The discovery of numerous cytokines produced by osteoblasts[49] and of transcripts of several of these (IL-3 and IL-8) in human bone cells[13] suggests that these molecules play an important role as messengers from osteoblasts to osteoclasts. These messages may stimulate osteoclastic activity. On the other hand, when released in reduced amounts (or not at all), as when osteoblasts are under estrogen domination,[42,52] the repression of the cytokine-induced increase in osteoclastic activity may account for the maintenance of the bone mineral mass in premenopausal women.[86] Osteoblasts respond to testosterone via specific receptors and, when under testosterone domination, also produce less IL-6.[10]

The detailed mechanisms by which gonadal hormones stimulate and maintain osteoblast-induced osteogenesis and inhibit osteoclastogenesis are not yet well understood. Some recent reports suggest steps by which these hormones might act. Thus, the inhibitory effect of parathyroid hormone on bone cell activity is diminished when estrogen or androgen is added to a cell culture.[40,41] Estradiol stimulates osteoblast proliferation, thymidine incorporation in vitro,[34] and synthesis of collagen mRNA and of collagen.[32]

If, as has become evident from cell culture experiments, gonadal hormones stimulate and maintain osteoblastic metabolism, a decrease in gonadal hormone levels would be accompanied by downregulation of osteoblasts, reduction of collagen synthesis and the diminution or even cessation of the cascade of events that lead to the formation of bone. Contrariwise, osteoclast activity would be enhanced if osteoclasts and/or their progenitor cells were to be relieved from gonadal hormone inhibition, thus being able to spread out over the bone surface and resorb bone at a maximum rate. In addition, whatever inhibition operated on precursor cells would also be relieved. Thus, in the absence of gonadal hormones, osteoblastic activity would be diminished and osteoblast generation would be reduced, whereas osteoclastic activity and osteoclastogenesis would approach a maximum. Those regions of bone where osteoblasts and osteoclasts are most numerous, as on trabecular surfaces, would be subject to the most intense destruction. Predictably, therefore, gonadectomy would lead to the most rapid bone loss;[4,89] the menopause, with its fairly drastic loss of ovarian function, would lead to rapid bone loss (Figure 4A), but to less loss than in the case of oophorectomy. The fairly gradual diminution of testosterone function in men would be — and is — accompanied by the relatively slow bone loss recorded for men (Figure 4B).

III. MODULATION OF SKELETAL FUNCTION

A. GENETIC

It seems obvious that many genes, mostly as yet unidentified, must be involved in specifying the processes that lead to skeletal assembly, shape, size, and turnover. One gene that has recently been identified as having an important potential role in bone density is linked to polymorphism in the vitamin D receptor gene. Morrison and collaborators[63] have shown that "allelic variants in the gene encoding the vitamin D receptor can be used to predict differences in bone density..." Postmenopausal women with a bone density two standard deviations below that of young women were found to exhibit a significantly higher incidence of the genotype associated with low bone density. It is not yet known whether this polymorphism results in alterations of receptor action and whether these can be linked to differences in bone mass. Nevertheless, the potential significance of this report is very great. To appreciate its significance, it is necessary to describe the function of vitamin D and its use in the therapy of osteoporosis.

B. HORMONAL — VITAMIN D

Originally classified as a vitamin, cholecalciferol (vitamin D) is now considered a hormone, because of its genomic action in specifying the synthesis of calbindin D_{9k} in the duodenal cell or calbindin D_{28k} in certain renal cells, primarily in the distal convoluted tubule (for details, see reference 28). The principal actions of vitamin D are to stimulate active calcium transport in the intestine[22] and the kidney,[17,23] thereby increasing the amount of dietary calcium that enters the body and decreasing the amount lost in the urine. Vitamin D, via its biologically active metabolite, 1,25-dihydroxyvitamin D, also stimulates bone cells, speeding the maturation and differentiation of osteoblasts, including the synthesis of osteocalcin (GLA protein).[77] The mechanisms by which vitamin D leads to enhanced bone calcium deposition[50] are not known, but, if genomic, must involve the vitamin D receptor.

Attempts to overcome osteoporosis, or at least to slow the course of bone mineral decrease, have, for many years, utilized vitamin D, either by itself or together with calcium supplementation. Results with vitamin D alone have been variable, some investigators reporting significant reductions in the fracture rate,[92] others failing to find any effect.[51] Dawson-Hughes et al., who reviewed several other publications on the effect of 1,25-dihydroxyvitamin D3 on the course of bone loss, concluded[31] that the more favorable outcomes, such as reducing fracture rates,[92] were associated with higher doses of the metabolite. Conceivably individuals who responded to vitamin D supplementation had a vitamin D receptor allele that required a higher than normal amount of vitamin D for bone density to come nearer to normal. Typically vitamin D supplementation of women with osteoporosis will increase calcium absorption and urinary calcium output, with no effect on the overall retention of calcium.[45] Indeed, in the study by Hall et al.,[45] bone turnover, i.e., the rates of bone calcium deposition and removal, diminished when the women ingested 3.75 mg vitamin D (150,000 international units) for six weeks prior to the study. It is of course possible that the two postmenopausal subjects in the Hall et al. study[45] did not have an allelic defect and increased vitamin D intake therefore was without effect. Sambrook et al.[81] have reported a positive effect of adding 1,25-dihydroxyvitamin D to calcium supplementation, in terms of the rate of bone loss from the lumbar spine, but their patients received corticosteroid therapy. The latter influences bone loss more from the spine than from other sites which do not show a vitamin D response. Conceivably, administration of vitamin D is less effective than administration of 1,25-$(OH)_2$-D_3, as the conversion of vitamin D to the dihydroxylated metabolite is regulated. Further study is needed, but the overall results reported for vitamin D and its congeners do not seem encouraging.

C. OTHER HORMONES

In addition to the specific calcitropic hormones, parathyroid hormone and calcitonin, a number of other hormones (thyroid, growth hormone, somatomedin, glucocorticoids, insulin, glucagon) play a role in modulating bone metabolism and therefore may also change the course of osteoporosis. The reader is referred to reviews by Rude and Singer,[80] Bronner,[18,19] and pertinent chapters in reference 35.

Both parathyroid hormone and calcitonin have been used in the treatment of osteoporosis, but with uncertain results. Some of the other hormones, like thyroid and somatomedin, act directly on bone cells, whereas others, like adrenal corticosteroids, by inhibiting the biosynthetic action of vitamin D, may act indirectly. To the extent that aging diminishes hormone synthesis and/or release, replacement therapy with hormones other than gonadal may be appropriate in some situations.

D. OTHER FACTORS
1. Exercise

Vigorous exercise is well known to lead to increased muscle and bone mass. Contrariwise, life under conditions of hypogravity is associated with loss of muscle and weight-bearing bone.[62] Given an adequate intake of calcium and appropriate levels of gonadal hormones, physical exercise will increase peak adult skeletal mass.[44] However, when gonadal hormone levels are depressed, as in postmenopausal osteoporosis, exercise alone will not arrest the decline in bone mass;[78] exercise combined with estrogen therapy is more effective than estrogen alone. The mechanism by which exercise enhances expression of the genetic program for bone mass is not known. Stretching and compression of bone due to weight-bearing exercise may be transduced by bone cells via increased metabolic activity.[47]

2. Caffeine

The 12th Framingham study examination[53] identified caffeine intake as a risk factor, especially for women under 65 years of age, but other studies[9] have failed to find such an effect. In men under 75 years of age, the Framingham study found no effect of caffeine intake; the risk of hip fractures was, however, nearly doubled in men 75 years and older, who drank two or more cups of coffee per day. How caffeine might act, whether directly on bone cells or indirectly, is not known.

3. Tobacco

Daniell[30] was the first to observe that smokers, 60 to 69 years of age, had lost cortical bone at an average rate of 1.02% per year, whereas nonsmokers lost only 0.69% per year, a statistically significant difference. Nonobese smokers lost significantly more bone than nonobese nonsmokers. There was, however, no statistically significant difference between obese smokers and obese nonsmokers; moreover, as also observed by others,[48] the obese population lost significantly less bone than nonobese.

While some investigators have failed to find that smoking affected the incidence of osteoporosis,[48,76] most[59,84,95] have shown that smoking does constitute a risk factor for osteoporosis.

4. Alcohol

A variety of studies[11,68,83,88] has confirmed that alcoholism is associated with diminished bone mass and density in both men and women. In men, chronic alcoholism was found by Spencer et al.[88] to lead to osteoporosis in half of the population of alcoholics under the age of 50 years, whereas this percentage is negligibly small in normal males (Figure 4B). Increasingly, evidence in human and animal studies points to a direct effect of alcohol on bone cells themselves,[36,54] with severe impairment of bone remodelling having been observed[11] in chronic alcoholics who have normal biochemical parameters of calcium metabolism.

IV. THERAPY CONSIDERATIONS

From what has been said above it follows that adequate calcium intake is necessary to permit full expression of the genetic program that leads to skeletal form, size and mass. It is also apparent that skeletal development is a complicated, multifactorial process that involves many hormones, with gonadal hormones, growth hormone and somatomedin playing a principal role. Bone mass begins to decrease after the third decade of life. The question therefore arises whether this can be arrested or slowed. Moreover, inasmuch as the decrease in bone mass implies that the formation rate is now smaller than the rate at which bone is being destroyed, one can also question whether therapy should consist of stimulating formation or inhibiting destruction, or both.

The data depicted in Figure 5A suggest that estrogen treatment can markedly slow the loss of bone in oophorectomized women, but from available information it seems unlikely that bone loss can be totally arrested. It seems likely, however, that with adequate replacement therapy and calcium intake, bone mass loss can be slowed to a minimum. The effect of this slowing, illustrated in Figure 2, is to delay significantly the point at which bone fracture becomes probable under an otherwise harmless impact. In the light of what is now known about the biology of bone cells (see above), gonadal hormone replacement would stimulate osteoblast function and number. This in turn would reduce the production of cytokines such as interleukin 6 which stimulate osteoclastogenesis.

An alternative approach is to attempt to influence osteoclast function directly. The principal means have been the administration of calcitonin[79] or the use of biphosphonates.[38] Calcitonin inhibits the osteoclast, causing it to round up and cease its metabolic activity, at least transiently.[27] Biphosphonates, at relatively high concentrations, alter the bone mineral to make it less soluble, thereby reducing osteoclastic activity. More recently formulated biphosphonates act at relatively low concentrations, probably by directly inhibiting the osteoclast. The long-term effects of inhibiting osteoclastic activity are not known. Over the short term, the reduction in osteolysis has caused bone mass loss to slow. Administration of calcitonin that is not isogenous can lead to immune resistance.

V. THE QUESTION OF CALCIUM INTAKE

Two questions arise in assessing the role of calcium intake in relation to osteoporosis: (1) are the recommended daily allowances (RDA) sufficient to meet the requirements for optimal skeletal growth, size and mass; and (2) how do actual intakes compare with the recommended daily intakes?

In countries that have Western-style diets, calcium intake varies somewhere between 15 and 30 mmol per day,[14] with boys and men consuming the higher levels, women and older teen-age girls typically consuming 15 mmol per day. Changes in dietary consumption patterns notwithstanding, the effects on calcium intake have been minimal. The 1985 USDA survey[93] reported that women 35 to 50 years consumed on the average 13.3 mmol calcium daily, not much lower than the value of 15 mmol/day reported in 1959.[14] Both values are significantly lower, however, than the recommended dietary daily allowances for women of 20 mmol.[66] Men aged 19 to 50 years, on the other hand, consumed 125% of their RDA for calcium when surveyed for one summer day in 1985.[94]

Since U.S. women consume less calcium than their RDA, it is instructive to calculate a probable minimal intake, based on typical balance data. Table 1 lists such data and indicates the minimum amount of calcium that needs to be absorbed to maintain the person's current calcium status. By dividing the minimum required absorption by the probable fractional absorption, one can arrive at an estimate of how much calcium should be consumed. In the case of the postmenopausal woman, it is uncertain whether boosting calcium intake will in the long run overcome the negative bone balance. The additional amount that would be needed is the negative calcium balance (−0.5 mmol) divided by the fractional absorption, i.e., 0.5/0.2 or 2.5 mmol more. The calculation disregards the fact that active absorption decreases with increased intake, but illustrates that even if women consumed their recommended calcium allowance, their intake would likely not meet their skeletal needs.

V. CONCLUDING SUMMARY

Sufficient calcium intake is needed to assure optimum expression of skeletal size, mass and density. The minimum amount of calcium required for building bone in childhood and adolescence and to minimize bone loss that begins in the fourth decade of life can be estimated from the rates of calcium loss in urine

TABLE 1
Estimating Calcium Requirements for U.S. Women

	Adolescent Girl	Woman	Postmenopausal Woman
Age, Yrs	14	30	60
Ca balance, mmol/d^{-1}	2.5	0.1	−0.5
Urinary Ca output, mmol/d^{-1}	5.0	3.75	2.5
Endogenous fecal Ca output, mmol/d^{-1}	5.0	3.5	3.0
Probable Ca absorption, %	40	30	20
Minimum amt of Ca to be absorbed, mmol/d^{-1}	12.5	7.35	5.5 or 5.0
Minimum Ca intake, mmol/d^{-1}	31.3	24.5	27.5 or 25
RDA, mmol/d^{-1}	30	20	20

Note: Minimum Ca absorbed = Ca balance + urinary + endogenous fecal Ca outputs

$$\text{minimum intake} = \frac{\text{minimum absorbed}}{\text{fractional absorption}}$$

For U.S. RDA, see reference 66.

From Bronner, F., *Mineral Metabolism — An Advanced Treatise,* Academic Press, New York, 1964, and Bronner, F., *Disorders of Mineral Metabolism,* Academic Press, New York, 1982.

and endogenous calcium loss in feces, but these rates increase with increased calcium intake. As a result, the estimate is approximate. If the estimated amount needed is divided by fractional calcium absorption, one arrives at an estimate of the needed calcium intake. However, calcium absorption involves two processes, an active, vitamin D-regulated process that is downregulated with age or when calcium intake is increased, and upregulated with low calcium intake or pregnancy (among others). The second process is a passive, paracellular process that is not subject to acute regulation. Hence, fractional absorption, the sum of the active and passive processes, will go down with increased calcium intake, approaching a constant level. Therefore, a recommended daily allowance, the U.S. RDA, of calcium is an estimate based on population statistics. Current RDA values[66] tend to be low for U.S. women, appropriate for U.S. men. Moreover, U.S. women tend to consume substantially less calcium than the current RDA. Their low calcium intakes, therefore, tend to result in lower peak skeletal mass, size and density and in accelerated bone loss after the menopause.

Of the many hormones that regulate bone size, mass, and density, the gonadal hormones and growth hormone and somatomedin play major roles. Gonadectomized individuals lose bone at a relatively fast rate that can be slowed to a virtual standstill by replacement therapy. Postmenopausal osteoporosis is characterized by significant and rapid trabecular bone loss, accompanied by low cortical bone loss that continues even when most trabecular bone has been lost. Gonadal hormone replacement in menopausal and postmenopausal women diminishes bone loss markedly, provided calcium intake is sufficient. Although evidence concerning the parallelism between gonadal hormone diminution and bone loss in men is now accumulating, there are no data yet on the effect of gonadal hormone replacement on bone in normal elderly men; data exist on the beneficial effect of hormone replacement in gonadectomized men.

The mechanisms by which bone-forming cells, osteoblasts, and bone-resorbing cells, osteoclasts, interact and respond to gonadal hormones and somatomedin are only beginning to be understood. Cytokines seem to play an important role in regulating the reciprocal behavior of bone cells. In the presence of gonadal hormones, osteoblasts are stimulated and their number increases, with the number of osteoblast-liberated cytokines that stimulate preosteoclasts to form osteoclasts diminished. In addition, estrogens may also act directly to inhibit osteoclasts. Thus, in the absence of gonadal hormones, osteoblastic activity and number are diminished, whereas osteoclastic activity is enhanced.

General factors that affect bone metabolism and may play a role in altering the rate of bone loss are, in addition to calcium, caffeine, alcohol and smoking. High intakes of caffeine and alcohol aggravate bone loss, probably by interacting directly with osteoblasts. While smoking aggravates bone loss, the mechanism is not known. Exercise, because it stimulates muscle growth, enhances muscle mass. Excessive exercise, as in professional female runners,[6] may suppress menses and then lead to osteoporosis. Astronauts, subjected to prolonged periods of hypogravity, use less muscular effort and therefore lose bone mass.[62]

The measures needed to minimize bone loss after the fourth decade include adequate calcium intake combined with gonadal hormone replacement, limited caffeine and alcohol intake, reduction or avoidance of smoking, and participation in moderate exercise.

Therapy for slowing bone loss should lead to the stimulation of osteoblasts and slowing of osteoclastic resorption. Research is needed to identify methods other than gonadal hormone therapy to stimulate osteoblast metabolism and multiplication. Treatment with calcitonin or biphosphonates has been shown to reduce or inhibit osteoclast metabolism, but the long-term effects of inhibiting osteoclastic bone resorption alone are not known.

REFERENCES

1. Abrams, S. A., Pubertal changes in calcium kinetics in girls assessed using ^{42}Ca, *Ped. Res.,* 34, 455, 1993.
2. Abrams, S. A., Esteban, N. V., Vieira, N. E., Sidbury, J. B., Speden, B. L., and Yergey, A. L., Developmental changes in calcium kinetics in children assessed using stable isotopes, *J. Bone Min. Res.,* 7, 287, 1992.

3. Abrams, S. A., Schanler, R. J., Yergey, A. L., Vieira, N. E., and Bronner, F., Compartmental analysis of calcium metabolism in very low birth weight infants, *Ped. Res.*, 36, 424, 1994.
4. Aitken, J. M., Hart, D. M., Anderson, J. B., Lindsay, R., and Smith, D. A., Osteoporosis after oophorectomy for non-malignant disease, *Brit. Med. J.*, 1, 325, 1973.
5. Albright, F., Bloomberg, F., and Smith, P. H., Postmenopausal osteoporosis, *Trans. Assoc. Amer. Phys.*, 55, 298, 1940.
6. Anon., Bone loss in amenorrheic athletes, *Nutr. Rev.*, 14, 361, 1986.
7. Avioli, L. V., Epidemiology of osteoporosis and its complications, in *Prevention of Postmenopausal Osteoporosis — Dream or Reality?* Peck, W. A., Ed., Parthenon Publishing Group, Park Ridge, NJ, 1990, 11.
8. Baran, D. T., Bergfeld, M. A., Teitelbaum, S. L., and Avioli, L. V., Effect of testosterone therapy on bone formation in an osteoporotic hypogonadal man, *Calcif. Tissue Res.*, 26, 103, 1978.
9. Barger-Lux, M. J., Heaney, R. P., and Stegman, M. R., Effects of moderate caffeine intake on the calcium economy of premenopausal women, *Amer. J. Clin. Nutr.*, 52, 722, 1990.
10. Bellido, T., Girasole, G., Jilka, R. L., Crabb, D., and Manolagas, S. C., Demonstration of androgen receptors in bone marrow stromal cells and their role in the regulation of transcription from the human interleukin-6 (IL-6) gene promoter, *J. Bone Min. Res.*, 8 Suppl. 1, S131, 1993.
11. Bikle, D. D., Genant, H. K., Cann, C., Recker, R. R., Halloran, B. P., and Strewler, G. J., Bone disease in alcohol abuse, *Ann. Int. Med.*, 103, 42-48, 1985.
12. Biller, B. M. K., Saxe, V., Herzog, D. B., Rosenthal, D. I., Holzman, S., and Klibanski, A., Mechanisms of osteoporosis in adult and adolescent women with anorexia nervosa, *J. Clin. Endoc. Met.*, 68, 548, 1989.
13. Birch, M. A., Ginty, A. F., Walsh, C. A., Fraser, W. D., Gallagher, J. A., and Bilbe, G., PCR detection of cytokines in normal human pagetic osteoblast-like cells, *J. Bone Min. Res.*, 8, 1155, 1993.
14. Bronner, F., Dynamics and function of calcium, in *Mineral Metabolism — An Advanced Treatise,* Comar, C. L. and Bronner, F., Eds., Vol. IIA, The Elements, Academic Press, New York, 1964, 341.
15. Bronner, F., Calcium homeostasis, in *Disorders of Mineral Metabolism,* Bronner, F. and Coburn, J.W., Eds., Vol. II, Calcium Physiology, Academic Press, New York, 1982, 43.
16. Bronner, F., Gastrointestinal absorption of calcium, in *Calcium in Human Biology,* Nordin, B. E. C., Ed., Springer, London, 1988, 93.
17. Bronner, F., Renal calcium transport: Mechanisms and regulation — an overview, *Amer. J. Physiol.*, 257, F707, 1989.
18. Bronner, F., The calcitropic hormones: Parathyroid hormone, calcitonin, and vitamin D, in *A Basic Science Primer in Orthopaedics,* Bronner, F. and Worrel, R. V., Eds., Williams and Wilkins, Baltimore, 1991, 91.
19. Bronner, F., Hormonal and local modifiers of bone metabolism other than calcitropic hormones, in *A Basic Science Primer In Orthopaedics,* Bronner, F. and Worrell, R. V., Eds., Williams and Wilkins, Baltimore, 1991, 105.
20. Bronner, F., Current concepts of calcium absorption: an overview, *J. Nutr.*, 122, 641, 1992.
21. Bronner, F. and Lemaire, R., Comparison of calcium kinetics in man and the rat, *Calcif. Tissue Res.*, 3, 238, 1969.
22. Bronner, F., Pansu, D., and Stein, W. D., An analysis of intestinal calcium transport across the rat intestine, *Amer. J. Physiol.*, 250, G561, 1986.
23. Bronner, F. and Stein, W. D., CaBPr facilitates intracellular diffusion for Ca pumping in distal convoluted tubule, *Amer. J. Physiol.*, 255, F558, 1988.
24. Bronner, F. and Stein, W. D., Modulation of bone calcium-binding sites regulates plasma calcium: an hypothesis, *Calcif. Tissue Int.*, 50, 483, 1992.
25. Bronner, F., Richelle, L. J., Saville, P. D., Nicholas, J. A., and Cobb, J. R., Quantitation of calcium metabolism in postmenopausal osteoporosis and in scoliosis, *J. Clin. Invest.*, 42, 898, 1963.

26. Bruns, M. E. H., Fausto, A., and Avioli, L. V., Placental calcium binding protein in rats: apparent identity with vitamin D-dependent calcium binding protein from rat intestine, *J. Biol. Chem.,* 253, 3186, 1978.

27. Chambers, T. J., McSheehy, P. M. J., Thompson, B. M., and Fuller, K., The effect of calcium-regulating hormones and prostaglandins on bone resorption by osteoclasts disaggregated from neonatal rabbit bones, *Endocrinology,* 60, 234, 1985.

28. Collins, E. D. and Norman, A. W., Vitamin D, in *Handbook of Vitamins,* Machley, L. J., Ed., 2nd ed., Dekker, New York, 1991, 59.

29. Colvard, D. S., Ericksen, E. F., Keeting, P. E., Wilson, E. M., Lubahn, D. B., French, F. S., Riggs, B. L., and Spelsberg, T. C., Identification of androgen receptors in normal human osteoblast-like cells, *Proc. Nat. Acad. Sci. U.S.A.,* 86, 854, 1989.

30. Daniell, H. W., Osteoporosis and the slender smoker. Vertebral compression fractures and loss of metacarpal cortex in relation to postmenopausal cigarette smoking and lack of obesity, *Arch. Intern. Med.,* 136, 298, 1976.

31. Dawson-Hughes, B., Harris, S., Kramich, C., Dallal, G., and Rasmussen, H. M., Calcium retention and hormone levels in black and white women on high- and low-calcium diets, *J. Bone Min. Res.,* 8, 779, 1993.

32. Ernst, M., Heath, J. K., and Rodan, G. A., Estradiol effects on proliferation, messenger ribonucleic acid for collagen and insulin-like growth factor-I, and parathyroid hormone-stimulated adenylate cyclase activity in osteoblastic cells from calvariae and long bones, *Endocrinology,* 125, 825, 1989.

33. Ernst, M. and Rodan, G. A., Increased activity of insulin-like growth factor (IGF) in osteoblastic cells in the presence of growth hormone (GH): positive correlation with the presence of the GH-induced IGF-binding protein BP-3, *Endocrinology,* 127, 807, 1990.

34. Ernst, M., Schmid, C. H., and Froesch, E. R., Enhanced osteoblast proliferation and collagen gene expression by estradiol, *Proc. Nat. Acad. Sci. U.S.A.,* 85, 2307, 1988.

35. Favus, M. J., Ed., *Primer on the metabolic bone diseases and disorders of mineral metabolism,* Second ed., Raven Press, New York, 1993, 441.

36. Feitelberg, S., Epstein, S., Ismail, F., and D'Amanda, C., Deranged bone mineral metabolism in chronic alcoholism, *Metabolism.,* 36, 322, 1987.

37. Finkelstein, J. S., Klibanski, A., Neer, R. M., Doppelt, S. H., Rosenthal, D. I., Segre, G. V., and Crowley, W. F., Jr., Increases in bone density during treatment of men with idiopathic hypogonadotropic hypogonadism, *J. Clin. Endocrin. Metab.,* 69, 776, 1989.

38. Fleisch, H., Biphosphonates: new developments in structure, mechanisms of action and clinical applications, in *Chemistry and Biology of Mineralized Tissues,* Slavkin, H. C. and Price, P., Eds., Excerpta Medica (Elsevier), Amsterdam, 1992, 499.

39. Finkelstein, J., Neer, R. M., Biller, B. M. K., Crawford, J. D., and Klibanski, A., Osteopenia in men with a history of delayed puberty, *New Engl. J. Med.,* 376, 600, 1992.

40. Fukayama, S. and Tashjian, A. H., Jr., Direct modulation by estradiol of the response of human bone cells (SaOS-2) to human parathyroid hormone and PTH-related protein, *Endocrinology,* 124, 397, 1989.

41. Fukayama, S. and Tashjian, A. H., Jr., Direct modulation by androgens of the response of human bone cells (SaOS-2) to human parathyroid hormone (PTH) and PTH-related protein, *Endocrinology,* 125, 1789, 1989.

42. Girasole, G., Jilka, R. L., Passeri, G., Boswell, S., Boder, G., Williams, D. C., and Manolagas, S. C., 17β-estradiol inhibits interleukin-6 production by bone marrow-derived stromal cells and osteoblasts in vitro: a potential mechanism for the antiosteoporotic effect of estrogens, *J. Clin. Invest.,* 89, 883, 1992.

43. Gotfredsen, A., Hadberg, A., Nilas, L., and Christiansen, C., Total body mineral in healthy adults, *J. Lab. Clin. Med.,* 110, 362, 1987.

44. Halioua, L. and Anderson, J. B., Lifetime calcium intake and physical activity habits: independent and combined effects on the radial bone of healthy premenopausal Caucasian women, *Amer. J. Clin. Nutr.,* 49, 534, 1989.

45. Hall, B. D., Macmillan, D. R., and Bronner, F., Vitamin D-resistant rickets associated with high fecal endogenous calcium output, A report of two cases. *Amer. J. Clin. Nutr.,* 22, 448, 1969.

46. Hannan, M. T., Felson, D. T., and Anderson, J. J., Bone mineral density in elderly men and women: results from the Framingham osteoporosis study, *J. Bone Min. Res.,* 7, 547, 1992.

47. Hasegawa, S., Sato, S., Saito, S., Suzuki, Y., and Brunette, D. M., Mechanical stretching increases the number of cultured bone cells synthesizing DNA and alters their pattern of protein synthesis, *Calcif. Tissue Int.,* 37, 431, 1985.

48. Hemenway, D., Colditz, G. A., Willett, W. C., Stampfer, M. J., and Speizer, F. E., Fractures and lifestyle: effect of cigarette smoking, alcohol intake and relative weight on the risk of hip and forearm fractures in middle-aged women, *Amer. J. Publ. Health,* 78, 1554, 1988.

49. Horowitz, M. C., Cytokines and estrogen in bone: antiosteoporotic effect, *Science,* 260, 626, 1993.

50. Hurwitz, S., Stacey, R. E., and Bronner, F., Role of vitamin D in plasma calcium regulation, *Amer. J. Physiol.,* 216, 254, 1969.

51. Jenson, G. F., Christiansen, C., and Transbol, I., Treatment of postmenopausal osteoporosis. A controlled therapeutic trial comparing estrogen/gestagen, 1-25-dihydroxyvitamin D_3 and calcium, *Clin. Endocrin.,* 16, 515, 1982.

52. Jilka, R. L., Hangoc, G., Girasole, G., Passeri, G., Williams, D. C., Abrams, J. S., Boyce, B., Broxmeyer, H., and Manolagas, S. C., Increased osteoclast development after estrogen loss: mediation by interleukin-6, *Science,* 257, 88, 1992.

53. Kiel, D. P., Felson, D. T., Hannan, M. T., Anderson, J. J., and Wilson, P. W. F., Caffeine and the risk of hip fracture: the Framingham study, *Amer. J. Epidemiol.,* 132, 675, 1990.

54. Labib, M., Abdel-Kader, M., Ranganath, L., Teale, D., and Marks, V., Bone disease in chronic alcoholism: the value of plasma osteocalcin measurement, *Alcohol Alcoholism,* 24, 141, 1989.

55. Lindsay, R. and Cosman, F., Estrogen therapy: benefits and risks in osteoporosis therapy, in *Prevention of Postmenopausal Osteoporosis. Dream or Reality?* Peck, W. A., Ed., Panthenon Publishing Group, Park Ridge, NJ, 1990, 29.

56. Margen, S., Chu, J. Y., Kaufman, N. A., and Calloway, D. H., Studies in calcium metabolism. 1. The calciuric effect of dietary protein, *Amer. J. Clin. Nutr.,* 27, 584, 1974.

57. Matkovic, V., Fontana, D., Tominac, C., Goel, P., and Chesnut, C. H. III, Factors that influence peak bone mass formation: a study of calcium balance and the inheritance of bone mass in adolescent females, *Amer. J. Clin. Nutr.,* 52, 878, 1990.

58. Matkovic, V., Kostial, K., Simonovic, R., Buzina, R., Brodarec, A., and Nordin, B. E. C., Bone status and fracture rate in two regions of Yugoslavia, *Amer. J. Clin. Nutr.,* 32, 540, 1979.

59. McNair, P., Christensen, M. S., Madsbad, S., Christiansen, C., Binder, C., and Transbol, C., I. Bone loss in patients with diabetes mellitus: effects of smoking, *Min. Elect. Metab.,* 3, 94, 1980.

60. Meunier, P. J., Treatment of vertebral osteoporosis with fluoride and calcium, in *Molecular and Cellular Regulation of Calcium and Phosphate Metabolism,* Peterlik, M., and Bronner, F., Eds., Wiley-Liss, New York, 1990, 221.

61. Moore, L. J., Machlan, L. A., Lim, M., Yergey, A. L., and Hansen, J. W., Dynamics of calcium metabolism in infancy and childhood, I. Methodology and quantification in the infant, *Ped. Res.,* 19, 329, 1985.

62. Morey-Holton, E. R. and Arnaud, S. B., Skeletal responses to space flight, *Adv. Space Biol. Med.,* 1, 37, 1991.

63. Morrison, N. A., Qi, J. C., Tokita, A., Kelly, P. J., Crofts, L., Nguyen, T. V., Sambrook, P. N., and Eisman, J. A., Prediction of bone density from vitamin D receptor alleles, *Nature,* 367, 284, 1994.

64. Murphy, S., Khaw, K. T., Cassidy, A., and Compston, J. E., Sex hormones and bone mineral density in elderly men, *Bone Min.,* 20, 133, 1993.

65. Nahoul, K. and Roger, M., Age-related decline of plasma bioavailable testosterone in adult men, *J. Steroid. Biochem.,* 35, 293, 1990.
66. National Research Council, Recommended dietary allowances, 10th ed., National Academy Press, Washington, DC, 1989, 174.
67. Nilas, L. and Christiansen, C., The pathophysiology of peri- and postmenopausal bone loss, *Brit. J. Obstet. Gynecol.,* 96, 580, 1989.
68. Nilsson, B. E. and Westlin, N. E., Changes in bone mass in alcoholics, *Clin. Orthop. Rel. Res.,* 90, 229, 1973.
69. Oursler, M. J., Osdoby, P., Pyfferoen, J., Riggs, B. L., and Spelsberg, T. C., Avian osteoclasts as estrogen target cells, *Proc. Nat. Acad. Sci. U.S.A.,* 88, 6613, 1991.
70. Oursler, M. J., Pederson, L., Fitzpatrick, L., Riggs, B. L., and Spelsberg, T. C., Human giant cell tumors of the bone (osteoclastomas) are estrogen target cells, *Proc. Nat. Acad. Sci. U.S.A.,* 91, 5227, 1994.
71. Pacifici, R., Brown, C., Puscheck, E., Friedrich, E., Slatopolsky, E., Maggio, D., McCracken, R., and Avioli, L. V., Effect of surgical menopause and estrogen replacement on cytokine release from human blood mononuclear cells, *Proc. Nat. Acad. Sci. U.S.A.,* 88, 5134, 1991.
72. Pansu, D., Bellaton, C. and Bronner, F., Developmental changes in the mechanisms of duodenal calcium transport in the rat, *Amer. J. Physiol.,* 244, G20, 1983.
73. Pansu, D., Duflos, C., Bellaton, C. and Bronner, F., Solubility and intestinal transit time limit calcium absorption in the rat, *J. Nutr.,* 123, 1396, 1993.
74. Parfitt, A. M., The physiologic and histomorphometric significance of bone histomorphometric data, in *Bone Histomorphometry: Techniques and Interpretation,* Recker, R. R., Ed., CRC Press, Boca Raton, FL, 1983, 53.
75. Perret, C., Desplan, C., and Thomasset, M., Cholecalcin (a 9-kDa cholecalciferol-induced calcium-binding protein) messenger RNA. Distribution and induction by calcitriol in the rat digestive tract, *Europ. J. Biochem.,* 150, 211, 1985.
76. Pocock, N. A., Eisman, J. A., Kelly, P. J., Sambrook, P. N., and Yates, M. G., Effects of tobacco use on axial and appendicular bone mineral density, *Bone,* 10, 329, 1989.
77. Price, P. A., GLA-containing proteins of mineralized tissues, in *Chemistry and Biology of Tissues,* Slavkin, H. and Price, P., Eds., Excerpta Medica, Amsterdam, 1992, 169.
78. Prince, R. L., Smith, M., Dick, I. M., Price, R. I., Webb, P. G., Henderson, N. K., and Harris, M. M., Prevention of postmenopausal osteoporosis. A comparative study of exercise, calcium supplementation and hormone-replacement therapy, *New Engl. J. Med.,* 325, 1189, 1991.
79. Riis, B. J., Overgaard, K., and Christiansen, C., The role of nasal salmon calcitonin in prevention and treatment of osteoporosis, in *Prevention of Postmenopausal Osteoporosis — Dream or Reality?* Peck, W. A., Ed., Parthenon Publishing, Park Ridge, NJ, 1990, 55.
80. Rude, R. and Singer, F., Hormonal modifiers of mineral metabolism other than parathyroid hormone, vitamin D, and calcitonin, in *Disorders of Mineral Metabolism,* Bronner, F. and Coburn, J. W., Eds., Vol. II, *Calcium Physiology,* Academic Press, New York, 1982, 481.
81. Sambrook, P., Birmingham, J., Kelly, P., Kempler, S., Nguyen, T., Pocock, N., and Eisman, J., Prevention of corticosteroid osteoporosis. A comparison of calcium, calcitriol and calcitonin, *New Eng. J. Med.,* 328, 1747, 1993.
82. Sammon, P. J., Stacey, R. E., and Bronner, F., Role of parathyroid hormone in calcium homeostasis and metabolism, *Amer. J. Physiol.,* 218, 479, 1970.
83. Saville, P. D., Changes in bone mass with age and alcoholism, *J. Bone Joint Surg.,* 47A, 492, 1965.
84. Seeman, E., Melton, L. J., O'Fallon, W. M., and Riggs, B. L., Risk factors for spinal osteoporosis in men, *Amer. J. Med.,* 75, 977, 1983.
85. Simmons, D. J. and Grynpas, M. D., Mechanisms of bone formation *in vivo,* in *Bone,* Vol. 1, *The Osteoblast and Osteocyte,* Hall, B. K., Ed., Telford Press, Caldwell, NJ, 1990.
86. Slemenda, C. N., Loncope, C., and Johnston, C. C., Endogenous sex steroids, bone mass and bone loss, *J. Bone Min. Res.,* 8 Suppl. 1, S142, 1993.

87. Spencer, H., Kramer L., and Osis, D., Do protein and phosphorus cause calcium loss? *J. Nutr.,* 118, 657, 1988.
88. Spencer, H., Rubio, N., Rubio, E., Indreika, M., and Seitam, A., Chronic alcoholism. Frequently overlooked cause of osteoporosis in men, *Amer. J. Med.,* 80, 393, 1986.
89. Stepan, J. J., Lachman, M., Zverina, J., Pacovsky, V., and Baylink, D. J., Castrated men exhibit bone loss: effect of calcitonin treatment on biomechanical indices of bone remodeling, *J. Clin. End. Metab.,* 69, 523, 1989.
90. Swartz, C. M. and Young, M. A., Male hypogonadism and bone fracture, *New. Engl. J. Med.,* 318, 996, 1988.
91. Termine, J. D., Cellular activity, matrix proteins and aging bone, *Exper. Gerontol.,* 25, 217, 1990.
92. Tilyard, M. W., Spears, G. F. S., Thomson, J., and Dovey, S., Treatment of postmenopausal osteoporosis with calcitriol or calcium, *New Engl. J. Med.,* 326, 357, 1992.
93. U.S. Department of Agriculture, CSFII nationwide food consumption survey. Continuing survey of food intakes by individuals. Women 19–50 years and their children, 1–5 years, 4 days 1985. NFCS, CSFII Report 85-4, U.S. Department of Agriculture, Hyattsville, MD, 1987, 182.
94. U.S. Department of Agriculture, CSFII nationwide food consumption survey. Continuing survey of food intakes by individuals. Men 19–50 years, 1 day 1985. NFCS, CSFII Report 853, U.S. Department of Agriculture, Hyattsville, MD, 1986, 9410.
95. Williams, A. R., Weiss, N. G., Ure, C. L., Ballard, J., and Daling, J. R., Effect of weight, smoking and oestrogen use on the risk of hip and forearm fractures in postmenopausal women, *Obstet. Gynecol.,* 60, 695, 1982.
96. Wyman, J., Facilitated diffusion and the possible role of myoglobin as a transport molecule, *J. Biol. Chem.,* 241, 115, 1966.
97. Yergey, A. L., Abrams, S. A., Vieira, N. E., Aldroubi, A., Marini, J., and Sidbury, J. B., Determination of fractional absorption of dietary calcium in humans, *J. Nutr.,* 124, 674, 1994.

Chapter 6

CALCIUM AND HEART DISEASE

**Chandana Saha, Ronglih Liao, Gowriharan Thaiyananthan,
and Judith K. Gwathmey**

CONTENTS

I. INTRODUCTION

The incidence of heart disease in particular diastolic dysfunction increases as a function of age. The aging heart demonstrates many of the adaptive biochemical and functional changes associated with cardiac hypertrophy and heart disease. In humans systolic and diastolic blood pressures increase with age. Trends may however differ between sex and race groups. Blacks and Hispanics tend to have a higher incidence of hypertensive heart disease. The current strategy is to identify pharmacologic interventions usually for a lifetime

0-8493-7849-4/95/$0.00+$.50

137

to control hypertension. This strategy is fraught with problems such as non-compliance, drug associated side effects, variable potency and efficacy between patient populations. Combinations of drugs administered often result in side effects and poorer compliance. With the increasing costs of pharmaceuticals and declining healthcare dollars of an aging population, scientists/physicians should also focus on the potential effects of nonpharmaceutical intervention and/or dietary interventions on heart disease.

Hypertension has been labelled the silent killer because it often strikes without clear warning. Patients often feel well and therefore are unaware of this killer until late in the disease process. Many persons do not realize that hypertension leads to and can often result in severe heart disease. Cardiac hypertrophy is an early manifestation of chronic hypertension and can progress to cardiac dilatation and failure. There is a high prevalence of hypertension and heart disease in the elderly, Blacks, and Hispanics.[30] Heart disease is the number one killer of Americans compared to all other causes of death including cancer, AIDS, and accidents.

Historically the approach that has been applied to the treatment of hypertension and heart disease is pharmacological. This approach has not overcome the problem and has resulted in only minor changes in morbidity and mortality in the population at large. Other approaches to effective treatment are therefore needed. Early in the history of treatment of hypertension the goal was to reduce blood volume e.g., diuretics and sodium restriction.[8,9] This thought so dominated the field of treatment and research on hypertension that other potential ions were not scrutinized as potential causative or preventative agents. It has however been demonstrated in several studies that the sodium content of food and salt has no relationship to blood pressure.[19,44,50] Long-term alterations in sodium balance do not solely account for the hypotensive effects and vasodilating actions of diuretics.[29,94] Thiazide diuretics elevate serum calcium concentration and may lower parathyroid hormone (PTH) levels; both elevated serum calcium and low PTH levels have been implicated in essential hypertension.[65,68,78,79,82] Thiazides induce a positive calcium balance in humans;[99] this may be a mechanism that induces smooth muscle relaxation, vasodilatation and a subsequent reduction in mean arterial pressure. Disturbances in calcium metabolism have been reported in humans and in animal models of hypertension. Disturbances have included chronic depression of serum ionized calcium concentrations, associated with elevated parathyroid hormone concentrations, altered membrane binding of calcium, and hypercalciuria. These observations along with experimental studies, have led to the suggestion that calcium metabolism is implicated in hypertension.[96] We will present findings from experimental studies with animals as well as supporting clinical and demographic findings in humans that support an important role for calcium metabolism in hypertension and heart disease. In this chapter we review the literature on the effects of dietary calcium and serum calcium concentrations on cardiovascular disease and hypertension in particular, and present ideas for future research and therapy.

II. ROLE OF CALCIUM METABOLISM IN EXCITATION–CONTRACTION COUPLING OF THE MYOCARDIUM AND SMOOTH MUSCLE ACTIVATION

A. HEART MUSCLE EXCITATION-CONTRACTION COUPLING

The heart maintains a 10,000-fold gradient between the extracellular calcium concentration, which is in the millimolar range and intracellular calcium concentration, which is in the nanomolar range.[106] This gradient exists in part because of selective permeability of the sarcolemmal membrane, the existence of voltage dependent calcium channels, calcium pumps and exchangers. With membrane depolarization there occurs an influx of a small amount of calcium (Figure 1). This calcium then activates the release of a much larger amount of calcium from the intracellular calcium store of the sarcoplasmic reticulum.[25] It is this much larger amount of calcium (micromolar concentration) that binds to contractile elements of the the myofilaments, causing myocardial contraction. Relaxation occurs when the cytosolic calcium concentration is lowered by being resequestered in the sarcoplasmic reticulum with the aid of the SR Ca^{2+} ATPase. This reaccumulated calcium is then extruded from the cell by two mechanisms: via the sarcolemmal Ca^{2+} ATPase which has high affinity but low capacity and by means of the electrogenic sodium-calcium exchanger which extrudes two calcium ions for three sodium ions. The exchanger has high capacity but low affinity. Receptor initiated phosphorylation of channels, pumps (e.g., the SR Ca^{2+} ATPase regulatory protein phospholamban) and thin filament regulatory subunits (e.g., troponin I and T) modulate contraction.

Elevated cytosolic calcium concentrations have been shown in spontaneous and oscillatory release of calcium from the sarcoplasmic reticulum.[16,97] Furthermore, pathological calcification as observed in myocardial infarcts induced by ischemic and other forms of myocardial injury indicates that calcium plays

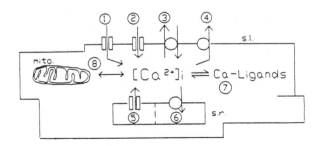

FIGURE 1. Schema of excitation–contraction coupling in cardiac muscle. The various cellular processes determine the intracellular calcium transient. 1. Voltage dependent calcium channels, 2. Leak channels for calcium; 3. Na^+/Ca^{2+} exchanger; 4. Sarcolemmal Ca^{2+} ATPase; 5. Ca^{2+} release channel of the sarcoplasmic reticulum (SR); 6. SR Ca^{2+} ATPase; 7. Ca-ligands = troponin C, calmodulin etc.; 8. mitochondria calcium transport. (Modified Webb, R. C. and Bohr, D. F., *Am. J. Physiol.*, 235, C227, 1978. With permission.)

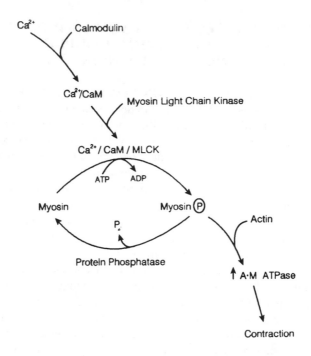

FIGURE 2. Schematic of smooth muscle contraction regulation through the myosin light-chain phosphorylation. Smooth muscle contractile elements are primarily activated by an increase in cytoplasmic calcium concentration. A.M = actin-myosin; P_i = inorganic phosphate. CaM = calcium calmodlin. MLCK = myosin light chain kinase. (From Wei, J. Y., Spurgeon, H. A., and Lakatta, E. G., *Am. J. Physiol.*, 246, H784, 1984. With permission.)

a role in the pathogenesis of contractile failure. Alterations in calcium metabolism and contractile activation have long been recognized in hypoxia and ischemia.[13,42,81]

B. SMOOTH MUSCLE CONTRACTION AND RELAXATION

Smooth muscle activation and relaxation differs somewhat from cardiac muscle activation (Figure 2).[79,85,109] Smooth muscle cells maintain the same calcium concentration gradient across the sarcolemma, with a small change in intracellular calcium concentration resulting in striking changes in cell function. The calcium messenger system in smooth muscle cells utilizes two key pathways: (1) the calmodulin-mediated cellular response, and (2) the *C*-kinase pathway that involves a diacylglycerol-mediated modulation of a Ca^{2+}-dependent protein kinase. Although calmodulin has no intrinsic enzymatic activity, it functions to bind calcium and facilitates intracellular signaling by promoting Ca^{2+}-dependent interactions with other cellular proteins, modifying their function. The interaction of an extracellular chemical stimulus, e.g., hormones, neurotransmitters, paracrine factors, with a surface receptor leads to activation of a membrane associated phospholipase. Phospholipase C catalyzes the hydrolysis of a membrane component phospholipids, and the subsequent intracellular release of second messengers, phosphatidylinositol, inositol phosphate and diacylglycerol (DG). The rise in DG leads to the intracellular translocation and activation of a calcium dependent protein kinase, *C*-kinase.

When smooth muscle is stimulated, intracellular calcium concentration rises and causes the calmodulin regulated activity of myosin light chain kinase to go up. This enzyme in turn phosphorylates myosin light chains of the thick filament of smooth muscle. The degree of phosphorylation of myosin light chain correlates with the development of smooth muscle shortening or load-bearing capacity. In contrast, catecholamines acting via β-adrenergic receptors on the cell surface relax smooth muscle. Activation of these receptors results in an increase in intracellular cyclic AMP. Under these conditions protein kinase A activity is increased. This in turn leads to the phosphorylation and activation of three critical intracellular sites (1) of the membrane associated Na^+/K^+ ATPase, resulting in a lowering of cytosolic calcium concentration; (2) of the calcium release channels of the endoplasmic reticulum, resulting in an increased reticular uptake of calcium and a lowering of cytosolic calcium, and (3) of the myosin light chain kinase, resulting in a decreased sensitivity to activation by calcium.

It is therefore apparent that intracellular calcium ions play a major and critical role as second messengers in the contraction and relaxation of both cardiac and smooth muscle. Calcium metabolism has been implicated in the abnormal vascular reactivity of smooth muscle in hypertension.[88,95] Dietary salt and high blood pressure have been linked to essential hypertension and abnormal calcium metabolism via an endogenous digitalis-like substance.[10]

III. ANIMAL STUDIES ON CALCIUM METABOLISM AND STUDIES ON HUMAN MYOCARDIUM

A. AGING MYOCARDIUM
1. Senescent Animals

The Fisher 344 rat has been extensively used as an animal model of the aging myocardium. In this model the senescent heart undergoes functional and biochemical changes similar to those seen in myocardial hypertrophy.[7,15,17,63] It is primarily characterized by diastolic dysfunction, i.e., a slowed contractile relaxation that has been attributed to the lower rate at which the SR pumps calcium (Figure 3A) and to the slower calcium transient as detected with the aid of aequorin, an intracellular calcium indicator.[59] SR Ca^{2+} ATPase activity is altered with age. The coupling of ATP hydrolysis to Ca^{2+} transport may therefore be altered with age (Figure 3B).[59] As also characteristic of the failing and hypertrophied heart, there is a prolonged duration of the action potential in the senescent heart of Fisher 344 rat.[107] Biochemically there is a decrease in myofibrillar Mg ATPase activity, a slowing of cross-bridge cycling dynamics, and a switch to the neonatal isotypes of key markers of myocardial energetics

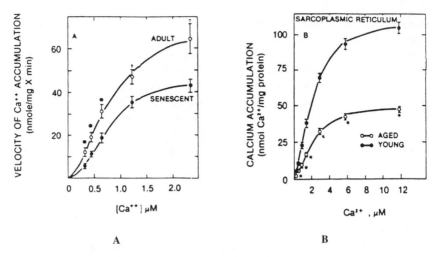

FIGURE 3. (A) The velocity of calcium uptake by cardiac sarcoplasmic reticulum isolated from 6 to 8 month-old (clear circle) and 24 to 25 month-old (filled circle) Wistan rats. (B) ATP-induced calcium accumulation by the SR as a function of calcium concentration from nine young (filled circle) and nine aged (clear circle) Fischer 344 rat hearts. (From Lakatta, E. G., *Circulation,* 75 Suppl. I, I-69, 1987. With permission.)

(e.g., lactate dehydrogenase and creatine kinase). Aged or senescent hearts would therefore appear to reflect abnormalities in calcium metabolism, as well as in myocardial energetics. These abnormalities have been implicated in ischemia-induced contractile failure and arrhythmogenesis in the senescent heart.[90] Similar to heart failure the senescent heart has a reduction in β-receptor density[52] as well as reduced responsiveness to α-adrenergic stimulation. In contrast there is increased responsiveness to cholinergic stimulation.[94] For a review of the pathophysiology of aging in animal and human myocardium see references 20, 37.

B. AGED HUMAN HEARTS

Older patients often have diastolic dysfunction in the absence of overt systolic failure. In humans maximal cardiac output decreases as a function of age and is associated with a decrease in myofibril protein synthesis. In aging human males the circulating atrial natriuretic factor (ANF) is elevated. In aging animals the heart has been shown to be the source of the ANF.

Older patients with primarily diastolic dysfunction are often treated with calcium channel blockers in an effort to improve myocardial relaxation. Calcium channel blockers have also often been used in the treatment of hypertension. Thus diastolic dysfunction may well be due, at least in part to abnormal calcium metabolism. Moreover, older patients in addition often suffer from hypertension and diabetes, both thought be associated with abnormal calcium metabolism.[20,37]

Calcium transients from patients with heart failure consist of two components. The first fast component is similar to the monophasic component seen in the nonfailing human myocardium and in normal animal hearts.[39] The second slower component may reflect abnormal calcium mobilization by failing myocytes and is associated with a slower relaxation response. When trabeculae carneae from nonfailing hearts from older patients (mean age 40.4 ± 6.5 years) that died from cerebrovascular events were loaded with the calcium indicator aequorin, changes in time course following stimulation were similar to those seen in failing human hearts.[36] However, unlike what happens in failing human myocardium, changing the calcium concentration of the medium resulted in a plateau above 4 mM $[Ca^{2+}]_o$, with no further increase in the amplitude of the second slower component as the calcium concentration rose. Also the relaxation time of the isometric twitch in these hearts was not slowed, unlike what happens in the failing human myocardium. These muscle preparations did, however, exhibit myocyte hypertrophy compared to heart preparations obtained from younger donors (mean age 24.0 ± 5.2 years). Thus, the nonfailing human heart without known cardiac disease can undergo hypertrophy with age.[36,77]

Cardiac risk factors such as, a rise in blood pressure and blood lipids are common in the elderly, though perhaps not inevitable. In the elderly, a diet consisting of an excess of calories, saturated fat, cholesterol or salt and one deficient in potassium, calcium and magnesium is thought to contribute to the incidence of hypertension.[56] The effect of chronic reduction in calcium intake as a function of age has not been rigorously investigated. The data in Table 1 indicate that total calcium, magnesium and phosphate did not change as a function of age. The effect of dietary intervention on the aging heart remains to be explored. Whether dietary calcium supplementation might prove beneficial alone or in combination with other dietary changes e.g., lower calories, salt and dietary fat, increased magnesium and potassium warrants investigation. As

TABLE 1
Serum Electrolyte Concentrations

	Ca^{2+} (mg/dl)	Mg^+ (meq/l)	PO_4^{-3} (mg/dl)	Ion Ca^{2+} (mg/dl)
Myopathic Old	9.02 ± 0.66	1.79 ± 0.45	3.69 ± 1.04	1.04 ± 0.11
Nonfailing Old	8.51 ± 2.22	1.58 ± 0.89	2.41 ± 0.61	ND
Myopathic Young	8.66 ± 0.83	1.94 ± 0.61	4.02 ± 1.24	1.06 ± 0.09
Nonfailing Young	8.05 ± 1.07	1.7 ± 0.30	3.05 ± 1.25	ND

Note: Myopathic old age 57.8 ± 3.81 (n = 41); myopathic young 41 ± 7.6 (n = 26); Nonfailing old = 60 ± 5.44 (n = 16); Nonfailing young 24.3 ± 6.06 (n = 4); ND = not determined. Mean ± SD; Ca^{2+} = serum total calcium concentration; Mg = magnesium; PO_4^{-3} = phosphate; Ion Ca^{2+} = free ionized calcium concentration.

the aging population continues to grow and with the projection that the aging population will constitute 20% of the population by the year 2000, the effects of aging on the heart and possible intervention will gain in importance.

C. HEART FAILURE

The effects of dietary calcium intake on heart failure have not been investigated. However, a leading hypothesis in heart failure is that because of decreased contractility there is a need for increased intracellular calcium. This has resulted in the development of inotropes that increase intracellular calcium concentrations, but these drugs have not proven very helpful in the treatment of heart failure. The demonstration that muscles from the hearts of patients with heart failure exhibit contractile failure as the stimulation rate is increased has led to investigations as to why patients with heart failure do not tolerate tachycardia. Elevated extracellular calcium concentrations cause the action potential in trabeculae carneae from failing human hearts to become shortened, perhaps reflecting unstable electromechanical coupling.[40] As proposed by Gwathmey[35] and demonstrated by Schwinger et al.[92] when the magnesium concentration in the bath was raised, the negative force interval relationship in the failing human myocardium was reversed (Figure 4).[92] These data suggest that membrane stabilization is important in the contractile dysfunction that is seen in the human myocardium from failing hearts. Magnesium also reduces calcium currents and therefore stabilizes the membrane and the intracellular calcium concentration.[43] Both extracellular magnesium and calcium serve to stabilize the sarcolemma and protect the glycocalyx against the calcium paradox (i.e., calcium overload and muscle contracture). If an increase in magnesium or calcium intake were to raise extracellular magnesium and calcium levels, diet may become important in the management of heart failure patients.

D. EXPERIMENTAL STUDIES ON HYPERTENSIVE RATS

Calcium plays a central role in normal cardiovascular function. Disturbances of calcium metabolism have been identified for most if not all etiologies of heart failure and hypertrophy.[38] Clear defects in calcium metabolism have been identified in hypertensive animals. The question remains whether alterations in calcium metabolism are pathogenic or simply reflect adaptive responses of the cardiovascular system.

Lower dietary calcium appears to be related to the occurrence of hypertension. Experiments with elevated dietary calcium (2.55%) in both spontaneously hypertensive (SHR) and Wistan–Kyoto (WKY) normotensive rats by Ayachi[4] have shown that the high calcium intake is associated with an attenuation of blood pressure, while the urinary excretion of Na^+, K^+, and Ca^{++} go up. Plasma ionized calcium has been reported to be decreased in the normotensive WKY rats and an enriched calcium diet (4%) can compensate for this reduction and restore normal levels.[73] A reduction of blood pressure due to increased dietary calcium in normotensive WKY as well as SHR has been associated

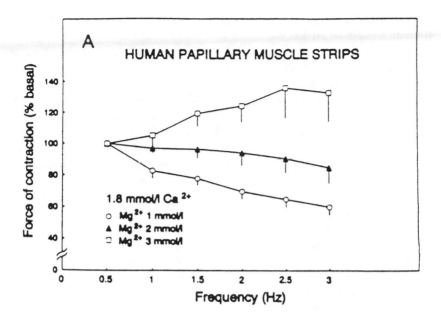

FIGURE 4. Force frequency relationship papillary muscle strips from failing human hearts studied under varying concentrations of magnesium. Notice the negative force-interval relationship at 1 mmol/l Mg$^+$ which was reversed at 3 mmol/l Mg$^+$. (From Schwinger, R. H. G., Böhm, M., Uhlmann, R., Schmidt, U., Überfuhr, P., Kreuzer, E., Reichart, B., and Erdmann, E., *Am. Heart. J.*, 126, 1018, 1993. With permission.)

with an increase in serum ionized calcium. This may indicate that calcium balance plays a role in blood pressure regulation.[66] Nevertheless, disturbances in the ratio of ionic to total plasma calcium have not been shown to be a primary factor in the development of hypertension.[110] On the other hand, an increase in calcium tissue content has been found associated with increased narrowing of hypertensive arterioles.[104]

Calcium plays an important role in vascular smooth muscle activity. High concentrations of calcium have been reported to diminish the magnitude of contraction of vascular smooth muscle;[11] this is often referred to as the "membrane-stabilizing effect"[50,87] and is dependent on the activity of the sodium potassium ATPase.[106] Ionic permeability in vascular smooth muscle cells depends on the extracellular calcium concentration. Thus for the higher turnover of K$^+$, Na$^+$ and Cl$^-$ in the aortae from SHR rats may be related to the decreased ability of the smooth muscle membrane to bind calcium for stabilization.[55] Observations made in normal and hypertensive humans and in experimental animals[67] indicate long-term variations in blood pressure that follow alterations in the metabolic balance of Ca^{++}, Mg^{++} and PO$_4^-$. Thus the reduction in the binding of calcium to membranes that occurs in the SHR animals and possibly in hypertensive humans may be reversed by dietary calcium supplementation that can bring about membrane stabilization and vascular smooth muscle relaxation.[14]

Aoki et al.[2,3] have suggested that the microsomal fractions of vascular smooth muscle from SHR animals can accumulate less calcium than such fractions from normotensive control rats. The low calcium binding capacity has been associated with a high ATPase activity. The latter, in turn, may induce an increase in vascular resistance and tone and thus result in elevated blood pressure as a compensatory response. Webb and Bhalla[105] have found that the calcium distribution in smooth muscle cells of SHR animals was altered because microsomal fraction of the muscle sequestered less calcium. Limas and Cohn[62] working with SHR and WKY rats have shown that calcium uptake and binding were reduced and ATP splitting acclerated in the SHR animals and that these abnormalities were associated with an age-dependent decrease in cyclic AMP-dependent protein kinase and a cyclic AMP-induced stimulation of SR calcium uptake. Studies with erythrocytes[21,84] and with adipocytes[83] suggest that the decrease in calcium binding may be a generalized phenomenon of the plasma membrane of cells from genetically hypertensive rats.

Hyperparathyroidism and increased PTH level are associated with high blood pressure in humans.[47,61] Calcium regulating hormones like PTH, calcitriol and calcitonin may play a role in blood pressure regulation. A new circulating hypertensive factor (parathyroid hypertensive factor, PHF) has been reported to exist in both SHR and human plasma, and parathyroidectomy eliminates this circulating factor, suggesting the parathyroid origin of PHF.[78] In addition, the calcitonin gene related peptide (CGRP) and parathyroid hypertensive factor (PHF) have been identified to be responsive to dietary calcium and thus may influence blood pressure.[45]

Regarding the influence of other electrolytes on blood pressure regulation by dietary calcium, Tamura[103] has shown that the regulatory effect of dietary calcium on blood pressure is independent of phosphate, but that the systolic blood pressure is positively correlated with serum magnesium levels. However, Evans et al.[24] did not find an effect of magnesium or an interactive effect of calcium and magnesium on blood pressure.

Many studies have revealed that dietary calcium attenuates sodium chloride dependent hypertension.[22,90] Several mechanisms have been proposed for this phenomenon. Scrogin et al.[93] have reported that high dietary intake of sodium chloride induces a rise in blood pressure and sympathoadrenal stress responses, as well as in vascular reactivity to norepinephrine. Dietary calcium supplementation reduces stress, but has no effect on blood pressure elevation due to sodium chloride.[93] These data would suggest that the hypotensive effects of dietary calcium are due to influences on sympathoadrenal activity rather than on vascular reactivity. In support of this mechanism Chen et al.[18] suggested that the hypotensive action of dietary calcium in sodium chloride induced SHR is mediated by decreased sympathetic activity. Recent study indicates that a modulation of α_1-adrenergic receptor activity is associated with the hypotensive action of dietary calcium.[46]

IV. HUMAN STUDIES ON POTENTIAL ROLE OF CALCIUM METABOLISM: IMPLICATIONS FOR DIETARY INTERVENTION

A. HEART FAILURE

The effects of dietary calcium on heart failure are unknown. Serum calcium concentrations in patients undergoing cardiac transplantation for end-stage heart failure do not differ from those donors of nonfailing hearts (Table 1). However, most heart failure patients on cardiac transplantation lists are electrolytically balanced. This may obscure differences in serum electrolytes, especially ionized calcium concentrations. Values obtained closer to the time of initial hospital admission tended to be lower for total calcium.

The number of calcium channels measured by radioligand binding has been reported to be reduced in idiopathic dilated cardiomyopathy; this suggests a possible need for higher serum calcium concentrations.[102] Other investigators however have found the numbers of calcium channels unchanged.[35,86] All investigators however agree that there is no change in calcium channel binding affinity (K_D) in the human myocardium.[27,35,86]

The effects of calcium on myocardial performance in humans have been investigated.[23,32,48,60] Left ventricular contractility was assessed using load and rate independent relationships between end-systolic wall-stress and rate corrected velocity for fiber shortening (Vcf_c). The latter was found to vary in near-linear fashion with the calcium ion concentration. These findings support the idea that variations in calcium are directly correlated with changes in myocardial contractility.

Ginsburg et al.[32] have shown that correction of serum ionized calcium correlated with myocardial contractility in a 16-year old patient with severe congestive heat failure and that calcium replacement normalized blood pressure and other hemodynamic parameters. For the next two weeks, cardiac output, blood pressure, and urine output were directly related to Ca^{2+} levels, with no change in total calcium or albumin and pH or evidence of abnormal parathyroid function. These findings point to the importance of determining ionized calcium levels in extremely ill patients.

B. HYPERTENSION

The observation that humans living in areas with "hard" water, i.e., high in calcium, had a lower incidence of heart disease sparked studies into the relationship between calcium intake and blood pressure. Several studies have noted an inverse relationship between dietary calcium intake and blood pressure.[76,101] This has led to the hypothesis that dietary calcium deficiency plays a role in hypertension.[69,71] The relationship between systolic and diastolic blood pressure and demographic, dietary, lifestyle and anthropometric variables was investigated in 10,419 adults age 18 and above who were not being treated for hypertension. Of the variables investigated calcium, sodium/calcium ratio, vitamin C and calcium/phosphorus ratio were significantly correlated with both systolic and diastolic pressure. However, the most important factors affecting blood pressure were body mass index and age.[99]

Abnormal calcium metabolism has been implicated in primary hypertension. Patients with hypertension exhibit high urinary calcium excretion and low serum ionized calcium concentrations. A high incidence of hypertension has also been found in patients with primary hyperparathyroidism and parathyroid hormone levels have been reported to be elevated in patients with primary hypertension.[61,78] Higher intakes of dietary calcium have been associated with lower systolic, and in some reports with lower diastolic, pressures. In Western cultures calcium intake often falls and systolic blood pressure rises with age. Dietary supplementation of calcium intake (1.5 g/d) and blood pressure was studied in 81 normotensive and 34 medicated hypertensive women age 35 to 65 years over a 4-year period. In the medicated hypertensive group there was a 13 mmHg decrease in systolic pressure and a 7 mmHg increase in unsupplemented women over the 4 years ($p < 0.02$).[54] In men a similar trend has been reported.[1] In a randomized placebo-controlled survey of simultaneous urinary electrolyte excretion and dietary intake in a matched population of hypertensives and normal patients, it was reported that urinary excretion of calcium in hypertensive patients was 63% higher. Importantly, there were no differences in urinary output of sodium, potassium, phosphate or magnesium. These hypertensive patients reported 22% less daily intake of calcium (728 ± 310 mg/d vs. 939 ± 338 mg/d). With dietary calcium supplementation (1000 mg/d), the higher urinary excretion of calcium was not different from placebo in hypertensives, although urinary excretion increased with supplementation in the normotensive patients and more closely resembled that of nonsupplemented hypertensive patients.[49]

In a double-blind study 90 mildly hypertensive subjects aged 16 to 29 years were randomly assigned to 1 g Ca/d or placebo. Calcium supplementation did not affect systolic pressure but diastolic pressures fell by 3.1 mmHg in the calcium supplemented group. Subjects with higher parathyroid hormone levels demonstrated an even greater decrease in diastolic pressure (5.4 to 6.1 mmHg). Subjects with lower serum total calcium benefited most from calcium supplementation.[34] It is important to consider that calcium supplementation had no effect on serum or intracellular electrolytes. Similar findings were reported in young adults who had been supplemented with 1 g Ca/d.[6]

In patients with mild to moderate hypertension, supplementation with 1000 mg/d for 8 weeks significantly lowered supine blood pressure (BP) by 3.8 mmHg, standing BP by 5.6 mmHg and supine diastolic by 2.3 mmHg.[70] The effect of calcium supplementation appeared to be time-dependent, progressive, and continuous. Urine and serum chemistry demonstrated no significant differences except that serum ionized calcium was significantly higher in hypertensives during calcium supplementation.

Women in the U.S. ingest significantly less calcium than their male counterparts and then calcium intake decreases with age. However, it has yet to be determined whether increasing dietary calcium as opposed to calcium supplementation will yield similar results.

As a result of the article published by McCarron et al.[72] several letters were written to the editors[26] challenging the conclusions that a major role had been demonstrated for dietary calcium in hypertension. Points raised were the selection criteria used for the patients in the McCarron et al. study,[72] the definition of hypertension, and the adequacy of the statistical analysis. Nevertheless, all corespondents agreed that sufficient data had been collected to justify further study.

One of the strong objections to studies by McCarron and others is that dietary intake can vary greatly on a day to day basis. However, in a study of 8000 Japanese men in Hawaii who showed little variance in their daily diets, a strong correlation with milk and potassium intake was noted. Only calcium from dairy products was associated with blood pressure. Milk consumption was inversely associated with both systolic and diastolic blood pressure ($p < 0.001$). In relative terms potassium intake showed the strongest association with both systolic and diastolic blood pressure.[87] On the basis of this study it is clear that multivariate analysis of highly intercorrelated variables make data interpretation and extrapolation difficult.

It has never been clearly shown that there is an independent role of any specific nutrient in hypertension. No nutrient has been studied in isolation.[87] Interestingly, in a study of men of Japanese ancestry living in Hawaii who had no history of cardiovascular disease or treated hypertension, it was found that of 61 dietary variables magnesium had the strongest association with blood pressure.[53]

According to the Health and Nutrition Survey I of the National Center for Health Statistics, adults whose calcium intake coverages 1500 mg Ca/d have a 45 to 50% lower incidence of hypertension than adults with a 500 mg/d intake. However, populations in countries where calcium intake is low tend to have blood pressures that are also low, with hypertension uncommon.[30] Consequently, the question of simple cause and effect remains. Perhaps it is too much to expect correlations across cultural, social, and ethnic lines.

V. CONCLUSIONS

Morgan and Suematsu have discussed the rationale for the use of calcium channel blockers in relation to the pathophysiology of hypertension and smooth muscle contraction.[75] Compelling data and arguments have been presented for a calcium overload state in hypertension in both animals and humans.[4,28]

In contradistinction, several investigators report an inverse relationship between dietary calcium intake and blood pressure. There nevertheless appears to be a heterogeneity in response;[33] therefore, the mechanism of a putative protective role for dietary calcium is still under scrutiny.[64] The potential hypotensive action of calcium supplementation is of special importance and interest for people with mild hypertension in whom drug treatment may be undesirable. Even though the idea of manipulating dietary calcium to control hypertension has been strongly criticized,[57] there are compelling data that suggest further investigation is warranted. There is evidence from both animal and human studies that indicates a role for dietary sodium in the genesis and treatment of hypertension.[41] It has been proposed that the antihypertensive action of calcium supplementation may involve natriuresis and diuresis, since renal calcium and sodium excretion are closely coupled.[8,10,71,94,99] At the same time it is difficult to reconcile the observation that intracellular calcium is elevated[88] with the use of dietary calcium supplementation which increases serum ionized calcium levels only minimally.

It is important to recognize that nutrients are not ingested in isolation. Conceivably the interaction of nutrients in the diet brings about synergistic benefits resulting from modulation due to hormones, paracrine factors, and neurotransmitters. This could also account for some of the heterogeneity of human blood pressure responses to variations in calcium intake.[58,74] Clearly, better defined end-points and biologic assessment of electrolyte, paracrine, and neurohumoral factors are needed to sort out whether changes in dietary calcium have a direct benefit or whether calcium functions indirectly as a sort of co-factor, in reducing blood pressure.

The picture in overt heart failure is clear, inasmuch as serum ionized calcium levels directly affect myocardial contractility. However, it remains unclear whether all patients with end-stage heart failure have significantly lower serum total calcium and/or ionized calcium concentrations.

REFERENCES

1. Ackley, S., Barrett-Connon, E., and Suarez, L., Dairy products, calcium, and blood pressure, *Am. J. Clin. Nutr.,* 38, 457, 1983.
2. Aoki, K., Ikeda, N., Yamashita, K., and Hotta, K., ATPase activity and Ca⁺⁺ interaction of myofibrils and sarcoplasmic reticulum isolated from the hearts of spontaneously hypertensive rats, *Jpn. Heart J.,* 15, 475, 1974.
3. Aoki, K.,Yamashita, K., Timita, N., Tazumi, K., and Hotta, K., ATPase activity and Ca⁺⁺ binding ability of subcellular membrane of arterial smooth muscle in spontaneously hypertensive rat, *Jpn. Heart J.,* 15, 180, 1974.
4. Atkinson, J., Vascular calcium overload. Physiological and pharmacological consequences, *Drugs,* 44, Suppl. 1, 111, 1992.
5. Ayachi, S., Increased dietary calcium lowers blood pressure in the spontaneously hypertensive rat, *Metabolism,* 28(12), 1234, 1979.
6. Belizan, J. M., Villar, J., Pineda, O., Gonzalez, A. E., Sainz, E., Garrera, G., and Sibrian, R., Reduction of blood pressure with calcium supplementation in young adults, *JAMA,* 249(9), 1161, 1983.
7. Besse, S., Assayag, P., Delcayre, C., Carre, F., Cheav, S. L., LeCarpentier, Y., and Swynghedauw, B., Normal and hypertrophied senescent rat heart: mechanical and molecular characteristics, *Am. J. Physiol.,* 265, H183, 1993.

8. Blaustein, M. P., Sodium ions, calcium ions, blood pressure regulation, and hypertension: a reassessment and a hypothesis, *Am. J. Physiol.,* 232(3), C165, 1977.

9. Blaustein, M. P., Role of a natriuretic factor in essential hypertension: a hypothesis, *Ann. Intern. Med.,* 98(2), 785, 1983.

10. Blaustein, M. P. and Hamlyn, J. M., Pathogenesis of essential hypertension. A link between dietary salt and high blood pressure, *Hypertension,* 18, III-184, 1991.

11. Bohr, D. F., Vascular smooth muscle: dual effect of calcium, *Science,* 139, 597, 1963.

12. Bond, M., Elevated cellular calcium in disease states: cause or effect? *Cell Calcium,* 9, 201, 1988.

13. Buja, L. M., Hagler, H. K., and Willerson, J. T., Altered calcium homeostasis in the pathogenesis of myocardial ischemic and hypoxic injury, *Cell, Calcium.,* 9, 205, 1988.

14. Bukosi, R. D. and McCarron, D. A., Altered aortic reactivity and lower blood pressure associated with high calcium intake, *Am. J. Physiol.,* 252, H976, 1986.

15. Buttrick, P., Malhotra, A., Factor, S., Geenen, D., Leinwand, L., and Scheuer, J., Effect of aging and hypertension on myosin biochemistry and gene expression in the rat heart, *Circ. Res.,* 68, 645, 1991.

16. Capogrossi, M. C., Silverman, H. S., Stern, M. D., and Lakatta, E. G., Pathophysiological effects of spontaneous sarcoplasmic reticulum Ca^{2+} release on myocardial function, in *Heart Failure: Basic Science and Clinical Aspects,* Gwathmey, J. K., Briggs, G. M., and Allen, P. D., Eds., Marcel Dekker, New York, 1993, 39.

17. Carrier, L., Boheler, K. R., Chasagne, C., de, la, Bastic, D., Wisnewsky, C., Lakatta, E. F., and Schwartz, K., Expression of sarcomeric actin isogenes in the rat heart with development and senescence, *Circ. Res.,* 70, 999, 1992.

18. Chen, Y. F., Wyss, J. M., Jin, H., and Oparil, S., Calcium loading prevents the Nickel induced exacerbation of hypertension and enhancement in sympathetic discharge in Nickel sensitive spontaneously hypertensive rats, *Clin. Res.,* 35, (Abstr.), 440A, 1987.

19. Cooper, R., Liu, K., Trevisan, M., Miller, W., and Stamler, J., Urinary sodium excretion and blood pressure in children: absence of a reproducible association, *Hypertension,* 5, 135, 1983.

20. Davidoff, J. A. and Gwathmey, K. J., Pathophysiology of cardiomyopathies: Part I. Animal models and humans, *Curr. Opinion Cardiol.,* 9, 357, 1994.

21. Devynck, M. A., Pernollet, M. G., Nunez, A. M., and Meyer, P., Analysis of calcium handling in erythrocyte membranes of genetically hypertensive rats, *Hypertension,* 3, 397, 1981.

22. Doris, P. A., Sodium and hypertension: effect of dietary calcium supplementation on blood pressure, *Clin. Exp. Hypertens.,* A, 7, 1441, 1985.

23. Drop, L. J. and Scheidegger, D., Plasma ionized calcium concentration: important determinant of hemodynamic response to calcium infusion, *J. Thorac. Cardiovasc. Surg.,* 79, 425, 1980.

24. Evans, G. H., Weaver, C. M., Harrington, D. D., and Babbs, C. F. Jr., Association of magnesium deficiency with the blood pressure-lowering effects of calcium, *J. Hypertens.,* 8, 327, 1990.

25. Fabiato, A., Myoplasmic free calcium concentration reached during the twitch of an intact isolated cardiac cell and during calcium induced release of calcium from the sarcoplasmic reticulum of a skinned cardiac cell from the adult rat or rabbit ventricle, *J. Gen. Physiol.,* 78, 457, 1981.

26. Feinleib, M., Lenfant, C., and Miller, S. A., Hypertension and calcium, *Science,* 226 (4673); 384, 1984.

27. Finkel, M. S., Patterson, R. E., Roberts, W. C., Smith, T. D., and Keiser, H. R., Calcium channel binding characteristics in the human heart, *Am. J. Cardiol.,* 62, 1281, 1988.

28. Fleckenstein-Grun, G., Frey, M., Thimm, F., Hofgartner, W., and Fleckenstein, A., Calcium overload — an important cellular mechanism in hypertension and arteriosclerosis, *Drugs,* 44 Suppl. 1, 23, 1992.

29. Freis, E. D., Salt in hypertension and the effects of diuretics, *Ann. Rev. Pharmacol. Toxicol.,* 19, 13, 1979.

30. Garcia-Palmieri, M. R., Costas, R., Cruz-Vidal, M., Sorlie, P. D., Tillotson, J., and Havlik, R. J., Milk consumption, calcium intake, and decreased hypertension in Puerto Rico. Puerto Rio Heart Health Program Study, *Hypertension,* 6, 322, 1984.
31. Garn, S. M. and Larkin, F. A., Calcium intake and hypertension, *Science,* 219 (4581), 112, 1983.
32. Ginsburg, R., Esserman, L. J., and Bristow, M. R., Myocardial performance and extracellular ionized calcium in a severely failing human heart, *Ann. Internal. Med.,* 98 (Part 1), 603, 1983.
33. Grobbee, D. E., Electrolytes and hypertension: results from recent studies, *Am. J. Med. Sci.,* 307 Suppl. 1, S17, 1994.
34. Grobbee, D. E. and Hofman, A., Effect of calcium supplementation on diastolic blood pressure in young people with mild hypertension, *Lancet,* 2 (8509), 703, 1986.
35. Gruver, E. J., Morgan, J. P., Stambler, B. S., and Gwathmey, J. K., Uniformity of calcium channel number and isometric contraction in human right and left ventricular myocardium, *Basic. Res. Cardiol.,* 89, 139, 1994.
36. Gwathmey, J. K., Bentivegna, L. A., Ransil, B. J., Grossman, W., and Morgan, J. P., Relationship of abnormal intracellular calcium mobilisation to myocyte hypertrophy in human ventricular myocardium, *Cardiovas. Res.,* 27, 199, 1993.
37. Gwathmey, J. K. and Davidoff, A. J., Experimental aspects of cardiomyopathy, *Curr. Opinion Cardiol.,* 8, 480, 1993.
38. Gwathmey, J. K., Liao, R., and Hajjar, R. J., Intracellular free calcium in hypertrophy and failure, in *Diastolic Relaxation,* Lorell, B. H. and Grossman, W., Eds., Kluwer Academic Publishers, Boston, 1994, 55.
39. Gwathmey, J. K. and Morgan, J. P., Calcium handling in myocardium from amphibian, avian, and mammalian species: the search for two components, *J. Comp. Physiol.,* B161, 19, 1991.
40. Gwathmey, J. K., Slawsky, M. T., Hajjar, R. J., Briggs, G. M., and Morgan, J. P., Role of intracellular calcium handling in force-interval relationships in human ventricular myocardium, *J. Clin. Invest.,* 85, 1599, 1990.
41. Haddy, F. J., Roles of sodium, potassium, calcium, and natriuretic factors in hypertension, *Hypertension,* 18 Suppl. III, III-179, 1991.
42. Hajjar, R. J., Ingwall, J. S., and Gwathmey, J. K., Mechanism of action of 2,3-butanedione monoxime on contracture during metabolic inhibition, *Am. J. Physiol.,* 267, H100, 1994.
43. Hall, S. K. and Fry, C. H., Magnesium affects excitation, conduction, and contraction of isolated mammalian cardiac muscle, *Am. J. Physiol.,* 263, H622, 1992.
44. Harlan, W. R., Hull, A. L., Schmouder, R. L., Landis, J. R., Thompson, F. E., and Larkin, F. A., Blood pressure and nutrition in adults. The national health and nutrition survey, *Am. J. Epidemiol.,* 120(1), 17, 1984.
45. Hatton, D. C. and McCarron, D. A., Dietary calcium and blood pressure in experimental models of hypertension: a review, *Hypertension,* 23(4), 513, 1994.
46. Hatton, D. C., Scrogin, K. E., Levine, D., Feller, D., and McCarron, D. A., Dietary calcium modulates blood pressure through α_1-adrenergic receptors, *Am. J. Physiol.,* 264, F234, 1993.
47. Hellstrom, J., Brike, G., and Edvall, C. A., Hypertension in hyperparathyroidism, *Br. J. Urol.,* 30, 13, 1958.
48. Henrich, W. L., Hunt, J. M., and Nixon, J. V., Increased ionized calcium and left ventricular contractility during hemodialysis, *N. Engl. J. Med.,* 310, 19, 1984.
49. Henry, H. J., Morris, C. D., and McCarron, D. A., Discordance of hypertensives' dietary Ca^{2+} intake and urinary Ca^{2+} excretion, *Kidney Int.,* 25(Abstr.), 201, 1984.
50. Holden, R. A., Ostfeld, A. M., Freeman, D. H. Jr., Hellenbrand, K. G., and D'Atri, D. A., Dietary salt intake and blood pressure, *JAMA,* 250, 365, 1983.
51. Hurwitz, L., Von Hagen, S., and Joiner, P. D., Acetylcholine and calcium on membrane permeability and contraction of intestinal smooth muscle, *J. Gen. Physiol.,* 50, 1157, 1967.

52. Jiang, M. T., Moffat, M. P., and Narayanan, N., Age-related alterations in the phosphory-
    lation of sarcoplasmic reticulum and myofibrillar proteins and diminished contractile
    response to isoproterenol in intact rat ventricle, *Circ. Res.,* 72, 102, 1993.
53. Joffres, M. R., Reed, D. M., and Yano, K., Relationship of magnesium intake and other
    dietary factors to blood pressure: the Honolulu Study, *Am. J. Clin. Nutr.,* 45, 469, 1987.
54. Johnson, N. E., Smith, E. L., and Freudenheim, J. L., Effects on blood pressure of calcium
    supplementation of women, *Am. J. Clin. Nutr.,* 42, 12, 1985.
55. Jones, A. W., Altered ion transport in large and small arteries from spontaneously
    hypertensive rats and the influence of calcium, *Circ. Res.,* 34, 35 Suppl. I, I-117, 1974.
56. Kannel, W. B., Nutritional contributors to cardiovascular disease in the elderly, *J. Am.
    Geriatr. Soc.,* 34, 27, 1986.
57. Kaplan, N. M. and Meese, R. B., The calcium deficiency hypothesis of hypertension: a
    critique, *Ann. Intern. Med.,* 105, 947, 1986.
58. Kristal-Boneh, E. and Green, M. S., Dietary calcium and blood pressure — a critical review
    of the literature, *Public Health Rev.,* 18(4), 267, 1990.
59. Lakatta, E. G., Do hypertension and aging have a similar effect on the myocardium?
    Circulation, 75 Suppl. I, I-69, 1987.
60. Lang, R. M., Fellner, S. K., Neumann, A., Bushinsky, D. A., and Borow, K. M., Left
    ventricular contractility varies directly with blood ionized calcium, *Ann. Intern. Med.,* 108,
    524, 1988.
61. Leug, M. C., Hypertension and primary hyperparathyroidism: a five year case review,
    South Med. J., 75, 1371, 1982.
62. Limas, C. J. and Cohn, J. N., Defective calcium transport by cardiac sarcoplasmic reticu-
    lum in spontaneously hypertensive rats, *Circ. Res.,* 40, I62, 1977.
63. Lompre, A. M., Lambert, F., Lakatta, E. G., and Schwartz, K., Expression of sarcoplasmic
    reticulum Ca^{2+}-ATPase and calsequestrin genes in rat heart during ontogenic development
    and aging, *Circ. Res.,* 69, 1380, 1991.
64. Luft, F. C., Putative mechanism of blood pressure reduction induced by increases in dietary
    calcium intake, *Am. J. Hypretens.,* 3, 156S, 1990.
65. McCarron, D. A., Low serum concentrations of ionized calcium in patients with hyperten-
    sion, *N. Engl. J. Med.,* 307, 226, 1982.
66. McCarron, D. A., Blood pressure and calcium balance in the Wistan-Kyoto rat, *Life
    Science,* 30(7, 8), 683, 1982.
67. McCarron, D. A., Calcium, magnesium and phosphorus balance in human and experimen-
    tal hypertension, *Hypertension,* 4 Suppl. III, III-27, 1982.
68. McCarron, D. A., Calcium and magnesium nutrition in human hypertension, *Ann. Intern.
    Med.,* 98(2), 800, 1983.
69. McCarron, D. A. and Morris, C. D., Dietary calcium in human hypertension, *Science,* 217,
    267, 1982.
70. McCarron, D. A. and Morris, C. D., Blood pressure response to oral calcium in persons
    with mild to moderate hypertension, *Ann. Intern. Med.,* 103(6: 1), 825, 1985.
71. McCarron, D. A. and Morris, C. D., The calcium deficiency hypothesis of hypertension,
    Ann. Intern. Med., 107, 919, 1987.
72. McCarron, D. A., Morris, C. D., Henry, H. J., and Stanton, J. L., Blood pressure and
    nutrient intake in the United States, *Science,* 224, 1392, 1984.
73. McCarron, D. A., Yung, N. N., Ugoretz, B. A., and Krutzik, S., Disturbances of calcium
    metabolism in the spontaneously hypertensive rat, *Hypertension,* 3 Suppl. I, I-162, 1981.
74. Mikami, H., Ogihara, T., and Tabuchi, Y., Blood pressure response to dietary calcium
    intervention in humans, *Am. J. Hypretens.,* 3(8: 2), 147S, 1990.
75. Morgan, K. G. and Suematsu, E., Effects of calcium on vascular smooth muscle tone, *Am.
    J. Hypertens.,* 3, 291S, 1990.
76. Neri, L. C. and Johansen, H. L., Water hardness and cardiovascular mortality, *Ann. N.Y.
    Acad. Sci.,* 304, 203, 1978.

77. Olivetti, G., Melissari, M., Capasso, J. M., and Anversa, P., Cardiomyopathy of aging human heart. Myocyte loss and reactive cellular hypertrophy, *Circ. Res.,* 68, 1560, 1991.
78. Pang, P. K., Benishin, C. G., and Lewanczuk, R. Z., Parathyroid hypertensive factor, a circulating factor in animal and human hypertension, *Am. J. Hypertens.,* 4, 472, 1991.
79. Parrott-Garcia, M. and McCarron, D. A., Calcium and hypertension, *Nutr. Rev.,* 42(6), 205, 1984.
80. Pawlowski, J., Physiology of vascular smooth muscle: clinical aspects of channel antagonists and direct acting vasodilating agents, in *Heart Failure: Basic Science and Clinical Aspects,* Gwathmey, J. K., Briggs, G. M., and Allen, P. D., Eds., Marcel Dekker, New York, 1993, 167.
81. Pesaturo, J. A. and Gwathmey, J. K., The role of mitochondria and sarcoplasmic reticulum calcium handling upon reoxygenation of hypoxic myocardium, *Circ. Res.,* 66, 696, 1990.
82. Popovtzer, M. M., Subryan, V. L., Alfrey, A. C., Reeve, E. B., and Schrier, R. W., The acute effect of chlorothiazide on serum-ionized calcium: evidence for a parathyroid hormone-dependent mechanism, *J. Clin. Invest.,* 55, 1295, 1975.
83. Postnov, Y. V. and Orlov, S. N., Evidence of altered calcium accumulation and calcium binding by the membranes of adipocytes in spontaneously hypertensive rats, *Pflügers. Arch.,* 385, 85, 1980.
84. Postnov, Y. V., Orlov, S. N., and Pokudin, N. I., Decrease in calcium binding by the red blood cell membrane in spontaneously hypertensive rats and in essential hypertension, *Pflugers. Arch.,* 379, 191, 1979.
85. Rasmussen, H., Cellular calcium metabolism, *Ann. Intern. Med.,* 98(2), 809, 1983.
86. Rasmussen, R. P., Minobe, W., and Bristow, M. R., Calcium antagonist binding sites in failing and nonfailing human ventricular myocardium, *Biochem. Pharmacol.,* 39, 691, 1990.
87. Reed, D., McGee, D., Yano, K., and Hankin, Diet, blood pressure, and multicollinearity, *Hypertension,* 7, 405, 1985.
88. Resnick, L. M., Cellular calcium and magnesium metabolism in the pathophysiology and treatment of hypertension and related metabolic disorders, *Am. J. Med.,* 93 Suppl. 2A, 2A-11S, 1992.
89. Rothstein, A., Membrane phenomena, *Ann. Rev. Physiol.,* 30, 15, 1968.
90. Saito, K., Sano, H., Furuta, Y., Yamonishi, J., Omatsu, T., Ito, Y., and Fukujaki, H., Calcium supplementation in salt-dependent hypertension, *Contrib. Nephrol.,* 90, 25, 1991.
91. Schmidlin, O., Garcia, J., and Schwartz, J. B., The effects of aging on the electrophysiologic responses to verapamil in isolated perfused rat hearts, *J. Pharmacol. Exp. Ther.,* 258, 130, 1991.
92. Schwinger, R. H. G., Böhm, M., Uhlmann, R., Schmidt, U., Überfuhr, P., Kreuzer, E., Reichart, B., and Erdmann, E., Magnesium restores the altered force-frequency relationship in failing human myocardium, *Am. Heart. J.,* 126, 1018, 1993.
93. Scrogin, E. K., Hatton, C., and McCarron, D. A., The interactive effects of dietary sodium chloride and calcium on cardiovascular stress responses, *Am. J. Physiol.,* 261, R945, 1991.
94. Shah, S., Khatri, I., and Freis, E. D., Mechanism of antihypertensives effect of thiazide diuretics, *Am. Heart. J.,* 95, 611, 1978.
95. Sharma, R. V. and Bhalla, R. C., Calcium and abnormal reactivity of vascular smooth muscle in hypertension, *Cell Calcium,* 9, 267, 1988.
96. Sowers, J. R., Zemel, M. B., and Standley, P. R., Calcium metabolism and dietary calcium in salt sensitive hypertension, *Am. J. Hypertens.,* 4(6), 557, 1991.
97. Stern, M. D., Capogrossi, M. C., and Lakatta, E. G., Spontaneous calcium release from the sarcoplasmic reticulum in myocardial cells: mechanisms and consequences, *Cell Calcium,* 9, 247, 1988.
98. Su, N. and Narayanan, N., Enhanced chronotropic and inotropic responses of rat myocardium to cholinergic stimulus with aging, *Can. J. Physiol. Pharmacol.,* 70, 1618, 1992.
99. Suki, W. N., Effects of diuretics on calcium metabolism, *Mineral. Electrolyte. Metab.,* 2, 125, 1979.

100. Stanton, J. L., Braitman, L. E., Riley, A. M., Khoo, C. S., and Smith, J. L., Demographic, dietary, life style, and anthropometric correlates of blood pressure, *Hypertension,* 4 Suppl. III, III-135, 1982.

101. Stitt, F. W., Clayton, D. G., Crawford, M. D., and Morris, J. N., Clinical and biochemical indicators of cardiovascular disease among men living in hard and soft water areas, *Lancet,* 1(795), 122, 1973,

102. Takahashi, T., Allen, P. D., Lacro, R. V., Marks, A. R., Dennis, A. R., Schoen, F. J., Grossman, W., and Marsh, J. D., Izumo, S., Expression of dihydropyridine receptor (Ca^{2+} channel) and calsequestrin genes in the myocardium of patients with end-stage heart failure, *J. Clin. Invest.,* 90, 927, 1992.

103. Tamura, H., Influence of a high calcium diet on the development of hypertension in the spontaneously hypertensive rat, *Jpn. J. Nephrol.,* 29, 107, 1987.

104. Tobian, L. and Chesley, G., Calcium content of arteriolar wall in normotensive and hypertensive rats, *Proc. Soc. Exp. Biol. Med.,* 121, 340, 1966.

105. Webb, R. C. and Bhalla, R. C., Altered calcium sequestration by subcellular fractions of vascular smooth muscle from spontaneously hypertensive rats, *J. Mol. Cell. Cardiol.,* 8, 651, 1976.

106. Webb, R. C. and Bohr, D. F., Mechanism of membrane stabilization by calcium in vascular smooth muscle, *Am. J. Physiol.,* 235, C227, 1978.

107. Wei, J. Y., Spurgeon, H. A., and Lakatta, E. G., Excitation-contraction in rat myocardium: alterations with aging, *Am. J. Physiol.,* 246, H784, 1984.

108. Wier, W. G., Excitation-contraction coupling in mammalian ventricle, in *Heart Failure: Basic Science and Clinical Aspects,* Gwathmey, J. K., Briggs, G. M., and Allen, P. D., Eds., Marcel Dekker, New York, 1993, 11.

109. Word, R. A. and Stull, J. T., Cellular regulation of smooth muscle contraction, in *Heart Failure: Basic Science and Clinical Aspects,* Gwathmey, J. K., Briggs, G. M., and Allen, P. D., Eds., Marcel Dekker, New York, 1993, 145.

110. Wright, G. L., Toraason, M. A., Barbe, J. S., and Crouse, W., The concentrations of ionic and total calcium in plasma of the spontaneously hypertensive rat, *Can. J. Physiol. Pharmacol.,* 58, 1494, 1980.

Chatper 7

VITAMIN E: DO WE NEED IT?

Lloyd A. Witting

CONTENTS

0-8493-7849-4/95/$0.00+$.50
© 1995 by CRC Press Inc.

I. INTRODUCTION

The above title should immediately indicate that this review has nothing to do with recommended daily allowances, deficiency signs, or normal nutrition. Rather, the question relates to the justification, or lack thereof, for recommendations for intakes of vitamin E, 400–800 IU/day, that cannot be achieved by diet and require pill popping supplementation. This should not be a surprise in an era where the Food and Nutrition Board[138] considers the scrapping of the Recommended Dietary Allowance in favor of a Safe Intake Range that is determined by toxicity.

With the control of infectious disease, improved sanitation and hygiene, and adequate nutrition there is relatively little mortality between infancy and what was once old age. Great improvements in average survival have focused attention on the problem that more people live longer, but no one lives longer. There comes a time when the incidence of "everything and anything" rises so rapidly with increasing age that a limit to maximum life span is encountered. While history chronicles individuals living to 95 to100 years of age in bygone eras, it is only within recent times that average survival has increased to the point where deteriorative processes are the major causes of death.

Mortality is due, at least in part, to the difficulties inherent in living in an oxygen containing environment. Utilization of oxygen involves free radical formation and aerobic life forms have developed elaborate, multilayered defense systems to protect against the occurrence of adventitious, free radical initiated tissue damage. This system is adequate to permit life, but not to sustain life indefinitely. Leakage of free radicals results in cumulative damage and oxidative stress that may overload the system. There has been a spectacular outpouring of interest in this area, and system failures have been proposed as the source of numerous problems including coronary heart disease, cancer, arthritis, cataracts, and even the generalized phenomenon of aging.[47,57,61,68,72,73,113,166,179,193-195,206,223,225,231,237,243,255,269]

Reactive oxygen species are produced enzymatically in the course of normal metabolism. Other enzyme systems such as superoxide dismutase, catalase, and glutathione peroxidase, are present to remove free radicals. Near the bottom of the multilayered defense system, vitamin E appears to act nonenzymatically, and rather nonspecifically, as a terminal stopgap responding to all manner of prior system lapses and failures resulting in free radical leakage into the lipid phase. Since free radicals originate in the aqueous phase, free radical leakage must originate in the aqueous phase. Depending on circumstances, however, oxidative damage might be expressed principally in the aqueous phase, the lipid phase, or to some degree in both.

Any lesion that is conjectured to be in any way related to free radical initiated tissue damage is, therefore, a candidate for vitamin E supplementation. Augmentation of the defense system at the lipid level is easily achieved with daily supplements of 400 to 800 IU of vitamin E. If any significant or measurable portion of the observed tissue damage or disease is due directly or indirectly to lipid peroxidation, there may be evidence of some beneficial or protective action. Observation of a beneficial effect may provide no constructive information as to the ultimate source or basic cause of the problem, other than that it may indeed be related in whole or part to free radical leakage. Approaching a problem from this perspective takes research into some rather nebulous areas and at times results in some rather fuzzy conclusions.

Since the multilayered defense system permits aerobic life at the "usual" level of free radicals, some leakage is "tolerable". For each specific lesion, research is needed to determine if a specific identifiable oxidative stress is the cause or if the imbalance between free radical production and control is related to some type of cumulative damage. Vitamin E and other components of the defense system have to some extent been used as tools to investigate and categorize lesions. Definitive treatment of the lesion requires knowledge of the cause of the lesion. In some instances, however, the beneficial effects in certain clinically important situations have been reported to be sufficient to consider the use of supplemental vitamin E for protective purposes. This in turn has led to interest in the possible antioxidant activity of certain drugs and in the design of drugs related structurally to vitamin E.

To put this topic in perspective, it is necessary to review first the multilayered defense system in terms of leakage rates and associated sequalae. Next, it is desirable to consider the biochemistry and nutrition of vitamin E in terms of the safety at high dosage levels, and to compare and contrast the mode of action with synthetic lipid antioxidants. The results of studies utilizing vitamin E supplements will then be examined. Studies in this area must frequently be evaluated in terms of "shotgun pattern". Results are not of the "all or none" type and it is usually important to note experiences with other components of the multilayered defense system.

II. THE MULTILAYERED DEFENSE SYSTEM PROTECTING AGAINST FREE RADICAL INITIATED TISSUE DAMAGE

A. IN THE BEGINNING — WITH EVOLUTION THERE CAME PROBLEMS

In complex systems, system integrity and continued function is typically ensured by inclusion of redundant safeguards. Biological systems are complex systems.

The earliest life forms were anaerobes in an anaerobic environment. With the advent of photosynthetic organisms, in the form of blue-green algae, free oxygen became available. The challenge of using atmospheric oxygen in metabolic processes, such as aerobic metabolism, was fraught with many dangers but offered the reward of increased energy yield from foodstuffs. Examination of modern organisms from bacteria to man reveals the presence of a rather standard armamentarium of multilayered defenses against adventitious damage by oxygen. To organisms lacking all of these defenses, such as strict anaerobes, oxygen is lethal.[171]

B. REGULATION OF FREE RADICALS

The earth's atmosphere contains approximately 20% oxygen. Our environment contains many flammable and combustible materials and yet the world around us does not spring spontaneously into flame. A mixture of hydrogen and oxygen is stable but the slightest spark results in an explosion. This is another way of saying that for reasons related to the triplet ground state of molecular oxygen, electron spins, and the conservation of angular momentum, such oxidations are free radical initiated.[147,221] Without the production of the initial free radical there is no reaction.

The reaction

$$2H_2 + O_2 \rightarrow 2H_2O \qquad\qquad 1.$$

proceeds via 4 electron transfers to produce the hydroperoxyl radical, $HO_2\cdot$, (or its conjugate base the superoxide anion, O_2^-), hydrogen peroxide, H_2O_2, the hydroxyl radical, $HO\cdot$, and water. The various reactive oxygen species discussed here are collectively referred to as free radicals. Historical usage and the desire to avoid a more cumbersome description results in inclusion of hydrogen peroxide.

In living organisms various enzymes produce the hydroperoxyl radical or hydrogen peroxide in the course of normal metabolic reactions.[93]

$$XH + O_2 \rightarrow X\cdot + HO_2\cdot \qquad\qquad 2.$$

$$XH_2 + O_2 \rightarrow X\cdot + H_2O_2 \qquad\qquad 3.$$

The respiratory chain transports electrons efficiently with little leakage of free radicals. If leakage does occur, however, enzymes are present to remove these free radicals.

Superoxide anions are removed by superoxide dismutase, (SOD).[93-95]

$$2O_2^- + 2H^+ \rightarrow H_2O_2 + O_2 \qquad\qquad 4.$$

and hydrogen peroxide is removed by glutathione peroxidase, (Gpx) or catalase.

$$H_2O_2 + 2GSH \rightarrow GSSG + 2H_2O \qquad\qquad 5.$$

In higher organisms, catalase may not be a critical enzyme in this system since, as reviewed by Aebi and Wyss,[2] humans with a genetic absence of catalase appear to lead a normal life. A comparison of enzyme kinetics suggests that a selenium-dependent Gpx is better suited to the scavenging of low concentrations of hydrogen peroxide associated with free radical leakage.[168] Ebselen (PZ 51), 2-phenyl-1,2-benzoiso-selenazol_3(2H)-one, a small molecule with antiinflammatory action in the lungs and other tissues, has been described as having glutathione peroxidase activity and antioxidant activity.[185,200] Many tissues also contain a nonselenium-dependent glutathione peroxidase. The relative proportions of the glutathione peroxidases and their total concentration differ markedly from tissue to tissue and species to species.[148]

It was the discovery of SOD by McCord and Fridovich[172] in 1969 that permitted the formulation of the comprehensive scheme for control of free radical initiated tissue damage.

For organisms lacking these protective enzymes, oxygen is lethal.[171] At the evolutionary edge are organisms with partial defenses, and oxygen is merely bacteriostatic rather than lethal.[39,116] Next come organisms such as *E. coli* that can grow either anaerobically or aerobically.[155] In the anaerobic cells an iron dependent SOD and a peroxidase with both hydroperoxidase and catalase activity provide standby protection. Exposure to oxygen induces high levels of a manganese-dependent SOD and a catalase. The presence of multiple forms of these enzymes is the rule rather than the exception. Maize has been reported to contain three catalases and five SODs.[226]

If these free radicals are not efficiently removed they may interact via a Fenton-type reaction catalyzed by chelated iron [27,258] to produce the extremely reactive hydroxyl radical HO^-.

$$Fe^{3+} + O_2^- \rightarrow Fe^{2+} + O_2 \qquad\qquad 6.$$

$$Fe^{2+} + H_2O_2 \rightarrow Fe^{3+} + HO^- + HO^- \qquad\qquad 7.$$

While superoxide is a relatively weak oxidant in aqueous solution,[224] the hydroxyl radical oxidizes essentially everything and anything. Superoxide inhibits catalase,[144] adversely affects many peroxidases,[180] and selectively damages certain metallo-protein enzymes,[98,99,156] but is not generally considered to be, per se, the source of dramatic, major oxidative damage. Suzuki and Ford,[252] however, have suggested that the hydroxyl radical is so reactive that most hits are wasted. On the basis of a mathematical model they suggest that it is far easier to recover after a 5% loss of every enzyme activity than after a 95% loss of a vital enzyme activity. Proteins are typically present in multiple copies and turn over relatively rapidly. It has been suggested[102] that in some systems up to 86% of free radicals are consumed via nonspecific protein damage.

The major identifiable free radical initiated tissue damage at the aqueous level tends to be oxidative damage to DNA, the master blueprint for life. In the absence of transition metal ions, neither superoxide nor hydrogen peroxide, (*in vitro* incubation) cause oxidative damage and strand breakage in DNA. The observed pattern of damage clearly points to the hydroxyl radical as the culprit.[6,7,219] This is predominantly a direct reaction, but can include reaction of DNA with secondary products of hydroxyl radical initiated lipid peroxidation, such as malondialdehyde or 4-hydroxy-2-nonenal.[110]

C. FREE RADICALS AND MEMBRANE LIPIDS

Having considered the production and destruction of free radicals, it is now appropriate to consider the leakage of free radicals into the lipid environment and the initiation of lipid peroxidation. The cell is a predominantly aqueous environment in which materials are made, synthesized, or destroyed, catabolized, and energy is produced or utilized. Coexistence of such diverse activities is possible, in part, because of the segregation and compartmentalization of specific activities within regions, subcellular organelles, bounded by lipid membranes. Lipid membranes may be described as boundary walls composed largely of phospholipids arranged in bilayers with the polar hydrophilic head groups oriented outwards and the hydrophobic fatty acid chains oriented inwards. The hydrophobic inner region acts as a barrier to the free movement of hydrophilic substances through the membrane. An attack upon membrane integrity has the potential to result in tissues damage. Damage to the membranes surrounding certain organelles, such as the lysosomes, which contain a wide variety of catabolic enzymes, can be particularly devastating.

Leakage of enzymatically produced free radicals into the lipid environment may adventitiously initiate lipid oxidation via a peroxidative reaction.

$$RH \xrightarrow{k_1} R^{\cdot} \qquad\qquad 8.$$

$$R^{\cdot} + O_2 \xrightarrow{k_2} RO_2^{\cdot} \qquad\qquad 9.$$

$$RH + RO_2^{\cdot} \xrightarrow{k_3} ROOH + R^{\cdot} \qquad\qquad 10.$$

This reaction resembles a wild fire. Once initiated, the process proceeds via a cyclic chain reaction. In theory a single initiation could conceivably result in the peroxidation of all of the fatty acids in the system. It is at this point that free radical leakage becomes a free radical cascade.

If lipid peroxidation is adventitiously initiated, tissue protection is afforded by several enzymes. Formation of peroxidized phospholipid bound fatty acids activates phospholipase A_2 which preferentially excises the peroxidized fatty acid.[265] Lipid hydroperoxides, ROOH, are then destroyed by a glutathione peroxidase.[149]

$$ROOH + 2GSH \rightarrow ROH + GSSG + H_2O \qquad 11.$$

Presumably the action of phospholipase A_2 makes the substrate more readily available to the enzyme in the aqueous phase. This problem of interaction of components of the hydrophobic lipid phase with components of the hydrophilic aqueous phase arises at other stages of the multilayered defense system as will be seen later. Schuckett et al.,[230] however, have described a distinct, selenium-dependent phospholipid hydroperoxide glutathione peroxidase associated with the membrane and reacting with substrate in the membrane. The dietary supply of sulfur amino acids has the potential to affect this defense as does the adequacy of local reducing equivalents to regenerate glutathione. As noted previously, many tissues also contain both a selenium-dependent and a nonselenium-dependent Gpx.[148]

If the rate of lipid peroxide production ever exceeds the rate of enzymatic hydroperoxide destruction, and if hydroperoxides accumulate, the process has the potential to become autocatalytic, to branch, and to expand exponentially via the reaction

$$2ROOH \rightarrow RO_2^{\cdot} + RO^{\cdot} + H_2O \qquad 12.$$

D. COMPETITIVE INHIBITION OF LIPID PEROXIDATION

The systems described above constitute the major enzymatic defenses against lipid peroxidation that are present in man and various animal species. If an exogenous source of one or another of a variety of lipid antioxidants is available, such a compound, (i.e., vitamin E) may act nonenzymatically in tissues to reduce the yield of lipid hydroperoxides per free radical initiation.

$$RO_2^{\cdot} + AH \xrightarrow{\ k_4\ } ROOH + A^{\cdot} \qquad 13.$$

A lipid antioxidant, AH, competes with phospholipid fatty acids, RH, for reaction with the lipid peroxy free radical, $RO_2^{\cdot}$. The antioxidant free radical, $A^{\cdot}$, leaves the system by dimerization or other reaction and thus terminates the cyclic chain reaction.[24,49]

E. EFFICIENCY CONSIDERATIONS IN THE AQUEOUS PHASE

Imlay and Fridovich[124] cite the electron transport chain in *E. coli* as being particularly "tight". However, with 6.2×10^6 molecules of oxygen consumed per cell per second, leakage of $3O_2^-/10^4$ electrons conducted, amounts to $1 \cdot 6$ $\times 10^7$ loose free radicals per cell per day. They then estimate that SOD acts to reduce this to a steady state level of 2×10^{-10} M.

In an interesting exercise Cutler[52] has shown that when tissue levels of SOD, corrected for specific metabolic rate, were plotted against the maximum life span potential for a variety of mammals, a rather good direct correlation was apparent. Does this mean that maximum life span potential is directly limited by tissue levels of SOD?

Another measure of free radical leakage is the level of oxidative damage to DNA.[219] Oxidized bases are excised and appear in the urine. Approximately 20 such compounds, including 8-hydroxydeoxyguanosine, thymine glycol, and 5-hydroxymethyluracil, have been reported.[64] The level of these 3 compounds in normal human urine is approximately 100 nmoles/day, leading to an estimate of 10^4 oxidative "hits" to DNA per cell per day.[210]

In the rat, oxidative damage to DNA has been described in terms of a steady-state level of 10^6 damaged nucleic acid residues per cell[87,210] with 10^5 new residues being damaged per day.[40,87] While the repair rate almost equals the damage rate, Fraga et al.[87] estimated that in rat kidney there is a net accumulation of 80 8-hydroxydeoxyguanosine residues per cell per day. Oxidized moieties such as 8-hydroxyguanosine and 8-hydroxyadenosine, while still present in intact DNA, may lead to mutations by inducing misreading of the base. Low levels of DNA damage may be efficiently repaired with a minimum of error.[29] This minimal error rate, however, may be a major cause of cancer and other deteriorative processes.

Some indication of the level of DNA damage occuring secondary to lipid peroxidation was recently reported by Chaudhary et al.[43a] They noted that human liver contained 5400 malondialdehyde modified deoxyguanosine residues per cell or 9 adducts per 10^7 bases.

In an SOD deficient mutant of *E. coli* there was, compared to the control, a 40-fold increase in the spontaneous mutation rate in air, and this was increased tenfold on exposure to oxygen.[263] With a mutant overexpressing the scavenging enzymes spontaneous mutagenesis was markedly suppressed.[104] This would suggest that all or some portion of spontaneous mutagenesis is the result of the "normal" level of free radical leakage.

Free radical attack may also result in DNA strand breakage. Emerit[74] has noted that the known human syndromes associated with chromosomal breakage, ataxia telangiectasia, Bloom's Syndrome, and Fanconi's Anemia, are marked by a high incidence of cancer at an early age and a shortened life span.

F. EFFICIENCY CONSIDERATIONS IN THE LIPID PHASE
1. Tissue Lipid Polyunsaturated Fatty Acid Content

Relative susceptibility of a given membrane to peroxidative damage is determined by the fatty acid composition of the component fatty acids. The rate, k_2, of reaction 9 is independent of fatty acid structure, but the rate, k_3, of reaction 10, the rate limiting propagation reaction, is strongly dependent

TABLE 1
Effect of the Number of Double Bonds in a Fatty Acid on the Relative Susceptibility to Peroxidation and Relative Tocopherol Requirement Generated

Number of Double Bonds	Relative Peroxidation Rate	Tocopheol Requirement
1	0.025	0.3
2	1	2
3	2	3
4	4	4
5	6	5
6	8	6

Adapted from Witting, L. A. and Horwitt, M. K., *J. Nutr.*, 82, 19, 1964.

on fatty acid structure.[121,159] As the number of double bonds in $CH_3(CH_2)_a$ $(CH=CHCH_2)_x(CH2)_bCO2-$ increases from 1 to 6, the relative values of k_3 increase[281] according to the series 0.025, 1, 2, 4, 6, 8 (Table 1). The potential for hydroperoxide accumulation increases with increasing membrane phospholipid fatty acid unsaturation.

The efficacy of a lipid antioxidant is determined by the relative magnitudes of the rate constants k_3 and k_4 for the competing propagation reaction, 10, and the termination reaction, 13. This relationship determines the average yield or cycle length of the chain reaction. Since the magnitude of k_4 is related to antioxidant structure and k_3 is related to the degree of fatty acid unsaturation, it follows that the efficacy of any given antioxidant decreases as fatty acid unsaturation increases. A nutritional study[281] in the rat suggested that comparable levels of termination (comparable average cycle chain lengths), were obtained with relative antioxidant levels corresponding to the series 0.3, 2, 3, 4, 5, 6 as the number of double bonds in the fatty acid was increased from 1 to 6, respectively (Table 1). One docosahexaenoic acid would, for instance, generate three times the antioxidant requirement of one octadecadienoic acid.

Average cycle chain lengths, molecules of lipid hydroperoxide formed per molecule of antioxidant consumed, tend to be difficult to determine. An *in vitro* study[282] estimated cycle chain length of approximately 83, 137, and 365 at relatively optimal levels of alpha-tocopherol in ethyl linoleate, linolenate, and arachidonate, respectively. At lower antioxidant concentrations the corresponding values exceeded 1000 and 1700 for ethyl linolenate and arachidonate, respectively. Using a liposome model system, a cyclic chain length of 10 to 100 was found for less highly unsaturated lipids.

Clearly, a lipid antioxidant does not prevent lipid autoxidation and lipid autoxidation can occur in the presence of a lipid antioxidant. Therefore, the subcellular architecture and separation of incompatible processes is under continuous attack. Tissue lipid polyunsaturated fatty acid content may also influence damage in the aqueous phase. It was reported[111] that oxidative damage to DNA in the rat mammary gland was directly proportional to the degree of unsaturation of the dietary fat. Antioxidant supplementation decreased the level of damage at each degree of unsaturation, but did not otherwise change the relationship.

2. Free Radical Leakage

Total body lipid peroxidation may possibly be estimated from exhaled ethane and pentane. These hydrocarbons are byproducts of the peroxidation of (n − 3) and (n − 6) polyunsaturated fatty acids, respectively. Although the quantity of (n − 6) PUFA in the body is much greater than that of (n − 3) PUFA, the latter are much more susceptible to peroxidation. Tappel and Dillard[254] reported values of 4 to 5 and 0.2 to 0.4 pmoles/kg/min for exhaled ethane and pentane, respectively. These levels are reduced by vitamin E supplementation. Others[141] have reported values for pentane exhalation that are an order of magnitude higher in controls and two orders of magnitude higher in cigarette smokers. Higher values have also been reported[141] in alcoholic and cholestatic liver disease, pulmonary disease, inflammatory bowel disease, autoimmune disease, neurologic disease, and after exercise. The yield of hydrocarbons has been estimated as little as 0.2 mM/M lipid peroxidized.[254]

These quantities of ethane and pentane are similar in order of magnitude, 400 to 500 and 20 to 40 nmoles/day, respectively, to the quantities of individual oxidatively damaged products of DNA excreted daily in the urine. Consideration of the low yield of hydrocarbons, however, would result in an estimate of 0.1 to 2.0 × 10^7 molecules of lipid peroxidized per cell per day, depending on whether the estimate was based on pentane or ethane. This is several orders of magnitude greater than the number of free radical hits on DNA per cell per day. However, since lipid peroxidation proceeds via a cyclic chain reaction, multiple peroxidized fatty acids arise per initiation and may account for the differences in estimates of hits on DNA and lipids. On the other hand, the difference may relate to the level of hits in the aqueous phase not producing identifiable or relevant damage.

In a study[283] of a vitamin E deficiency sign, nutritional muscular dystrophy, in the rat it was estimated that the onset of creatinuria occurred after the peroxidation of 0.116 to 0.133 μg of polyunsaturated fatty acids per gram of muscle or about 4 × 10^7 molecules of fatty acid per cell. Obviously these estimates are only estimates. The suggestion is interesting however, in that pathological tissue, damage could be noted when the cumulative lipid peroxidation amounted to a few times the "normal" amount estimated to occur daily.

G. NUTRITIONAL INPUTS

Enzyme defenses against free radical initiated tissue damage are surprisingly dependent on nutritional status. The most prevalent SOD in higher organisms is a cuprozinc enzyme. A copper deficiency[275] has been shown to influence tissue levels of this enzyme. A mild zinc deficiency[63] enhances the free radical initiated liver damage associated with carbon tetrachloride intoxication. Zinc supplementation or combined zinc and copper supplementation may be undesirable since at only three to ten times the requirement, zinc reduces copper absorption. Selenium restriction[45] results in lowered tissue levels of the selenium-dependent Gpx and the appearance of deficiency signs in experimental animals. Selenium supplementation is limited by the toxicity of this trace element at only ten times the requirement. Protective action is also affected by the dietary availability of sulfur amino acids and tissue reducing capacity to regenerate glutathione.

This layer of the multilayered defense system is also dependent on nutritional status with regard to sulfur amino acids and the capacity of the tissue to regenerate glutathione. In addition, the susceptibility of tissue lipids to peroxidation is determined by the dietary input of polyunsaturated fatty acids. There is a requirement for a dietary input of a lipid antioxidant, vitamin E, and the magnitude of this requirement is determined by the polyunsaturated fatty acid content of the tissue phospholipids.

H. THE INTEGRATED MULTILAYERED DEFENSE SYSTEM

While the overall system functions adequately to permit life, it is obviously leaky and less than totally effective. The redundancy of the system, multiple layers of defense with a single goal — containment of free radicals — creates a research nightmare. It is apparent that a weakness at a primary defense level might overload an otherwise adequate secondary defense level and result in tissue damage. Supplementation at the overloaded defense level or even at some intermediate defense level might prevent tissue damage without leading to an awareness of or addressing the primary weakness. Efforts to sort out cause and effect and input–outcome relationships without an understanding of the total system were the sources of confusion and controversy in the 1960s. In the 1980s and 1990s, system redundancy became a potential blessing. A shotgun approach to augmentation, a shot of "this and that" fired speculatively into the system may very well have a beneficial effect. With the above background it is now possible to consider the subject of vitamin E.

III. BIOCHEMISTRY AND NUTRITION OF VITAMIN E

A. VITAMIN E — A VITAMIN?

In 1920 it was noted[167] that when a ration meeting all of the then known dietary requirements was fed to rats, conception occurred normally, but the fetuses died *in utero* and were reabsorbed. Subsequently Evans and Bishop[78] described a material from plant tissues which prevented resorption gestation after gestation and termed it vitamin E. It is now known that a related series of eight compounds, tocopherols and tocotrienols, are produced via the shikimic acid pathway. The compound with the highest biological activity in this assay is *d*-alpha-tocopherol, 2,5,7,8-tetramethyl-2-(4′,8′,12′-trimethyltridecyl)-6-chromanol, or 5,7,8-trimethyltocol. Other less active compounds differ in the number of methyl groups on the chromane ring, β-tocopherol or 5,8-dimethyltocol, γ-tocopherol or 7,8-dimethyl tocol, and δ-tocopherol or 8-methyltocol, and in the occurrence of unsaturation at positions 3′,7′ and 11′ in the phytyl sidechain. A number of other deficiency signs are known in various species which are also responsive to supplementation with vitamin E.

Description of the tocopherols as a vitamin was consistent with the general trend of biochemistry and nutrition in the 1920s. Subsequently, however, some scientists attempted to define vitamins in terms that could not be reconciled with the properties of the tocopherols. It was argued that a vitamin functioned as the prosthetic group of an enzyme or at the very least functioned somehow in an enzymatic reaction. Furthermore, vitamins have rather stringent structural requirements for biological activity.

By 1937 the *in vitro* antioxidant properties of the tocopherols were recognized.[191] In 1939 Evans et al.[79] reported that many of the more than 100 compounds tested, having some structural similarity to vitamin E, were active in the resorption gestation assay. Dam et al.[54,55] reported in 1948 and 1951 that partial protection against the appearance of vitamin E deficiency signs could be attained with compounds structurally unrelated to vitamin E. By 1958 Draper et al.[67] had maintained rats for three generations on a vitamin E-deficient diet supplemented with the synthetic lipid antioxidant N,N′-diphenyl-para-phenylenediamine, DPPD. Other synthetic lipid antioxidants such as ethoxyquin, butylated hydroxyanisole, BHA, and butylated hydroxy toluene, BHT, have been shown to have vitamin E-like activity *in vivo* under certain circumstances and in certain species.

B. ABSORPTION, TRANSPORT, DISTRIBUTION, AND TURNOVER OF VITAMIN E

The relative biological activities of α-, β-, γ-, and δ-tocopherol and α- and β-tocotrienol have been stated as 1.00, 0.50 ,0.10, 0.03, 0.30, and 0.05, respectively.[33,153,161,186] This bears no relationship to the relative antioxidant activities observed *in vitro*. It is possible by dietary manipulations to obtain human erythrocytes containing graded levels of total tocopherols consisting of different proportions of alpha- and gamma-tocopherol.[284] Based on the peroxide hemolysis test, when present at the same tissue site, both vitamers exert similar protective activity. The observed differences in biological activity must, therefore, arise somewhere between the mouth and the tissues.

Using intestinal loops, differential absorption, $\alpha > \gamma > \beta >> \delta$, of the various tocopherols was noted.[203] After direct injection[46] into the blood stream the rate of disappearance was $\delta > \beta > \gamma > \alpha$. The basis for the differences in rates of clearance may arise from the existence of a tocopherol binding protein in the liver.[41] After intestinal absorption, the tocopherols are equally incorporated into chylomicrons. In the liver, discrimination occurs, presumably based on the presence of the binding protein in the hepatocytes, and alpha-tocopherol is preferentially incorporated into very low density lipoproteins (VLDL), and distributed to the tissues.[259,260] Excess vitamin E is rapidly excreted in the bile and appears in the feces[140] In an extremely rare genetic defect of vitamin E metabolism, a failure to incorporate alpha-tocopherol into VLDL has been reported.[241,261] This defect is associated with a neuromyopathy and a spinocerebellar degeneration.

Alpha-tocopherol is absorbed with lipids and any impairment of lipid absorption reduces tocopherol absorption. Tracer level quantities of alpha-tocopherol, 40 μg/day, are well absorbed, 50 to 80%, but absorption may drop to as little as 5% at higher intakes, 200 mg/day.[158] It has been suggested that tissue levels increase in proportion to the logarithm of the dose.[279] A tenfold increase in intake is needed to double the plasma level. Mason[164] found that tissue levels could be increased three- to fivefold at intakes of 10 to 10,000 times the minimum daily requirement. Only the liver appears to store tocopherol and this has been reported to be limited to the parenchymal cells.[20] Since tocopherol typically occurs within a biological membrane, there appear to be practical limits to the level of incorporation. *In vitro* tocopherol has frequently been noted to be an antioxidant at low concentrations and a prooxidant at high concentrations.

Alpha-tocopherol is distributed largely in membrane lipids, particularly those of the mitochondria, 60%, and the endoplasmic reticulum, 30%. Synthetic lipid antioxidants such as BHT and ethoxyquin, 60%, are found largely in the cytosol.[50]

Tissue depletion of alpha-tocopherol follows a biphasic curve.[115] Initial rapid depletion is followed by a stubborn retention of residual vitamin E. This is consistent with the general inability to produce a deficiency in adult animals or man. Such cases as are observed are normally associated with malabsorption of extremely prolonged duration or lengthy periods of total parenteral nutrition not providing a source of vitamin E.

C. TOXICITY

In an investigation of chronic toxicity and possible carcinogenicity, Wheldon et al.[274] fed rats 500, 1000, and 2000 mg/kg/day of alpha-tocopheryl acetate for 2 years with no increase in tumors. Hemorrhages were observed in male rats after 15 to 18 weeks, but were controlled by supplementation with vitamin K. In a study[1] of acute toxicity, excess vitamin E increased prothrombin time, thromboplastin times, and liver weight. Polymorphonuclear cells showed an enhanced phagocytic rate but decreased bactericidal activity.[178] The influence on blood clotting appears to arise through inhibition of vitamin K epoxide reductase.[136]

Studies in premature infants have yielded mixed results. A double blind study[205] of vitamin E in premature infants failed to document protection against retrolental fibroplasia and reported a significant increase in retinal hemorrhages. Vitamin E has been reported to increase and decrease periventricular hemorrhages in very low birth weight babies.[205,243a] Recent meta-analyses of 20 studies of retrolental fibroplasia and 6 studies of intraventricular hemorrhage claimed beneficial effects of vitamin E in both.[262] Problems have been reported with plasma levels >5 mg/dL, which are thought to inhibit macrophage activity and increase the incidence of necrotizing enterocolitis and sepsis.[131]

Compared to the other fat-soluble vitamins, vitamin E is essentially nontoxic. This is presumably related to the rapid decrease in absorption with increased intake and excretion of excess into the bile and thence to the feces. The existence of large numbers of faddists voluntarily taking huge supplements of vitamin E for years on end attests to the absence of major side effects. Bendich[14] and Bendich and Machlin[15,16] have extensively reviewed the literature on vitamin E supplementation. Numerous reports have described groups taking 200 to 2400 IU/day for years. In a Parkinson's disease pilot study,[80] a limited number of patients received 3000 mg vitamin E/day for periods of up to 7 years. In a long term study[199] of Parkinson's disease, 800 patients were started on a double blind protocol providing 2000 IU/day of vitamin E plus Deprenyl or placebo in 1987. The lack of change in various parameters has been documented for liver, kidney, and thyroid function, red and white blood cell counts, platelets, serum lipids, and blood clotting indices. Subjective complaints such as headache, gastrointestinal upsets, muscle weakness, and hypertension have also been discounted based on placebo comparisons. Herbert et al.[119] noted in preliminary information gathered on a large scale work-site study that 27% of the subjects were already taking a vitamin supplement including vitamin E.

D. RECYCLING OF VITAMIN E

Compared to the other free radicals mentioned herein, the tocopherol free radical is extremely stable.[35] McCay et al.[169] have described the production of this radical for use in electron paramagnetic resonance studies and maintained the material for several hours in a hydrophobic medium. The operation of the multilayered defense system would benefit greatly from the existence of a mechanism to regenerate the antioxidant from the free radical. Unfortunately, all of the reactants that might facilitate regeneration are present in the aqueous phase while alpha-tocopherol is in the hydrophobic lipid membrane. Various physical chemistry studies have suggested that the chromane ring is near the aqueous interface and thus might be positioned to react with both hydrophobic and hydrophilic substances.[71,204]

In 1961 Uri[264] suggested that a transient tocopherol semiquinone might be reduced by ascorbic acid, which could be regenerated by reaction with glutathione, which in turn could be regenerated by NADPH. In recent years this suggestion has resurfaced as a reaction of a chromanoxy free radical with ascorbic acid and glutathione. There is considerable, compelling evidence that the postulated reaction with ascorbic acid can be demonstrated *in vitro*.[132,187,196,197,232,233] Evidence has also been presented for an *in vitro* tie of the recycling process to glutathione and lipoic acid.[9]

An early nutritional study claimed chicks deficient in vitamin E benefited from ascorbic acid supplementation.[12] Subsequently, in the rat, vitamin C synthesis was found to be adversely affected by a vitamin E deficiency.[139] More numerous reports have indicated either no synergistic effect[152,184] between vitamin C and vitamin E or an exacerbation[44] of a vitamin E deficiency sign by vitamin C. The logical model for studies of the possible interactions of vitamin E and vitamin C requirements is the guinea pig. Using three dietary levels of vitamin C and two levels of vitamin E, Burton et al.[36] reported that ascorbate deficiency had no effect on the rate of tocopherol turnover or loss in the guinea pig. Regardless of the quality of the *in vitro* studies, for recycling to be generally accepted, there must be more convincing *in vivo* evidence.[251]

Even without a role in the recycling of vitamin E, ascorbate may have an important place in the multilayered defense system. Fraga et al.[88] restricted ascorbate intake (from 250 mg/day to 5 mg/day) in humans, and when the level in seminal fluid had decreased 50% the production of damaged DNA nucleic acid residues doubled.

E. VITAMIN E AND POLYUNSATURATED FATTY ACIDS

With the advent of gas chromatography in the late 1950s, it became possible to study the effect of dietary polyunsaturated fatty acid composition on tissue lipid fatty acid composition. By judicious selection of deficiency signs it was possible to study the vitamin E requirement at sites where a relatively simple dietary lipid-tissue lipid relationship prevailed.[284] In tocopherol-deficient chicks, the incidence of encephelomalacia increased from 0 to 100% as the level of dietary linoleate was increased from 0.7 to 9.6% of calories, and the levels of brain mitochondrial (n – 6) polyunsaturated fatty acids increased from 10 to 26%. Plots of incidence vs. percentage dietary linoleate or percentage mitochondrial (n – 6) polyunsaturated fatty acids suggested direct linear relationships.

An example[281] of a titration of a deficiency sign with graded levels of vitamin E was reported in a study of the onset of creatinuria as a sign of nutritional muscular dystrophy in the rat. The dietary fats used in this study were specially formulated. Each fat was of the same total unsaturation but differed in how this was provided — six parts monoenoic acid, or three parts dienoic acid plus three parts saturated fatty acid, or two parts trienoic acid plus four parts saturated fatty acid, or one part hexaenoic acid plus five parts saturated fatty acid. The delay in the onset of creatinuria provided by each dietary level of α-tocopherol was the same for each dietary fat except for the fat containing monoenoic fatty acids. On the basis of these data it was suggested that the vitamin E requirement generated by a dietary fat, except for monoenoic acids, is directly related to total unsaturation (Table 1).

The inability to detect peroxidized fatty acids in the tissues, other than adipose tissue, of vitamin E-deficient animals was viewed in the 1960s as a basis for disputing the antioxidant mode of activity.[34,62] Now these findings are viewed as a tribute to efficacy of Gpx. With the advent of more sensitive techniques, however, it became possible to detect peroxidized fatty acids not only in tissues from deficient animals, but also in the tissues from supplemented animals.[69]

It was also expected that lipid peroxidation could be demonstrated by a selective loss of the most highly polyunsaturated fatty acid(s) from tissue lipids. If this is arachidonic acid, peroxidative loss stimulates increased synthesis from linoleate with a net increase in arachidonate. Only when the diet contained significant quantities of (n – 3) fatty acids was it possible to demonstrate the progressive and selective loss of polyunsaturated fatty acids *in vivo*.[283]

F. OTHER ANTIOXIDANTS

1. Synthetic Lipid Antioxidants

The use of certain synthetic lipid antioxidants, with vitamin E-like activity, in some of the augmentation studies requires a brief digression into the biochemistry and nutrition of these compounds, particularly BHT, BHA, ethoxyquin, and DPPD.

Certain lipid antioxidants may lower the vitamin E requirement by a mechanism not necessarily related to antioxidant activity. The microsomal drug metabolizing system is a remarkable complex of enzymes that is responsible for coping with all manner of toxic substances and xenobiotics. However, these extraordinary capabilities are associated with probably the worst free radical leakage in the body. McCay et al.[170] have suggested that this system alone must account for a significant portion of the normal vitamin E requirement. Phase I drug metabolizing enzymes generally oxidize substrates and in the process inadvertently convert a number of compounds to strong, active carcinogens. Phase II enzymes lead to conjugation with polar, water soluble moieties, such as glutathione, glucuronic acid, or sulfate, which hinder further catabolism but facilitate excretion. BHT and BHA, but not vitamin E, induce a proliferation of Phase II enzymes.[126,133] This induction may be sufficient to result in an increase in liver weight. Since free radical leakage is related to oxidation, rather than conjugation, this shift in the balance of drug metabolizing enzymes via enzyme induction may lower the requirement for lipid antioxidants.

Action of a synthetic lipid antioxidant as an antioxidant may result in increased toxicity and the induction of an enzyme for detoxification. The hydroperoxide of BHT is known to be formed by hepatic microsomes. BHT hydroperoxide is 20 times as toxic as BHT by ip injection,[286] and promotes tumor formation in mouse skin.[253] Other investigators[108] have suggested that the quinone methide is the active compound. BHA, BHT, and ethoxyquin, but not vitamin E, induce increased transcription of a quinone reductase gene.[82] This would suggest that these antioxidants are not recycled nonenzymatically and are detoxified in the aqueous phase.

Since BHT has been legally used as a food additive since the 1950s, this is a logical candidate for inclusion in augmentation studies.[134,136] The allowable daily intake of BHT as determined by the World Health Organization and the European Economic Community is 0.125 and 0.05 mg/kg, respectively. These levels are based in part on blood clotting problems in the rat and increased thyroid weight in the pregnant pig.

BHA has similar effects in the same species, and produces carcinomas of the fore stomach in animals having fore stomachs[127,165] (rat, hamster, and mouse) but not in animals lacking this anatomical feature (guinea pig, monkey, and beagle dog). BHA is rapidly demethylated to *tert*-butyl hydroquinone,[51] which is excreted as the sulfate or glucuronide. Cycling of *tert*-butyl hydroquinone and the corresponding quinone is thought to increase oxidative stress.[51]

When fed as 1 to 2% of the diet for 104 weeks, BHT produced dose related hepatocellular adenomas in male mice.[125] Hepatocellular carcinomas were also produced in rats fed 500 mg/kg/day of BHT.[192] Tumors, however, appeared only late in life and the experimental animals lived longer than the controls. Since BHT, or its active metabolite(s) is a tumor promoter in carcinogen-treated animals, it has been suggested that this might have represented promotion of latent tumors. The simultaneous anticarcinogenic and tumor promoting activities are illustrated in the work of Williams et al.[276] They found simultaneous inhibition of liver carcinogenicity and enhancement of bladder carcinogenicity in animals fed acetylaminofluorene and BHT.

DPPD was used in the classic multigeneration study of Draper et al.[67] However, this synthetic lipid antioxidant is sufficiently toxic in pregnant female rats that heroic efforts were required to reach the third generation.

Vitamin E and various synthetic lipid antioxidants have been reported to have in common the inhibition of protein kinase C, which acts as the receptor for phorbol esters and related tumor promoters.[3,85,162]

2. Miscellaneous Antioxidants

In a manner of speaking, almost anything that reacts with a free radical might be described as an antioxidant. As noted by Frei et al.,[89] various small molecules, such as uric acid, bilirubin, and ubiquinol-10, and large molecules such as albumin, transferin, and lactoferin, may react with free radicals. Basically these are materials present in more than one copy, that turn over relatively rapidly, and their damage by free radicals does not cause a deficiency or lesion. In plasma, proteins may account for 86% of free radical consumption.[102] While, perhaps quite important in the overall context of reducing free radical initiated tissue damage, these materials are not germane to the present discussion.

Carotenoids, on the other hand, represent a special minor case.[145] Singlet oxygen is a product of certain photooxidations and a limited number of enzyme reactions. The carotenoids are among the most efficient singlet oxygen quenchers, and therefore occupy a small, specialized layer in the multilayered defense system.

IV. AUGMENTATION WITH VITAMIN E

A. EARLY CLINICAL RESEARCH ON VITAMIN E

When vitamin E was discovered, malnutrition was not uncommon. Each new vitamin could be applied to a condition, such as scurvy, beriberi, or pellagra, occurring in man. Based on studies in animals vitamin E should have been appropriate for reproductive problems and muscular dystrophy. In retrospect it is now obvious that since, for all practical purposes, vitamin E deficiency does not normally occur in man and is almost impossible to produce in the adult, there were no deficiency signs to treat. Those conditions in humans resembling deficiency signs in animals had distinctly different causes. The very active search for clinical conditions responding to vitamin E supplementation was, therefore, in principle doomed to failure. This did not prevent, however, publication of numerous reports, frequently based on anecdotal evidence, that vitamin E was beneficial in essentially any ailment known to man.[236]

In the early 1960s various transient difficulties were encountered in the efforts to separate and distinguish the nutritional roles of selenium and vitamin E. Combined with the resistance from some quarters to the acceptance of the main role of the vitamin as a biological antioxidant, vitamin E was a rather controversial topic, even in terms of experimental animal nutrition.

In 1962 Marks[163] noted that in the previous 25 years over 2000 papers on the clinical use of vitamin E had appeared in the medical literature. At that time there seemed to be good evidence to support the value of supplementation in moderate intermittent claudication due to arteriosclerosis, in fat malabsorption syndromes, and in premature infants receiving artificial foods. A very lengthy review by Farrell[81] in 1980 found some basis for supplementation in malabsorption syndromes, retrolental fibroplasia, abetalipoproteinemia, and prematurity, but questioned the basis for use in intermittent claudication, ischemic heart disease, aging, and other conditions. Farrell concluded rather succinctly that most of the published studies regarding vitamin E supplementation were not adequately controlled and would not withstand careful scientific scrutiny. It would probably be fair to say that clinical research on vitamin E, the "shady lady" of nutrition, has, in the recent past, not enjoyed a good reputation or been viewed as particularly credible.

It is against this dubious background that the evidence presented by another generation of investigators linking vitamin E supplementation to the amelioration of clinical problems must be considered. In view of the extremely large number of clinical and epidemiological studies reported, it is not possible to review each in detail. Emphasis has, therefore, been placed on those studies most directly relevant to the existence or nonexistence of justification for prolonged, high level vitamin E supplementation. Such data tend to come from intervention trials and certain cohort studies where a significant minority of the participants were found, after the fact, to be gobbling vitamin pills.

B. CANCER

The multilayered defense system protecting against free radical initiated tissue damage may also provide some protection against carcinogenesis. However, until such time as the etiology of cancer is better understood, it is not possible to explain or reconcile the diverse reports.

Cancer is readily produced, albeit in an incompletely understood manner, in experimental animals by the administration of a variety of chemical carcinogens. Test systems are available, therefore, to evaluate other chemicals for possible protective effects. In the 1960s, dietary antioxidants were found to have such protective effects.[271] In certain cases this occurs through a shift in the balance between activation of a procarcinogen to a carcinogen and detoxification by the microsomal drug metabolizing enzymes induced by varoius synthetic lipid antioxidants.[43,137] As noted previously, vitamin E does not induce a comparable proliferation. Synthetic lipid antioxidants, such as BHA or BHT, may also promote or even cause cancer. The example was cited earlier of the simultaneous inhibition of hepatic carcinogenesis and enhancement of bladder carcinogenesis in rats fed BHT and acetylaminofluorene.[276]

In animal experiments vitamin E has been reported to inhibit,[234] to have no effect upon,[244] and to promote carcinogenesis.[257] Both tumor regression and tumor growth have been attributed to vitamin E.[235] Epidemiological data will next be reviewed to determine relevance to man.

There is a very large accumulation of data on cancer incidence that can be screened for clues to possible protective materials. A review of 156 epidemiological studies by Block[23] concluded that 128 supported a role for fruits and vegetables in reducing the risk of cancer. This has often been interpreted as a response to increased intakes of vitamins A, C, E, and carotenes in these foodstuffs. These materials have, unfortunately, been frequently referred to collectively as the antioxidant vitamins.

1. Types of Epidemiological Studies

The classical retrospective epidemiological study looks at historic data for populations with different incidences of cancer at all sites and at specific sites and then searches out, via multiple regression analysis, possible factors, such as high or low vitamin E intake, that can account for the difference. This approach depends on the completeness and quality of the public health records surveyed. If enough variables are considered, some will be found to be related directly or inversely to incidence in a statistically significant manner purely by chance. Confounding variables also routinely occur in epidemiological studies. Examples might include smoking or taking supplements of other vitamins.

Case control studies involve comparing a collection of cancer cases to a control group with regard to such variables as vitamin E intake or preferably serum vitamin E levels. Definition of a suitable control group can be a significant problem. There has been a regrettable tendency to utilize hospitalized patients who do not have cancer. The difficulties associated with selection of a control group on the basis of dietary recall questionnaires are well known. Questions have also been raised regarding the relevance that analytical values obtained on a sick individual have to the person's status during the period of cancer development.

Cohort studies are prospective studies where intakes are determined by diet recall or inferred by serum analysis, and cumulative incidence at each tumor site is compared between high and low intake groups. Cohort studies may be used to investigate numerous topics simultaneously. Input data on all manner of variables may be compared in terms of possible relationship to all subsequent health problems including cancer, coronary heart disease, or other degenerative process. Typically the limiting factor is the cost of the initial screenings and analyses. Concern has been expressed that initial values, serum levels, may be depressed by developing but undetected cancer. This would suggest possible exclusion from the study of individuals with cancer detected early in the follow-up period.

Nested case control studies might be considered the economy version of cohort studies. Appropriate samples are collected from all participants and stored, but only those samples from cancer cases and selected controls are subsequently analyzed. Unfortunately, losses of vitamin E are seen in serum samples stored at $-20°C$ and this was the storage temperature selected in five out of nine studies tabulated by Knekt.[142]

Intervention studies, which may be double-blind with placebo, are the human equivalent of experimental animal studies and as such are most apt to yield definitive results. Such studies are typically enormously expensive to carry out, largely because of the need to monitor for undesirable side effects. With vitamin E this is not necessary and very large groups may be studied relatively inexpensively. Very large groups are desirable in intervention trials to permit evaluation of the response at sites other than lung, breast, and colon. Cancers of these organs may be strongly correlated with enhancing factors such as smoking, hormonal levels, and fecal retention time, and may, therefore, not constitute appropriate outcome criteria for vitamin E supplementation.

The high dosages, 400 to 800 IU of vitamin E per day, needed to raise tissue levels are known to be well tolerated. Combination or factorial studies including vitamins A and C are possible by replacing vitamin A with β-carotene.

2. Results of Epidemiological Studies

Since this review is concerned with the possible justification for high intakes of vitamin E, most available epidemiological data are not relevant, as it is difficult to provide as much as 1.5 times the recommended dietary allowance for vitamin E in normal diets. The tenfold increase in intake needed to double plasma levels must obviously be achieved through prolonged supplementation. It is interesting, however, to consider these reports briefly in terms of the data upon which intervention studies have been based.

Case control and nested case control studies in general have reported that cancer patients tend to have lower mean values for plasma or serum vitamin E than do controls.[151,175,188,220,270] Such differences, while repeatedly noted in numerous studies of colorectal cancer and lung cancer, were generally not statistically significant.

A cohort study[96] in San Francisco reported an inverse relationship between prescribed vitamin E and all sites of cancer combined. Other cohort studies[245] not involving supplemental vitamin E have yielded variable results. Numerous very large cohort studies are now in progress throughout the world. Such studies typically follow health problems in general. The spread of self-supplementation with vitamin E has begun to impinge upon such studies in regard to incidence of cancer and, as noted elsewhere, coronary heart disease. The Iowa Women's Health Study[28] is a prospective cohort study of 35,215 women aged 55 to 69. A comparison of the highest and lowest quintiles for vitamin E intake over a five-year period showed a 68% lower risk of colon cancer in the high intake individuals. High intake was largely associated with supplementation.

A recent four-year intervention trial[105] concluded that supplemental vitamin E (400 mg/day) did not protect against colorectal cancer. This was a 2 × 2 factorial study providing β-carotene (25 mg/day); vitamin C (1 g/day) plus vitamin E; β-carotene plus vitamins C and E, and a placebo. The 864 subjects had already developed one benign polyp of the colon and none of the treatments reduced the risk of developing additional polyps. Two previous studies[58,112] had also shown no effect for vitamins C and E, whereas one study had reported a positive response.[215]

Another intervention trial[117] reported that vitamin E (50 mg/day) had no effect on lung cancer incidence (875 new cases) among 29,133 male smokers during a 5 to 8 year follow-up. This was a 2 × 2 factorial study providing vitamin E; β-carotene (20 mg/day); vitamin E plus β-carotene; and placebo. β-Carotene supplementation was associated with an 18% increase in lung cancer incidence and an increase in ischemic heart disease. The authors raised the question of the possible harmful effect of this supplement. While the quantity of supplemental vitamin E was sufficient to increase the serum level 50%, it was much lower than the 400 to 800 IU/day recommended by others. In terms of the quantity of supplemental vitamin E needed to lower exhaled pentane from smokers to control levels,[121a] a higher level of supplementation would have been desirable.

C. ATHEROSCLEROSIS

Atherosclerosis research has been frustrated for decades by the missing link between the predisposing factor, elevated serum cholesterol, and the disease, clogged arteries. How and why does the initial fatty streak containing cholesterol-laden foam cells arise in the arteries?

Frei et al.[90] noted that blood plasma contains no significant catalase or peroxidase activity. An extracellular form of SOD, while present, appears to be bound to the extracellular surfaces of epithelial cells. Selenium-dependent Gpx is present, but the plasma level of glutathione is insufficient to permit effective function.[37a] The repeated recommendation by the atherosclerosis research community calling for substitution of polyunsaturated fats for saturated dietary fats has created a subpopulation whose blood lipids have a greatly enhanced susceptibility to peroxidative damage.[177] Recent promotion of (n − 3) fatty acids from fish oil has further exacerbated this situation. Even when fish oil contains added vitamin E and synthetic lipid antioxidant, the plasma level of vitamin E may be below the normal range.[222]

The major carrier of cholesterol in the blood stream is low density lipoprotein, LDL. Esterbauer et al.[75] has estimated that the lipid associated with an LDL molecule contains six molecules of alpha-tocopherol. This is a rather enormous amount of vitamin E corresponding to ratios of vitamin E to total fatty acid and vitamin E to polyunsaturated fatty acid of 1:482 and 1:218, respectively. Membrane lipids typically contain one molecule of vitamin E to 1000 to 3000 fatty acids. Isolation of lipoproteins must be carried out in the presence of metal chelators, such as EDTA, to prevent rapid oxidative damage. Without such protection the isolated LDL is cytotoxic to cultured cells.[120]

Cellular interaction with LDL is mediated by an LDL receptor.[31] Chemical modification, i.e., acetylation, of the lysine residues of LDL results in recognition by a scavenger receptor.[31] In 1984 there were reports[182,249] that vascular endothelial and smooth muscle cells, *in vitro,* in the presence of metal ions could alter LDL by free radical initiated lipid peroxidation. Minimally oxidized LDL, as judged by the thiobarbituric acid test, while still recognized by the LDL receptor, was cytotoxic.[181] The lipid extract of such material contains most of the cytotoxic activity. *In vitro,* such oxidative degradation can readily be carried to the point of loss of polyunsaturated fatty acids and appearance of secondary lipid peroxidation products, such as malondialdehyde and 4-hydroxy-2-nonenal.[76] These aldehydes can react with the free amino groups of lysine residues in LDL.[250] Subsequently, immunological techniques permitted the detection of malondialdehyde and 4-hydroxy-2-nonenal-modified LDL in lesions in Watanabe heritable hyperlipidemic rabbits.[109,216]

Suddenly lipid peroxidation became a major topic in atherosclerosis research.[130,247,248] The nonsaturable character of the scavenger receptor[31] may be a factor in foam cell formation. How or why LDL lipid peroxidation occurs, however, is an interesting question. A number of studies involving vitamin E and synthetic lipid antioxidants that have evolved from this area of research are germane to this review. These experiments tend to fall into three groups which consider the effect of supplementation on the stability of LDL to *in vitro* lipid peroxidation, the development of atherosclerotic lesions, and the incidence of atherosclerosis (epidemiology).

When plasma levels of alpha-tocopherol were increased 1.7 to 2.5 times by supplementation, the LDL levels of vitamin E also increased 1.7 to 3.1 times.[60] Jialal and Grundy[129] compared the effect of a daily supplement of 800 IU of vitamin E for 3 months with the same supplement plus 1 g/day of vitamin C and 30 mg/day of β-carotene. Upon subjecting LDL to *in vitro* lipid peroxidation, a protective effect was noted which was entirely attributable to vitamin E. A comparable experiment by Reaven et al.[209] involving daily supplements of 60 mg β-carotene, 1600 mg vitamin E, and 2 g vitamin C also attributed all of the observed protective action to vitamin E. Belcher et al.[13] found that vitamin E provided protection after only two weeks supplementation, whereas vitamin C had no effect.

Probucol, long used as a drug in the treatment of atherosclerosis, has an antioxidant structure.[146] The LDL from hypercholesterolemic patients treated with probucol was described as highly resistant to oxidative modification *in vitro*.[201] BHT, DPPD,[242] nordihydroguaiaretic acid, and idapamide supplementation also seems to protect LDL against *in vitro* oxidation.[77] Such experiments measure a difference in protection of LDL from lipid peroxidation *in vitro* and are meaningful only if LDL peroxidation occurs *in vivo* and the observed differences are physiologically significant.[38]

Vitamin E has been reported to inhibit early aortic lesion development in the Watanabe heritable hyperlipidemic rabbit by 32%.[277] In another study, the extent of plaque formation was comparable, but the amount of cholesterol in the lesion was less in the vitamin E supplemented rabbits.[278] The narrowing (stenosis) of the carotid arteries in monkeys[268] was followed for 36 months by ultrasound. With vitamin E supplementation, stenosis progressed more slowly and to a lesser degree. When vitamin E was added to the diet of monkeys, previously unsupplemented for a period of 24 months, the degree of narrowing was reduced. A protective effect of vitamin E was reported in the Japanese quail[65] and in the nonovulatory hen.[239] It has been reported that probucol has a beneficial antioxidant effect *in vivo* that is separate from its plasma cholesterol lowering effect.[146] Some degree of protection has also been attributed to BHT[19] and DPPD[242] in animal studies.

1. Epidemiology

The possible protective role of vitamin E in coronary heart disease has received considerable support from the ongoing epidemiological studies.[118] In 16 European study populations, an inverse relationship was found between plasma vitamin E and mortality.[101] Multiple regression analysis yielded a much higher correlation with vitamin E, 0.62, than had been obtained previously in 33 population groups with the classical risk factors, total cholesterol, blood pressure, and smoking, 0.20.

Interim reports from the Male Health Professionals Follow-up Study,[211] involving 39,910 men, and the Nurses' Health Study,[246] involving 87,245 women, make several interesting points. Significant numbers of participants in each group, approaching 20%, were apparently taking supplemental vitamin E. A comparison of those taking supplements with those at the low end of normal intake, indicated a 37 to 41% reduction in relative risk of coronary heart disease. Manifestation of the protective effect of vitamin E required intake of amounts of the vitamin far beyond the levels attainable in any reasonable diet, i.e., five to ten times the Recommended Daily Allowance, for a protracted period, at least two years. As noted elsewhere in this review, the number of individuals taking supplemental vitamin E has been reported to influence the incidence of cancer in another large cohort study.[28] A recent review by Gey[101a] provides over 400 references and numerous unpublished updates on this subject of coronary heart disease and relevant epidemiological studies.

In 1991 the National Heart, Lung, and Blood Institute convened a workshop to consider the topic of antioxidants in the prevention of atherosclerosis. It was reported[248] that the evidence for the oxidative modification of LDL was very strong. However, the relationship between oxidative modification of LDL and atherosclerosis, while felt to be reasonably strong, was not found to be totally conclusive. Among the dietary factors evaluated, epidemiological support was considered moderately strong for vitamin E, weak for selenium and vitamin C, and intermediate for β-carotene. Support for β-carotene derives largely from the Harvard study. At that time the consensus favored a clinical trial involving the nontoxic materials, vitamin E, vitamin C, and β-carotene. Such a trial would be inexpensive, involve negligible risk, not require monitoring for side effects, and could include a very large number of participants. It was noted that a $2 \times 2 \times 2$ factorial study of vitamin E, β-carotene, and aspirin was in progress in a group of 40,000 women and might provide guidance. Consideration of a trial with antioxidant drugs, which might have side effects, was not considered justified at that time. Such constructive evidence as has appeared regarding the possible beneficial effects of antioxidants has spurred efforts to develop relevant drugs.

D. NEUROLOGICAL DISORDERS

Since the rare cases of vitamin E deficiency in man are accompanied by neurological damage[241] it is not surprising that a variety of other neurological disorders have been considered potential targets for supplementation. Reduced plasma vitamin E levels were reported in patients with epilepsy who were treated with antiepileptic drugs.[189] In a double-blind, placebo controlled study,[190] patients refractory to antiepileptic drugs were given D-α-tocopheryl acetate in addition to the usual drugs. These patients were reported to show a significant improvement in seizure rate. A phosphate diester of vitamins C and E has been reported to be useful in an animal model.[183]

Supplementation with vitamin E, 3000 IU/day, and vitamin C, 3000 mg/day, was reported to extend the period before treatment with levodopa or a dopamine agonist became necessary in patients with Parkinson's disease.[80] However, in a multicenter controlled clinical trial that involved 800 patients, there was no evidence that dl-α-tocopheryl acetate, 2000 IU/day, slowed or ameliorated the progression of Parkinson's disease.[199]

The long-term use of neuroleptic drugs for the control of psychotic behavior may result in tardive dyskinesia. On an abnormal involuntary movement scale patients receiving α-tocopherol showed a significant improvement over placebo.[157]

E. CATARACTS

The eye is exposed directly to the environment and is subject to attack by oxidants and radiation. Vitamin E deficiency in rabbits,[59] rats,[32] and turkeys[83] promotes cataract formation. Supplementation with vitamin E has been reported to reduce or delay the progression of cataracts in streptozotocin-diabetic rats,[217] galactose-fed rats,[48] and cataract prone mice.[107] BHT[5] delays cataract formation in the galactose-fed rat. Cataract formation has been reported to be associated with lipid peroxidation.[17,18,266,288] Vitamin E, superoxide dismutase (SOD), and catalase each increased survival time of isolated corneas. Cataract formation in rat lenses in tissue culture was prevented by vitamin E or glutathione.[267]

The incidence of senile cataracts increases rapidly with advancing age, 4.5% at 52 to 64, 18% at 65 to 74 and 45% at 75 to 85. Delaying the onset of cataract formation could result in large savings in treatment and transplant costs.[262] Various epidemiological studies have suggested a protective effect for supplementary quantities of vitamin E and vitamin C.[128,212,213,256,263] Leske et al.[152] reported a protective effect for vitamin E, but no synergistic effect for vitamin C. Two intervention trials in China reported[243a] no protective effect for α-tocopherol or β-caotene against cataract formation, but the supplement of vitamin E was rather low, 30 mg/day. A recent review by Trevithick et al.[262] provides extensive coverage of the topic of free radical phenomena and the eye.

F. SKIN

Skin is exposed to sunlight and hence ultraviolet radiation in addition to various environmental pollutants. It would, therefore, seem reasonable to expect free radical initiated tissue damage of the skin. Vitamin E has been recommended for various dermatological conditions since 1936. Conditions included are radiation dermatitis,[92] fibrotic skin disease,[114,202] lupus erythematosus,[272] acne,[53] psoriasis,[227] wound healing,[70] venous stasis ulcer,[208] and cancer.[238] Studies in this area tend to be old and involve rather small groups of subjects. This topic has been extensively reviewed by Fuchs and Packer.[97]

G. ISCHEMIA–REPERFUSION

When blood flow to an area is reduced or blocked, ischemia (hypoxia) results. While prolonged ischemia can cause tissue damage and eventually results in cell death, only minor morphological modifications are noted in the short-term. It is obviously desirable to reinstitute blood flow as rapidly as possible, but reperfusion may cause damage in various tissues[26] (heart, kidney, brain, liver, small intestine, and pancreas) due to a rather sudden burst of free radical production.[22,25] With the increasing frequency of bypass surgery and organ transplants, this problem has attracted considerable interest. After cardiac surgery arrythmias, loss of contractility, and necrosis may detract from an otherwise successful procedure.

Research in this area can utilize animals and involve experiments of limited duration. A simple clamp may be sufficient to produce the desired ischemia and a wide variety of materials may be added to the reperfusing solution. Free radicals can be measured by techniques such as electron spin resonance,[100] and the perfusate[22,290] may be analyzed after passing through the previously ischemic area. Needless to say, the literature on this topic is extensive.

Rather convincing evidence is available for the production of free radicals.[25] The source of the free radicals, however, is still a subject of debate. One possible source is the xanthine oxidase activity induced by ischemia.[172a] Infusion of the enzyme and its substrate, hypoxanthine, has been reported to mimic the damage seen upon reperfusion after ischemia.[102a] This hypothesis[56] has been studied with the aid of the xanthine oxidase inhibitor, allopurinol, with mixed results. At high concentrations allopurinol is a free radical scavenger. Another possible source is the polymorphonuclear leukocytes activated by the free arachidonic acid which accumulates during ischemia due to inactivation of lysophosphatidyl choline acyltransferase.

A wide variety of materials have been tested for possible protective activity. Superoxide dismutase (SOD)[4,10,86,290] appears to provide some protection, but is cleared from the blood stream in 5 to 10 minutes. SOD linked to other materials to slow turnover has also been investigated.[11] The use of SOD and catalase has been reviewed by Greenwald.[106] Various small sulfur compounds, N-acetylcysteine, 2-mercaptopropionylglycine,[289] and Captopril,[174,273] have been reported to provide beneficial effects. Protective effects have also been attributed to dihydrolipoic acid,[91] trimetazidine,[42] a 21-aminosteroid,[30] and certain monohydroxamates.[103]

Vitamin E supplementation has been reported[8,84] to reduce reperfusion damage to the heart and to reduce the size of the subsequent myocardial infarct. Epidemiological data also support the possible beneficial effect of supplemental quantities of vitamin E in ischemic heart disease.[101] It has been reported that 300 mg vitamin E/day for 14 days is needed to double the myocardial level of α-tocopherol.[178] Supplementation at the time of surgery may not be timely since peak releases of conjugated diene (peroxidized lipid) occur at 3 and 60 min after reperfusion.[214] Intravenous administration of Trolox, a water soluble variant of vitamin E without the phytyl sidechain, has reduced myocardial infarction in dogs.[150] This compound has also greatly reduced liver necrosis in rats after hepatic ischemia.[285]

In kidney transplant patients, intravenous infusion of a multivitamin solution containing antioxidants prior to reperfusion was reported to improve renal function in the first four to five days after surgery.[207] Several drugs modeled in part on the vitamin E structure have also shown protective action in other tissues. One of these is IFRI-0048, 2,3-dihydro-5-methoxy-4,6,7-trimethyl-2-benzofuran acetic acid,[37] and the other is the lazaroid U78517F, a 2-methylaminochromane derivative.[112]

H. ARTHRITIS

Inflammatory joint disease in some ways resembles the ischemia–reperfusion process.[66] During exercise the capillary bed is occluded and reperfusion occurs on cessation of exercise.[21] Prior to the discovery of SOD, a material, Orgotein, isolated from bovine liver was found to be useful in treating joint disease in horses. The active component of Orgotein was subsequently identified as SOD.[122] In randomized double-blind studies SOD was found to be superior to a placebo in osteoarthritis but not in rheumatoid arthritis.[86] Subjective effects, reduction in pain and increase in walking ability, persisted up to six months after withdrawal of treatment.

Evidence of lipid peroxidation, conjugated dienes and thiobarbituric acid reactive materials, were found in synovial fluid and sera.[160,219] Exhaled pentane was elevated in patients with rheumatoid arthritis and correlated with disease activity.[123] Supplementation with 400 IU α-tocopherol/day for 6 weeks allowed the amount of nonsteroidal antiinflammatory drugs that were being administered to be reduced.[229] In three double-blind studies vitamin E was as effective as Diclofenac-Na in the treatment of rheumatoid arthritis[143,154] and osteoarthritis.[228] Vitamin E has also been found to be beneficial in animal models.[135,287]

I. EXERCISE
Increased oxygen consumption during exercise may be associated with increased lipid peroxidation.[198] Vitamin E supplementation, 400 IU/day, has been reported to prevent increased pentane exhalation in mountain climbers.[240]

V. VITAMIN E — DO WE NEED IT?

The logic for prescribing or recommending supplementation with vitamin E is persuasive — a potential for low-cost protection against a wide panoply of ills without the threat of side effects or the need for ongoing monitoring. What more could a physician ask for? The message has been pervasive and the apparent number of willing listeners is astonishing. Based on data from at least four very large cohort studies, the number of individuals taking vitamin E supplements is approaching 20% and still climbing. Obviously these are motivated participants in health studies and may not represent the population as a whole. Through shear number these vitamin E gobblers have converted cohort studies into quasi-intervention trials.

Large scale intervention studies that provide supplemental vitamin E have not, thus far, been particularly successful. This may be due in part is to the choice of an inappropriate disease or because the level of supplementation was not adequate. Obviously not every condition benefits from vitamin E supplementation. Where beneficial results have been noted there are indications that this requires relatively large amounts to have been ingested for a prolonged period. The adherents of what appeared not long ago to be the worst quackery imaginable may now be providing evidence that perhaps vitamin E no longer deserves the title of the "shady lady" of nutrition.

In the multilayered defense system protecting against free radical initiated tissue damage, prolonged, high-level vitamin E supplementation is something of a last ditch stopgap, ameliorating effect without regard to cause. Enhanced protection may buy time, but ultimately the real answer to the problem lies in determining and responding to the source of excess free radical production and leakage.

REFERENCES

1. Abdo, K. M., Rao, G., Montgomery, C. A., Dinowitz, M., and Kanagalingam, K., Thirteen week toxicity study of d-α-tocopheryl acetate (vitamin E) in Fischer 344 rats, *Food Chem. Toxic.*, 24, 1043, 1986.
2. Aebi, H. E. and Wyss, S. R., Acatalasemia, in *The Metabolic Basis of Inherited Disease*, Stanbury, J. B., Wyngaarden, J. B., Fredrickson, D. S., and Brown, M. S., Eds., McGraw Hill, New York, 1978, 1792.
3. Alexandre, A., Doni, M. G., Padoin, E., and Deana, R., Inhibition by antioxidants of agonist evoked cytosolic Ca^{++} increase, ATP secretion and aggregation of aspirinated platelets, *Bichem. Biophys. Res. Commun.*, 139, 509, 1986.
4. Ambrosco, G., Becker, L. C., Hutchins, G. M., Weisman, H. F., and Weisfeldt, M. L., Reduction in experimental infarct size by recombinant human superoxide dismutase: insights into the pathophysiology of reperfusion injury, *Circulation*, 74, 1424, 1986.
5. Ansari, H. H., Schulter, A., and Srivastava, S. K., Antioxidant (BHT) significantly delays galactose cataract formation in rats, *Invest. Ophthamol. Vis. Sci.*, 28, Suppl., 192, 1987.
6. Arouma, O. I., Halliwell, B., and Dizdaroglu, M., Iron ion-dependent modification of bases in DNA by the superoxide radical-generating system hypoxanthine/xanthine oxidase, *J. Biol. Chem.*, 264, 13024, 1989.
7. Arouma, O. I., Halliwell, B., Gajewski, E., and Dizdaroglu, M., Damage to the bases in DNA induced by hydrogen peroxide and ferric iron chelates, *J. Biol. Chem.*, 264, 20509, 1989.
8. Axford-Gatley, R. A. and Wilson, G. S., Reduction of experimental myocardial infarct size by oral administration of α-tocopherol, *Cardiovasc. Res.*, 28, 89, 1991.
9. Bast, A. and Haenen, G. R. M. M., Regulation of lipid peroxidation by glutathione and lipoic acid: involvement of liver microsomal vitamin E free radical reductase, in *Antioxidants in Therapy and Preventive Medicine*, Emerit, I., Packer, I., and Auclair, C., Eds., Plenum Press, New York, 1990, 111.
10. Becker, G. L., Corry, R. J., and Autor, A. P., Oxygen free radical induced damage in kidneys subjected to warm ischemia and reperfusion: protective effect of superoxide dismutase, *Ann. Surg.*, 202, 628, 1985.
11. Beckman, J. S., Minor, R. L., Jr., White, C. W., Repine, J. E., Rosen, G. M., and Freeman, B. A., Superoxide dismutase and catalase conjugated to polyethylene glycol increases endothelial cell activity and antioxidant resistance, *J. Biol. Chem.*, 263, 6884, 1988.
12. Behrens, W. A. and Madere, R., Ascorbic and dehydroascorbic acids status in rats fed diets varying in vitamin E levels, *Int. J. Vit. Nutr. Res.*, 59, 360, 1989.
13. Belcher, J. D., Balla, J., Balla, G., Jacobs, D. R., Gross, M., Jacobs, H. S., and Vercelloti, G. M., Vitamin E, LDL, and endothelium. Brief oral vitamin supplementation prevents oxidized LDL-mediated vascular injury in vitro, *Arterio. Thromb.*, 12, 1779, 1993.
14. Bendich, A., Safety issues regarding the use of vitamin supplements, *Ann. N.Y. Acad. Sci.*, 669, 300, 1992.
15. Bendich, A. and Machlin, L. J., Safety of oral intakes of vitamin E, *Am. J. Clin. Nutr.*, 48, 612, 1988.

16. Bendich, A. and Machlin, L. J., The safety of oral intakes of vitamin E: data from clinical studies from 1986-1991, in *Vitamin E in Health and Disease,* Packer, L. and Fuchs, J., Eds., Marcel Dekker, New York, 1992, 411.

17. Bhuyan, K. C., Bhuyan, D. K., Kuck, J. F. R., Kuck, K. D., and Kern, H. L., Increased lipid peroxidation and altered membrane functions in Emory mouse cataract, *Curr. Eye Res.,* 2, 597, 1983.

18. Bhuyan, K. C. and Bhuyan, D. K., Molecular mechanisms of cataractogenesis: 3. Toxic metabolites of oxygen as initiators of lipid peroxidation and cataracts, *Curr. Eye Res.,* 3, 67, 1984.

19. Bjorkhen, I., Henriksson-Freyschress, A., Breuer, O., Diczfalusy, U., Borglund, L., and Henriksson, P., The antioxidant butylated hydroxytoluene protects against atherosclerosis, *Arterioscl. Thromb.,* 11, 15, 1991.

20. Bjorneboe, A., Nenseter, M., Hagen, B. F., Bjorneboe, G.-E., Prydz, C., and Drevon, C. A., Distribution and subcellular localization of α-tocopherol in rat liver cells, in *Transport and Distribution of α-Tocopherol in Rats,* Bjorneboe, A., Ed., National Institute of Forensic Toxicology, Oslo, Norway, 1988, 1.

21. Blake, D. R., Merry, P., Unsworth, J., Kidd, B., Outhwaite, J. M., Ballard, R., Morris, C. J., Gray, L., and Lunec, J., Hypoxic-reperfusion injury in the inflamed human joint, *Lancet,* 8653, 289, 1989.

22. Blasig, I. E., Shuter, S., Garlick, A., and Slater, T., Relative time profiles for the free radical trapping, coronary flow, enzymatic leakage, arrhythmias, and function during myocardial reperfusion, *Free Rad. Biol. Med.,* 16, 35, 1994.

23. Block, G., Patterson, B., and Subor, X., Fruit, vegetables and cancer prevention: a review of the epidemiological evidence, *Nutr. Cancer,* 18, 1, 1992.

24. Boguth, W. and Niemann, H., Electron spin resonance of chromanoxy free radicals from α, ζ_2, β, γ, δ-tocopherol and tocol, *Biochim. Biophys. Acta,* 248, 121, 1971.

25. Bolli, R., Jeroudi, M. O., Patel, B. S., Dubose, C. M., Lai, E. K., Roberts, R., and McCay, P. B., Direct evidence that oxygen-derived free radicals contribute to post ischemic myocardial dysfunction in the intact dog, *Proc. Natl. Acad. Sci. U.S.A.,* 86, 4695, 1989.

26. Bolli, R., Jeroudi, M. O., Patel, B. S., Aruoma, P., Halliwell, B., Lai, E. K., and McCay, P. B., Marked reduction of free radical generation and contractile dysfunction by an antioxidant therapy begun at the time of reperfusion. Evidence that myocardial "stunning" is a manifestation of reperfusion injury, *Circ. Res.,* 65, 607, 1989.

27. Bors, W., Saran, M., Lengfelder, E., Spottl, R., and Michel, C., Relevance of the superoxide anion radical in biological systems, *Curr. Top. Radiat. Res. Q.,* 9, 309, 1974.

28. Bostwick, R. M., Potter, J. D., McKenzie, D. R., Sellers, T. A., Kushi, L. H., Steinmetz, K. A., and Folsom, A. R., Reduced risk of colon cancer with high intake of vitamin E: the Iowa Women's Health Study, *Cancer Res.,* 53, 4230, 1993.

29. Breimer, L. H., Repair of DNA damage induced by reactive oxygen species, *Free Rad. Res. Commun.,* 14, 159, 1993.

30. Broughler, J. M., Hall, E. D., Jacobsen, E. S., McCall, J., and Means, E. D., The 21- amino steroids. Potent inhibitors of lipid peroxidation for the treatment of central nervous system trauma and ischemia, *Drugs Future,* 14, 143, 1989.

31. Brown, M. S. and Goldstein, J. L., Lipoprotein metabolism in the macrophage; implications for cholesterol deposition in atherosclerosis, *Ann. Rev. Biochem.,* 52, 223, 1983.

32. Bunce, G. E. and Hess, J. L., Lenticular opacities in young rats as a consequence of maternal diets low in trytophane and/or vitamin E, *J. Nutr.,* 106, 222, 1976.

33. Bunyan, J., McHale, D., Green, J., and Marcinkiewicz, S., Biological potencies of ε- and ζ_1-tocopherol and 5-methyltocol, *Brit. J. Nutr.,* 15, 253, 1961.

34. Bunyan, J., Murrell, E. A., Green, J., and Diplock, A. T., On the existance and significance of lipid peroxides in vitamin E-deficient animals, *Br. J. Nutr.,* 21, 475, 1967.

35. Burton, G. W. and Ingold, K. U., Vitamin E as an in vitro and in vivo antioxidant, *Ann. N.Y. Acad. Sci.,* 570, 7, 1989.

36. Burton, G. W., Wronska, U., Stone, L., Foster, D. O., and Ingold, K. U., Biokinetics of dietary RRR-α-tocopherol in the male guinea pig at three dietary levels of vitamin C and two levels of vitamin E, *Lipids,* 25, 199, 1990.

37. Campo, G. M., Squadrito, F., Iocalano, M., Altavilla, D., Catapali, G., Zingaretti, B., Scuri, R., and Caputi, N. A., Reduction of myocardial infarct size in rat by IFRI-0048 a selective analogue of vitamin E, *Free Rad. Biol. Med.,* 16, 427, 1994.

37a. Cantin, A. M., North, S. L., Hubbard, R. C., and Crystal, R. G., Normal alveolar epithelial lining fluid contains high levels of glutathione, *J. Appl. Physiol.,* 63, 152, 1987.

38. Carew, T. E., Schwenke, D. C., and Steinberg, D., Antiatherogenetic effect of Probucol unrelated to its hypocholesterolemic effect: evidence that antioxidants in vivo can selectively inhibit low density lipoprotein degradation in macrophage-rich fatty streaks and slow progression of atherosclerosis in the Watanabe heritable hyperlipidemic rabbit, *Proc. Natl. Acad. Sci. U.S.A.,* 84, 7725, 1987.

39. Carlsson, J., Wrethen, J., and Beckman, J., Superoxide dismutase in Bacteroides fragilus and related Bacteroides species, *J. Clin. Microbiol.,* 6, 280, 1977.

40. Cathcart, R., Schwiers, E., Saul, R. L., and Ames, B. N., Thymineglycol and thymidine glycol in human and rat urine: a possible assay for oxidative DNA damage, *Proc. Natl. Acad. Sci. U.S.A.,* 81, 5633, 1984.

41. Catigani, G. L., An α-tocopherol binding protein in rat liver cytoplasm, *Biochem. Biophys. Res. Commun.,* 67, 66, 1975.

42. Catroux, P., Cambar, J., Benchekraun, N., Robert, J., Clauser, J., Clauser, P., and Harvey, C., Antilipoperoxidant effect of trimetaazidine in post ischemic acute renal failure in the rat, in *Antioxidants in Therapy and Preventive Medicine,* Emerit, I., Packer, L., and Auclair, C., Eds., Plenum Press, New York, 1990, 383.

43. Cha, Y.-N. and Heine, H., Comparative effects of dietary administration of 2(3)-tert-butyl-4-hydroxyanisole and 3,5-di-tert-butyl-4-hydroxytoluene on several hepatic enzyme activities in mice and rats, *Cancer Res.,* 42, 2609, 1982.

43a. Chaudhary, A. K., Nokubo, M., Reddy, G. R., Yeola, S. N., Morrow, J. D., Blair, I. A., and Marnett, Detection of endogenous malondialdehyde-deoxyguanosine adducts in human liver, *Science,* 265, 1580, 1994.

44. Chen, L. H., An increase in vitamin E requirement induced by high supplementation of vitamin C in rats, *Am. J. Clin. Nutr.,* 34, 1036, 1981.

45. Chow, C. K. and Tappel, A. L., Response of glutathione peroxidase to dietary selenium in rats, *J. Nutr.,* 104, 444, 1974.

46. Chow, C. K., Csallany, A. S., and Draper, H. H., Relative turnover rates of tocochromanols in rabbit plasma, *Nutr. Rep. Int.,* 4, 45, 1971.

47. Crastes de Paulet, A., Douste-Blazy, L., and Paoletti, R., *Free Radicals Lipoproteins and Membrane Lipids,* Plenum Press, New York, 1990.

48. Creighton, M. O., Ross, W. M., Stewart-DeHaas, P. J., Sawal, M., and Trevithick, J. R., Modelling cataractogenesis VII. Effects of vitamin E treatment on galactose-induced cataracts, *Exp. Eye Res.,* 40, 213, 1985.

49. Csallany, A. S., A reapraisal of the structure of a dimeric metabolite of — tocopherol, *Int. Z. Vitaminforsch.,* 41, 376, 1971.

50. Csallany, A. S. and Draper, H. H., Determination of N,N'-diphenyl-*p*-phenylenediamine in animal tissues, *Proc. Soc. Exp. Biol. Med.,* 104, 739, 1960.

51. Cummings, S. W., Ansari, G. A. S., Guengerich, F. P., Crouch, L. S., and Prough, R. A., Metabolism of 3-tert-butyl-hydroxyanisole by microsomal fractions and isolated hepatocytes, *Cancer Res.,* 45, 5617, 1985.

52. Cutler, R. G., Antioxidants and the longevity of mammalian species, in *Molecular Biology of Aging,* Woodhead, A. D., Blackett, A. D., and Hollander, A., Eds., Plenum Press, New York, 1985, 15.

53. Dainow, P. I., La vitamin E dans le traitment de l'acne, *Dermatologica,* 106, 197, 1953.

54. Dam, H., Kruse, I., Prange, I., and Sondergaard, E., Influence of dietary ascorbic acid, nordihydroguaiaretic acid, and cystine on vitamin E deficiency symptoms in chicks, *Biochim. Biophys. Acta,* 2, 501, 1948.

55. Dam, H., Kruse, I., Prange, I., and Sondergaard, E., Substances affording a partial protection against certain vitamin E deficiency symptoms, *Acta Physiol. Scand.,* 22, 299, 1951.

56. Das, D. K. and Engelman, R. M., Mechanisms of free radical generation during reperfusion of ischemic myocardium, in *Oxygen Radicals: Systemic Events and Disease Processes,* Das, D. K. and Essman, W. B., Eds., Karger, Basel, Switzerland, 1990, 97.

57. Davies, K. J. A., *Oxidative Damage and Repair: Clinical, Biological and Medical Aspects,* Pergamon Press, Tarrytown, N.Y., 1992.

58. De Cosse, J. J., Miller, H. H., and Lesser, M. L., Effect of wheat fiber and vitamins C and E on rectal polyps in patients with familial adenomatous polyposis, *J. Natl. Cancer Inst.,* 81, 1290, 1989.

59. Devi, A., Raina, P. L., and Singh, A., Abnormal protein and nucleic acid metabolism as a cause of cataract formation induced by nutritional deficiency in rabbits, *Br. J. Ophthamol.,* 49, 271, 1965.

60. Dieber-Rotheneder, M., Puhl, H., Waeg, G., Striegl, G., and Esterbauer, H., Effect of oral supplementation with D-alpha-tocopherol on the vitamin E content of human low density lipoproteins and resistance to oxidation, *J. Lipid Res.,* 32, 1325, 1991.

61. Diplock, A. T., Machlin, L. J., Packer, L., and Pryor, W. A., *Ann. N.Y. Acad. Sci.,* 570, 1, 1989.

62. Diplock, A. T., Cawthorne, M. A., Murrell, E. A., Green, J., and Bunyan, J., Measurements of lipid peroxidation and α-tocopherol destruction in vitro and in vivo and their significance in connexion with the biological function of vitamin E, *Br. J. Nutr.,* 22, 465, 1968.

63. DiSilvestro, R. A. and Carlson, G. P., Effects of mild zinc deficiency, plus or minus acute phase response on CCl$_4$ hepatotoxicity, *Free Rad. Biol. Med.,* 16, 57, 1994.

64. Dizdaroglu, M., Chemical determination of free radical-induced damage to DNA, *Free. Rad. Biol. Med.,* 10, 225, 1991.

65. Donaldson, W. E., Atherosclerosis in cholesterol-fed Japanese quail: evidence for amelioration by dietary vitamin E, *Poultry Sci.,* 61, 2097, 1982.

66. Dowling, E. J., Winrow, V. R., Merry, P., and Blake, D. R., Oxidants, joint inflammation, and anti-inflammatory strategies, in *Antioxidants in Therapy and Preventive Medicine,* Emerit, I., Packer, L., and Auclair, C., Eds., Plenum Press, New York, 1990, 463.

67. Draper, H. H., Goodyear, S., Barbee, K. K., and Johnson, B. C., A study of the nutritional role of antioxidants in the diet of the rat, *Brit. J. Nutr.,* 12, 89, 1958.

68. Dratz, E. A. and Jesaitis, A. J., *Molecular Basis of Oxidative Damage by Leukocytes,* CRC Press, Boca Raton, FL, 1992.

69. Dratz, E. A., Farnsworth, C. C., Loew, E. C., Stephens, R. J., Thomas, D. W., and van Kuijk, F. J. G. M., Products of in vivo peroxidation are present in tissues of vitamin E-deficient rats and dogs, *Ann. N.Y. Acad. Sci.,* 570, 46, 1989.

70. Ehrlich, H., Tarver, H., and Hunt, T., Inhibitory effects of vitamin E on collagen synthesis and wound repair, *Ann. Surg.,* 175, 235, 1972.

71. Ekiel, I. H., Hughes, L., Burton, G. W., Jovall, P. I., Ingold, K. U., and Smith, I. C. P., Structure and dynamics of α-tocopherol in model membranes and in solutions: a broadline and high resolution NMR study, *Biochemistry,* 27, 1432, 1988.

72. Emerit, I. and Chance, B., *Free Radicals and Aging,* Birkauser Verlag, Basel, Switzerland, 1992.

73. Emerit, I., Packer, L., and Auclair, C., *Antioxidants in Therapy and Preventive Medicine,* Plenum Press, New York, 1990.

74. Emerit, I., Reactive oxygen species, chromosome mutation and cancer: possible role of clastogenic factors in carcinogenesis, *Free Rad. Biol. Med.,* 16, 99, 1994.

75. Esterbauer, H., Dieber-Rotheneder, M., Striegl, G., and Waeg, G., Role of vitamin E in preventing the oxidation of low density lipoprotein, *Am. J. Clin. Nutr.,* 53, 314S, 1991.
76. Esterbauer, H., Jurgens, G., Quehenberger, O., and Koller, E., Autoxidation of human low density lipoprotein: loss of polyunsaturated fatty acids and vitamin E and generation of aldehydes, *J. Lipid. Res.,* 28, 495, 1987.
77. Esterbauer, H., Waeg, G., Puhl, H., Dieber-Rotheneder, M., and Tatzber, F., Inhibition of LDL oxidation by antioxidants, in *Free Radicals and Aging,* Emerit, I. and Chance, B., Eds., Birkhauser Verlag, Basel, Switzerland, 1992, 145.
78. Evans, H. M. and Bishop, K. S., On the existence of a hitherto unrecognized dietary factor essential for reproduction, *Science,* 56, 650, 1922.
79. Evans, H. M., Emerson, O. H., Emerson, G. A., Smith, L. I., Ungrade, H. E., Prickard, W. W., Austin, F. L., Hoehn, H. H., Opie, J. W., and Wawzonek, S., Chemistry of vitamin E. XII Specificity and relation between chemical structure and vitamin E activity, *J. Org. Chem.,* 4, 376, 1939.
80. Fahn, S., A pilot trial of high-dose alpha-tocopherol and ascorbate in early Parkinson's disease, *Ann. Neurol.,* 32, S128, 1992.
81. Farrell, P. M., Deficiency states, pharmacological effects and nutrient requirements, in *Vitamin E,* Maclin, L. J., Ed., Marcel Dekker, New York, 1980, 520.
82. Favreau, L. V. and Pickett, C. B., NAD(P)H: Quinone reductase gene which responds with increased transcriptional activity to metabolites of BHA, tert-butyl hydroquinone, TBHQ, also responds to BHT and ethoxyquin but not vitamin E, *J. Biol. Chem.,* 266, 4556, 1991.
83. Ferguson, T. M., Rigdon, R. H., and Couch, J. R., Cataracts in vitamin E deficiency, *Arch. Ophthamol.,* 55, 346, 1956.
84. Ferrari, R., Cecori, C., Curelli, S., Cargoni, A., Condorelli, E., and Raddino, R., Role of oxygen in ischemia and reperfusion damage: effect of tocopherol, *Vitaminol. Enzymol.,* 7, 61, 1988.
85. Ferriola, P. C., Cody, V., and Middleton, E. Jr., Protein kinase C inhibition by plant flavinoids: kinetic mechanisms and structure activity relationships, *Biochem. Pharmacol.,* 38, 1617, 1989.
86. Flohe, L., Superoxide dismutase for therapeutic use: clinical experience, dead ends and hopes, *Mol. Cell Biol.,* 84, 123, 1988.
87. Fraga, C. G., Shigenaga, M. K., Park, J.-W., Degan, P., and Ames, B. N., Oxidative damage to DNA during aging, 8-Hydroxy-2'-deoxyguanosine in rat organ DNA and urine, *Proc. Natl. Acad. Sci. U.S.A.,* 87, 4533, 1990.
88. Fraga, C. G., Motchnik, P. A., Shigenaga, M. K., Helbock, H. J., Jacob, R., and Ames, B. N., Ascorbic acid protects against endogenous oxidative DNA damage in human sperm, *Proc. Natl. Acad. Sci. U.S.A.,* 88, 11003, 1991.
89. Frei, B., Stocker, R., and Ames, B. N., Small molecule antioxidant defenses in human extracellular fluids, in *Molecular Biology of Free Radical Scavenging Systems,* Scandalios, J. G., Ed., Cold Spring Harbor Laboratory Press, Plainview, N.Y., 1992, 23.
90. Frei, B. Stocker, R., and Ames, B. N., Antioxidant defenses and lipid peroxidation in human blood plasma, *Proc. Natl. Acad. Sci. U.S.A.,* 85, 9748, 1988.
91. Freisleben, H. J., Beyersdorf, F., Assadnazari, H., Seewalt, X., Simon, J., Hanselmann, A., and Zimmer, G., Dihydrolipoic acid is protective against reperfusion injury, in *Lipid Soluble Antioxidants: Biochemistry and Clinical Applications,* Ong, A. S. H. and Packer, L., Eds., Birkhauser Verlag, Basel, Switzerland, 1992, 515.
92. Frey, J. G., Uber die kombintionsbehandlung von rontgenspatschaden der haut mit kurzwellen un vitamin E, *Strahlentherapie,* 95, 440, 1954.
93. Fridovich, I., The biology of oxygen radicals, *Science,* 201, 875, 1978.
94. Fridovich, I., Superoxide dismutase, *Ann. Rev. Biochem.,* 44, 147, 1975.
95. Fridovich, I., Oxygen radicals, hydrogen peroxide, and oxygen toxicity, in *Free Radicals in Biology,* Vol. 1, Pryor, W. A., Ed., Academic Press, New York, 1976, 239.
96. Friedman, G. D. and Selby, J. V., Epidemiological screening for potentially carcinogenic drugs, *Agents Actions,* 29 Suppl. 83, 1990.

97. Fuchs, J. and Packer, L., Vitamin E in dermatological therapy, in *Vitamin E in Health and Disease,* Packer, L. and Fuchs, J., Eds., Marcel Dekker, New York, 1993, 739.
98. Gardner, P. R. and Fridovich, I., Superoxide sensitivity of the *Escherichia coli* 6-phosphonogluconate dehydratase, *J. Biol. Chem.,* 266, 1478, 1991.
99. Gardner, P. R. and Fridovich, I., Superoxide sensitivity of the *Escherichia coli* aconitase, *J. Biol. Chem.,* 266, 19328, 1991.
100. Garlick, P. B., Davies, M. J., Hearse, D. J., and Slater, T. F., Direct detection of free radicals in the perfused heart using electron spin resonance, *Circ. Res.,* 61, 757, 1987.
101. Gey, K. F., Puska, P., Jordan, P., and Moser, U. K., Inverse correlation between plasma vitamin E and mortality from ischemic heart disease, *Am. J. Clin. Nutr.,* 53, 326S, 1991.
101a. Gey, K. F., Vitamin E and other essential antioxidants regarding coronary heart disease: risk assessment studies, in *Vitamin E in Health and Disease,* Packer, L. and Fuchs, J., Eds., Marcel Dekker, New York, 1993, 589.
102. Ghiselli, A., Serafini, M., and Ferro-Luzzi, A., New approaches for measuring plasma or serum antioxidant capacity: a methodological note, *Free Rad. Biol. Med.,* 16, 135, 1994.
102a. Granger, D. N., Role of xanthine oxidase and granulocytes in ischemia- reperfusion injury, *Am. J. Physiol.,* 255, H1269, 1988.
103. Green, E., Rice-Evans, D., Davies, M. J., Salah, N., Evans, H., and Rice-Evans, P., The efficacy of monohydroxamates as free radical scavenging agents compared with di- and tri-hydroxamates, *Biochem. Pharmacol.,* 45, 357, 1993.
104. Greenberg, J. T. and Demple, B., Overproduction of peroxide scavenging enzymes in *Escherichia coli* suppresses spontaneous mutagenesis and sensitivity to redox-cycling agents in OxyR-mutants, *EMBO J.,* 7, 2611, 1988.
105. Greenberg, E. R., Baron, J. A., Tosteson, T. D., Freemam, D. H. Jr., Beck, G. J., Bond, J. H., Collachio, T. A., Coller, J. A., Frankl, H. D., Haile, R. W., Mandel, J. S., Nierenberg, D. W., Rothstein, R., Snove, D. C., Stevens, M. M., Summers, R. W., and van Stolk, R. U., A clinical trial of antioxidant vitamins to prevent colorectal adenoma, *N. Engl. J. Med.,* 331, 141, 1994.
106. Greenwald, R., Superoxide dismutase and catalase as therapeutic agents for human disease, a critical review, *Free Rad. Biol. Med.,* 8, 201, 1990.
107. Gupta, P. P., Pandey, D. J., Sharma, Y. R., Srivastava, R. K., and Mishra, S. S., Prevention of experimental cataracts by alpha tocopherol, *Indian J. Exp. Biol.,* 22, 620, 1984.
108. Guyton, K. Z., Dolan, P. M., and Kensler, T. W., Quinone methide mediates in vitro induction of ornithine decarboxylase by the tumor promoter butylated hydroxytoluene hydroperoxide, *Carcinogenesis,* 15, 817, 1994.
109. Haberland, M. E., Fong, D., and Cheng, L., Malondialdehyde-altered protein occurs in atheroma of Watanabe heritable hyperlipidemic rabbits, *Science,* 241, 215, 1988.
110. Hadley, M. and Draper, H. H., Isolation of a guanine-malondialdehyde adduct from rat and human urine, *Lipids,* 25, 81, 1990.
111. Haegele, A. D., Briggs, S. P., and Thompsom, H. J., Antioxidant status and dietary lipid unsaturation modulate oxidative DNA damage, *Free Rad. Biol. Med.,* 16, 111, 1994.
112. Hall, E. D., Broughler, J. M., Yonkers, P. A., Smith, S. L., Linseman, K. l., Means, E. D., Scheich, H. F., Von Voightlander, P. F., Lahti, R. A., and Jacobsen, E. J., U78517F, A potent inhibitor of lipid peroxidation with activity in experimental brain injury and ischemia, *J. Pharm. Exper. Ther.,* 258, 686, 1991.
113. Halliwell, B. and Gutteridge, J. M. C., *Free Radicals in Biology and Medicine,* 2nd ed., Clarendon Press, Oxford, England, 1989.
114. Hanfstaengel, E., Zur behandlung der Dupuytrenscen Palmarfascienkontraktur mit vitamin E, *Med. Klin. Wochenschr.,* 373, 1951.
115. Harmon, E. M., Witting, L. A., and Horwitt, M. K., Relative rates of depletion of α-tocopherol and linoleic acid after feeding polyunsaturated fats, *Am. J. Clin. Nutr.,* 18, 243, 1966.
116. Hatchikian, E. C. and Henry, J. A., An iron containing superoxide dismutase from the strict anaerobe Desulfovibrio desulfuricans (Norway 4), *Biochimie,* 59, 153, 1977.

117. Heinonen, D. P. and Albanes, D., The effect of vitamin E and β-carotene on the incidence of lung cancer and other cancers in male smokers, *N. Engl. J. Med.,* 330, 1029, 1994.

118. Hennekens, C. H. and Gaziano, J. M., Antioxidants and heart disease: epidemiologic and clinical evidence, *Clin. Cardiol.,* Suppl. 16, 110, 1993.

119. Herbert, E. R., Hurley, T. G., Hsieh, J., Rogers, E., Stoddard, A. M., Sorensen, G., and Nicols, R. J., Determinants of plasma vitamins and lipids: the working well study, *Am. J. Epidem.,* 140, 132, 1994.

120. Hessler, J. R., Morel, D. W., Lewis, L. J., and Chisholm, G. M., Lipoprotein oxidation and liopoprotein-induced cytotoxicity, *Arteriosclerosis,* 3, 215, 1983.

121. Holman, R. T., Autoxidation of fats and related substances, in *Progress in the Chemistry of Fats and Other Lipids,* Vol. 2, Holman, R. T., Lundberg, W. O., and Malkin, T., Eds., Academic Press, New York, 1954, 51.

121a. Hoshino, E., Sahariff, R., Van Gossum, A., Allard, J. P., Pichard, C., Kurian, R., and Jeejeebhoy, K. N., Vitamin E suppresses increased lipid peroxidation in cigarette smokers, *J. Parenteral Enteral Nutr.,* 14, 300, 1990.

122. Huber, W., Orgotein — (bovine Cu-Zn, SOD) an anti-inflammatory protein drug: discovery, toxicology, and pharmacology, *Europ. J. Rheum. Inflamm.,* 4, 173, 1981.

123. Humad, S., Zarling, M., Clapper, M., and Skasey, J. L., Breath pentane excretions as a marker of disease activity in rheumatoid arthritis, *Free Rad. Res. Commun.,* 5, 101, 1986.

124. Imlay, J. A. and Fridovich, I., Assay of metabolic superoxide production in *Escerichia coli, J. Biol. Chem.,* 266, 6957, 1991.

125. Inai, K., Kobuke, T., Nambu, S. Takemoto, T., Kou, E., and Nishina, H., Hepatocellular tumorigenicity of butylated hydroxytoluene administered orally to B6C3F$_1$ mice, *Jap. J. Cancer Res.,* 79, 49, 1988.

126. Ito, N. and Hirose, M., The role of antioxidants in chemical carcinogenesis, *Jpn. J. Cancer Res.,* 78, 1011, 1987.

127. Ito, N., Hagiwara, A., Shibata, M., Ogiso, T., and Fukushima, S., Induction of squamous cell carcinoma in the forestomach of F344 rats with butylated hydroxyanisole, *Gann,* 73, 332, 1982.

128. Jacques, P. F. and Chylack, L. T. Jr., Epidemiologic evidence of a role for the antioxidant vitamins and carotenoids in cataract prevention, *Am. J. Clin. Nutr.,* 53, 352S, 1991.

129. Jialal, I. and Grundy, S. M., Effect of combined supplementation with alpha- tocopherol, ascorbate and beta-carotene on low-density lipoprotein oxidation, *Circulation,* 88, 2780, 1993.

130. Jialal, I. and Grudy, S. M., Influence of antioxidant vitamins on LDL oxidation, *Ann. N.Y. Acad. Sci.,* 669, 237, 1992.

131. Johnson, L., Bowen, F. W., Abasi, S., Herrmann, N., Weston, M., Sacks, L., Porat, R., Stahl, G., Peckham, G., and Delivori, M., The relationship of prolonged pharmacologic serum vitamin E levels to incidence of sepsis and necrotizing enterocolitis in infants with birth weight 1500 grams or less, *J. Pediatr.,* 75, 619, 1985.

132. Kagan, V. E., Serbinova, E. A., and Packer, L., Recycling and antioxidant activity of tocopherol homologs of differing chain length in liver microsomes, *Arch. Biochem. Biophys.,* 282, 221, 1990.

133. Kahl, R., Synthetic antioxidants: biochemical actions and interference with radiation, toxic compounds, chemical mutagens and chemical carcinogens, *Toxicology,* 33, 185, 1984.

134. Kahl, R., Butylated hydroxytoluene toxicity, in *Lipid Soluble Antioxidants: Biochemistry and Clinical Applications,* Ong, A. S. H. and Packer, L., Eds., Birkhauser Verlag, Basel, Switzerland, 1992, 590.

135. Kamimura, M., Antiinflammatory activity of vitamin E, *J. Vitaminol.,* 18, 204, 1972.

136. Kappus, H. and Kahl, R., Comparative toxicology of BHA, BHT and vitamin E, in *Antioxidants, Free Radicals and Polyunsaturated Fatty Acids in Biology and Medicine,* Diplock, A. T., Gutteridge, J. M. C., and Shukla, V. K. S., Eds., International Food Science Center, Lystrup, Denmark, 1993, 73.

137. Kensler, T. W., Egner, P. A., Trudh, M. A., Bueding, E., and Groopman, J. D., Modification of aflatoxin B_1 binding to DNA in vivo in rats fed phenolic antioxidants, ethoxyquin, and a dithiolthione, *Carcinogenesis,* 6, 759, 1985.

138. King, J. C. and the Food and Nutrition Board, How should the recommended dietary allowance be revised? A concept paper from the Food and Nutrition Board, *Nutr. Rev.,* 52, 216, 1994.

139. Kitabchi, A. E., McCay, P. B., Carpenter, M. P., Feinberg, R. H., Trucco, R. E., and Caputto, R., The site of inhibition of ascorbic acid synthesis by liver preparations from rats deprived of vitamin E, *Biochem. Biophys. Res. Commun.,* 1, 216, 1959.

140. Klatskin, G. and Molander, D. W., The chemical determination of tocopherols in feces and the fecal excretion of tocopherol in man, *J. Lab. Clin. Med.,* 39, 802, 1952.

141. Kneepkens, C. M. F., Lepage, G., and Ray, C. V., The potential of the hydrocarbon breath test as a measure of lipid peroxidation, *Free Rad. Biol. Med.,* 17, 127, 1994.

142. Knekt, P., Epidemiology of vitamin E: evidence for anticancer effects in humans, in *Vitamin E in Health and Disease,* Packer, L. and Fuchs, J., Eds., Marcel Dekker, New York, 1993, 513.

143. Kolarz, G., Scherak, O., Shouhoumi, M. E. L., and Blankenhorn, G., Hochdosierte vitamin E bei chronischer polyarthritis, *Akt. Rheumatol,* 15, 233, 1990.

144. Kono, Y. and Fridovich, I., Superoxide radical inhibits catalase, *J. Biol. Chem.,* 257, 5751, 1982.

145. Krinsky, N. I., The protective function of carotenoid pigments, *Photophysiology,* 3, 123, 1968.

146. Kuzuya, M. and Kuzuya, F., Probucol as an antioxidant and antiatherogenic drug, *Free Rad. Biol. Med.,* 14, 67, 1993.

147. Lapidot, A. and Irving, C. S., The electronic structure of coordinated iron, in *Molecular Oxygen in Biology,* Hayaishi, O., Ed., North-Holland, Amsterdam, 1974, 33.

148. Lawrence, R. A. and Burk, R. F., Species, tissue, and subcellular distribution of non Se-dependent glutathione peroxidase, *J. Nutr.,* 108, 211, 1978.

149. Lawrence, R. A. and Burk, R. F., Glutathione peroxidase activity in selenium deficient rat liver, *Biochem. Biophys. Res. Commun.,* 71, 952, 1976.

150. Lee, K., Caniff, P., Hamel, D., Silver, P., and Ezrion, A., Trolox but not superoxide dismutase or ascorbic acid limits myocardial infarction in dogs, *Clin. Pharmacol. Ther.,* 47(2), 174, 1990.

151. LeGardeur, B. Y., Lopez, S. A., and Johnson, W. D., A case-control study of serum vitamins A, E, and C in lung cancer patients, *Nutr. Cancer,* 14, 133, 1990.

152. Leske, M. C., Chylack, L. T., and Wu, S. Y., The lens opacities case-control study: risk factors in cataracts, *Arch. Ophthalmol.,* 109, 244, 1991.

153. Leth, T. and Sondergaard, H., Biological activity of vitamin E compounds and natural materials by the resorption-gestation test and chemical determination of vitamin E activity in food and feeds, *J. Nutr.,* 107, 2236, 1977.

154. Link, P. and Dreher, R. D., D-α-Tocopherol acetate (vitamin E) versus Diclofenac-Na in der therapie der aktivierten arthrose, *Dtsch. Artzemagazin,* 22, 48, 1990.

155. Liochev, S. I. and Fridovich, I., Superoxide Radical in *Escherichia coli,* in *Molecular Biology of Free Radical Scavenging Systems,* Scandalios, J. G., Ed., Cold Spring Harbor Laboratory Press, Plainview, NY, 1992, 213.

156. Liochev, S. I. and Fridovich, I., The role of $O_2{}^-$ in the production of HO in vitro and in vivo, *Free Rad. Biol. Med.,* 16, 29, 1994.

157. Lohr, J. R., Cadet, J. L., Lohr, M. A., Jeste, D. V., and Wyatt, R. J., Alpha tocopherol in tardive dyskinesia, *Lancet,* 1, 913, 1987.

158. Losowsky, M. S., Kelleher, J., Walker, B. E., Davies, T., and Smith, C. L., Intake and absorption of tocopherol, *Ann. N.Y. Acad. Sci.,* 203, 212, 1972.

159. Lundberg, W. O., *Autoxidation and Antioxidants,* Vol. I, Interscience, New York, 1961.

160. Lunec, J., Halloran, S. P., White, A. G., and Dormandy, T. L., Free radical oxidation (peroxidation) products in serum and synovial fluid in RA, *J. Rheum.,* 8, 233, 1981.

161. Machlin, L. J. and Gordon, R. S., Linoleic acid as a causative agent of encephalomalacia, *Proc. Soc. Exptl. Biol. Med.,* 103, 659, 1960.

162. Mahoney, C. V. and Azzi, A., Vitamin E inhibits protein kinase C activity, *Biochem. Biophys. Res. Commun.,* 154, 694, 1988.

163. Marks, J., Critical appraisal of the therapeutic value of α-tocopherol, *Vitam. Horm.,* 20, 574, 1962.

164. Mason, K., Distribution of vitamin E in the tissues of the rat, *J. Nutr.,* 23, 71, 1942.

165. Masui, T., Hirose, M., Imaida, K., Fukushima, S., Tamano, S., and Ito, N., Sequential changes in the forestomach of F344 rats, Syrian golden hamsters, and B6C3F$_1$ mice treated with butylated hydroxyanisole, *Jpn. J. Cancer. Res.,* 77, 1083, 1986.

166. Matkovics, B., Karmazsin, L., and Kalasz, H., *Radicals, Ions and Tissue Damage,* Academiai Kaido, Budapest, Hungary, 1990.

167. Mattill, H. A. and Conklin, R. E., The nutritional properties of milk with special reference to reproduction in the albino rat, *J. Biol. Chem.,* 44, 137, 1920.

168. McCay, P. B., Gibson, D. D., Fong, K.-L., and Hornbrook, K. R., Effect of glutathione peroxidase activity on lipid peroxidation in biological membranes, *Biochim. Biophys. Acta,* 431, 459, 1976.

169. McCay, P. B., Bruggemann, G., Lai, E. K., and Powell, S. R., Evidence that alpha-tocopherol functions cyclically to quench free radicals in hepatic microsomes, *Ann. N.Y. Acad. Sci.,* 570, 32, 1989.

170. McCay, P. B., Poyer, J. L., Pfeifer, P. M., May, H. E., and Gillian, J. M., A function of α-tocopherol: stabilization of the microsomal membrane from attack during TPNH dependent oxidations, *Lipids,* 6, 297, 1971.

171. McCord, J. M., Keele, B. B. Jr., and Fridovich, I., An enzyme based theory of obligate anaerobiosis: the physiological function of superoxide dismutase, *Proc. Natl. Acad. Sci. U.S.A.,* 68, 1024, 1971.

172. McCord, J. M. and Fridovich, I., Superoxide dismutase: an enzyme function for erythrocuprein (hemocuprein), *J. Biol. Chem.,* 244, 6049, 1969.

172a. McCord, J. M., Roy, R. S., and Schaeffer, S. W., Free radicals and myocardial ischemia: the role of xanthine oxidase, *Adv. Myocardiology,* 5, 183, 1985.

173. McKeown-Eyssen, G., Holloway, C., Jazmajr, V., Bright-See, E., Dion, P., and Bruce, W. R., A randomized trial of vitamins C and E in the prevention of recurrance of colorectal polyps, *Cancer Res.,* 48, 4701, 1988.

174. Mehta, P. M., Przyklenk, K., and Kloner, R. R., Cardioprotective effects of Captopril in myocardial ischemia, ischemia/reperfusion, and infarction, *Eur. Heart J.,* 11, 94, 1990.

175. Menkes, M. S., Comstock, G. W., Vuilleumier, J. P., Helsing, K. J., Rider, A. A., and Brookmeyer, R., Serum beta-carotene, vitamins A and E, selenium, and the risk of cancer, *N. Engl. J. Med.,* 315, 1250, 1986.

176. Meydani, S. N., Hayek, M., and Coleman, L., Influence of vitamins E and B$_6$ on immune response, *Ann. N.Y. Acad. Sci.,* 669, 125, 1992.

177. Meydani, M., Natiello, F., Goldin, B., Woods, M., Schaefer, E., Blumberg, J. B., and Gorbach, S. L., Effect of long-term fish oil supplementation on vitamin E status and lipid peroxidation in women, *J. Nutr.,* 121, 484, 1991.

178. Mickle, D. A. G., Weisel, R. D., Burton, G. W., and Ingold, K. U., Effect of orally administered α-tocopheryl acetate on human myocardial α-tocopherol levels, *Cardiovasc. Drugs Ther.,* 5, 309, 1991.

179. Miquel, J., Quintanilha, A. I., and Wber, H., *CRC Handbook of Free Radicals and Antioxidants in Biomedicine,* CRC Press, Boca Raton, FL, 1989.

180. Mitodiewa, D. and Dunfield, H. B., The reaction of horseradish peroxidase, lactoperoxidase, and myeloperoxidase with enzymatically generated superoxide, *Arch. Biochem. Biophys.,* 272, 245, 1989.

181. Morel, D. W., Hessler, J. R., and Chisholm, G. M., Low density lipoprotein cytotoxicity induced by free radical peroxidation of lipid, *J. Lipid. Res.,* 24, 1070, 1983.

182. Morel, D. W., Di Corleto, P. E., and Chisholm, G. M., Endothelial and smooth muscle cells alter low density lipoproteins in vitro by free radical oxidation, *Arteriosclerosis,* 4, 357, 1984.

183. Mori, A., Yokoi, I., and Kabuto, H., Effects of vitamin E and its derivative in post traumatic epilepsy and seizures, in *Vitamin E in Health and Disease,* Packer, L. and Fuchs, J., Eds., Marcel Dekker, New York, 1993, 851.

184. Mulholland, C. W. and Strain, J. J., Effect of antioxidant vitamin supplementation on peroxyl radical trapping ability of plasma, *Proc. Nutr. Soc.,* 50, 133A, 1991.

185. Muller, A., Cadenas, E., Graf, P., and Sies, H. A., A novel biologically-active selenoorganic compound 1. Glutathione peroxidase activity in vitro and antioxidant capacity of PZ 51 (Ebselen), *Biochem. Pharmacol.,* 33, 3235, 1984.

186. Newberne, P. M., Bresnahan, M. R., and Kula, N. J., Effects of two synthetic antioxidants, vitamin E and ascorbic acid on the choline deficient rat, *J. Nutr.,* 97, 219, 1969.

187. Niki, E., Tsuchiya, J., Tanimura, R., and Kamiya, Y., Regeneration of vitamin E from α-chromanoxy radical by glutathione and vitamin C, *Chem. Lett.,* 789, 1982.

188. Nomura, A. N.Y., Stemmermann, G. N., Heilbrun, L. K., Salkeld, R. M., and Vuilleumier, J. P., Serum vitamin levels and the risk of cancer of specific sites in men of Japanese ancestry in Hawaii, *Cancer. Res.,* 45, 2369, 1985.

189. Ogunmekan, A. O., Vitamin E deficiency and seizures in animals and man, *Can. J. Neurol.,* 6, 43, 1979.

190. Ogunmekan, A. O. and Hwang, P. A., A randomized double-blind placebo controlled clinical trial of D-α-tocopheryl acetate (vitamin E) as add-on therapy for epilepsy in children, *Epilepsia,* 30, 84, 1989.

191. Olcott, H. S. and Emerson, O. H., Antioxidants and the autoxidation of fats. IX. Antioxidant properties of the tocopherols, *J. Am. Chem. Soc.,* 59, 1008, 1937.

192. Olsen, P., Meyer, O., Billie, N., and Wurtzen, G., Carcinogenicity study on butylated hydroxytoluene in Wistar rats exposed in utero, *Food Chem. Toxicol.,* 24, 1, 1986.

193. Ong, A. S. H. and Packer, L., *Lipid Soluble Antioxidants: Biochemistry and Clinical Applications,* Birkauser Verlag, Basel, Switzerland, 1992.

194. Packer, L. and Fuchs, J., *Vitamin E in Health and Disease,* Marcel Dekker, New York, 1992.

195. Packer, L., Prilipko, L., and Christen, Y., *Free Radicals in the Brain,* Springer Verlag, Heidelberg, Germany, 1992.

196. Packer, L., Maguire, J. J., Melhorn, R. J., Serbinova, E. A., and Kagan, V. E., Mitochondria and microsomal membranes have a free radical reductase activity that prevents chromanoxyl radical accumulation, *Biochem. Biophys. Res. Commun.,* 159, 229, 1989.

197. Packer, L., New horizons in vitamin E research — the vitamin E cycle, biochemistry, and clinical applications, in *Lipid Soluble Antioxidants: Biochemistry and Clinical Applications,* Ong, A. S. H. and Packer, L., Eds., Birkhauser, Verlag, Basel, Switzerland, 1992, 1.

198. Packer, L., Vitamin E, physical exercise, and tissue damage in animals, *Med. Biol.,* 62, 105, 1984.

199. Parkinson Study Group, Effects of tocopherol and Deprenyl on the progression of disability in early Parkinson's disease, *N. Engl. J. Med.,* 328, 176, 1993.

200. Parnham, A. J. and Graf, E., Selenoorganic compounds and the therapy of hydroperoxide-linked pathological conditions, *Biochem. Pharmacol.,* 36, 3095, 1987.

201. Parthasarathy, S., Young, S. G., Witztum, J. L., Pittman, R. C., and Steinberg, D., Probucol inhibits oxidative modification of low density lipoprotein, *J. Clin. Invest.,* 77, 641, 1986.

202. Pascher, F., Sawicky, H. H., Mabel, M. D., Silverberg, M. G., Braitman, M., and Kanof, N. B., Therapeutic assays of the skin and cancer unit of the New York Universities hospitals, Assay V. Tocopherols (vitamin E) for discoid lupus erythematosus and other dermatoses, *J. Invest. Dermatol.,* 17, 261, 1951.

203. Pearson, C. K. and Barnes, M. McC., Absorption of tocopherols by small intestinal loops of the rat in vivo, *Int. Z. Vitaminforsch.,* 40, 19, 1970.

204. Perly, B., Smith, I. C. P., Hughes, L., Burton, G. W., and Ingold, K. U., Estimation of the location of α-tocopherol by ¹³C-NMR spectroscopy, *Biochim. Biophys. Acta,* 819, 131, 1985.

205. Phelps, D. L., Rosenbaum, A. L., Isenberg, S. J., Leake, R. D., and Darcy, F. J., Tocopherol efficacy and safety for preventing retinopathy of prematurity: a randomized, controlled, double-masked trial, *Pediatrics,* 79, 489, 1987.

206. Poli, G., Albano, E., and Dianzani, M. U., *Free Radicals from Basic Science to Medicine,* Birkhauser Verlag, Basel, Switzerland, 1993.

207. Rabl, H., Khoschsorur, G., Colombo, T., Peritsch, P., Rauchenwald, M., Koltringer, P., Tatzber, F., and Esterbauer, H., A multivitamin infusion prevents lipid peroxidation and improves transplantation performance, *Kidney Int.,* 43, 912, 1993.

208. Ramasastray, S. S., Angel, M. F., Narayanan, K., Basford, R. A., and Futrell, J. W., Biochemical evidence of lipoperoxidation in venous stasis ulcer: beneficial role of vitamin E as antioxidant, *Ann. N.Y. Acad. Sci.,* 570, 56, 1989.

209. Reaven, P. D., Khouw, A., Beltz, W. F., Parthasarathy, S., and Witztum, J. L., Effect of dietary antioxidant combinations in humans. Protection of LDL by vitamin E but not by beta-carotene, *Aterioscler. Thromb.,* 13, 590, 1993.

210. Richter, C., Park, J.-W., and Ames, B. N., Normal oxidative damage to mitochondrial and nuclear DNA is extensive, *Proc. Natl. Acad. Sci. U.S.A.,* 85, 6465, 1988.

211. Rimm, E. B., Stampfer, M. J., Ascherio, A., Giovannuci, E., Colditz, G. A., and Willett, W. C., Vitamin E consumption and the risk of coronary heart disease in men, *N. Engl. J. Med.,* 328, 1450, 1993.

212. Robertson, J. McD., Donner, A. P., and Trevithick, J. R., A possible role for vitamins C and E in cataract prevention, *Am. J. Clin. Nutr.,* 53, 346S, 1991.

213. Robertson, J. McD., Donner, A. P., and Trevithick, J. R., Vitamin E intake and risk of cataracts in humans, *Ann. N.Y. Acad. Sci.,* 570, 372, 1989.

214. Romaschin, A. D., Rebyka, I., Wilson, G. J., and Mickle, D. A. G., Conjugated dienes in ischemia and reperfused myocardium: an in vivo signature of oxygen free radical mediated injury, *J. Mol. Cell Cardiol.,* 19, 289, 1987.

215. Roncucci, L., Di Donato, P., Carati, L., Ferrari, A., Perini, M., Bertoni, G., Paris, B., Svanoni, F., and Girola, M., Antioxidant vitamins or lactulose for the prevention of the recurrence of colorectal adenomas, *Dis. Colon Rectum.,* 36, 227, 1993.

216. Rosenfield, M. E., Palinski, W., Yla-Herttuala, S., Butler, S., and Witztun, J. L., Distribution of oxidation specific lipid-protein adducts of apolipoprotein B in atherosclerotic lesions of varying severity from WHHL rabbits, *Arteriosclerosis,* 10, 336, 1990.

217. Ross, W. M., Creighton, M. O., Stewart-DeHaas, P. J., Sanwal, M., Hirst, M., and Trevithick, J. R., Modelling cataractogenesis. 3. In vivo effects of vitamin E on cataractogenesis in diabetic rats, *Can. J. Ophthalmol.,* 17, 61, 1982.

218. Rowley, D. A. and Halliwell, B., DNA damage by superoxide-generating systems in relation to the mechanism of action of the anti-tumor antibiotic adriamycin, *Biochim. Biophys. Acta,* 761, 86, 1983.

219. Rowley, G., Gutteridge, J. M. C., Blake, D. R. Farr, M., and Halliwell, B., Lipid peroxidation in RA, thiobarbituric acid reactive material and catalytic iron salts in synovial fluid from rheumatoid patients, *Clin. Sci.,* 66, 691, 1984.

220. Salonen, J. T., Salonen, R., Lappetelainen, R., Maenpaa, P. H., Alfthan, G., and Pusksa, P., Risk of cancer in relation to serum concentrations of selenium and vitamins A and E: matched case-control analysis of prospective data, *Br. Med. J.,* 290, 417, 1985.

221. Samuel, D. and Steckel, F., The physico-chemical properties of oxygen, in *Molecular Oxygen in Biology,* Hayaishi, O., Ed., North-Holland, Amsterdam, The Netherlands, 1974.

222. Sanders, T. A. B. and Hinds, A., The influence of a fish oil high in docosahexaenoic acid on plasma lipoprotein and vitamin E concentrations and hemostatic function in healthy male volunteers, *Brit. J. Nutr.,* 68, 163, 1992.

223. Sauberlich, H. E. and Maclin, L. J., Beyond deficiency: new views on the function and health effects of vitamins, *Ann. New York Acad. Sci.,* 669, 1, 1992.

224. Sawyer, D. I. and Valentine, J. S., How super is superoxide?, *Acc. Chem. Res.,* 14, 393, 1981.
225. Scandalios, J. G., *Molecular Biology of Free Radical Scavenging Systems,* Cold Spring Harbor Laboratory Press, Plainview, N.Y., 1992.
226. Scandalios, J. G., The antioxidant enzymes genes CAT and SOD of maize: regulation, functional significance, and molecular biology, *Isozymes: Curr. Top. Biol. Med. Res.,* 14, 19, 1987.
227. Schade, W., Zur therapie der psoriasis vulgaris, *Hautarzt.,* 3, 373, 1952.
228. Scherak, O., Kolarz, G., Schodl, C., and Blankenhorn, G., Hochdosierte vitamin E therapie bei patienten mit aktivierter arthrose, *Z. Rheumatol.,* 49, 369, 1990.
229. Schmidt, K. H. and Bayer, W., Efficacy of vitamin E as a drug in inflammatory diseases, in *Antioxidants in Therapy and Preventive Medicine,* Emerit, I., Packer, L., and Auclair, C., Eds., Plenum Press, New York, 1990, 147.
230. Schuckett, R., Brigelius-Fluhe, R., Maiorino, M., Riveri, A., Reumkens, J., Straburger, W., Wolf, B., and Flohe, L., Phospholipid hydroperoxide glutathione peroxidase is a selenoenzyme distinct from the classical glutathione peroxidase as evident from cDNA and amino acid sequencing, *Free Rad. Res. Commun.,* 14, 343, 1991.
231. Scott, G., *Atmospheric Oxidation and Antioxidants,* Vol. 3. Elsevier Science Publishers, Amsterdam, The Netherlands, 1993.
232. Serbinova, E. A., Kagan, V. E., Han, D., and Packard, L., Free radical recycling and intramembrane mobility in the antioxidant properties of α-tocopherol and α-tocotrienol, *Free Rad. Biol. Med.,* 10, 263, 1991.
233. Sharma, M. K. and Buettner, G. R., Interaction of vitamin C and vitamin E during free radical stress in plasma: an ESR study, *Free Rad. Biol. Med.,* 14, 649, 1993.
234. Shklar, G., Schwartz, J. L., Trickler, D. P., and Reid, S., Prevention of experimental cancer and immunostimulation by vitamin E (immunosurveillance), *J. Oral Pathol. Med.,* 19, 60, 1990.
235. Shklar, G., Schwartz, J. L., Trickler, D. P., and Niukian, K., Regression by vitamin E of experimental oral cancer, *J. Natl. Cancer Inst.,* 78, 987, 1987.
236. Shute, W. E., *Health Preserver,* Roedale Press, Emmaus, Pa, 1977.
237. Simic, M. G., Taylor, K. A., Ward, J. F., and Sonntag, C., *Oxygen Radicals in Biology and Medicine,* Plenum Press, New York, 1988.
238. Slaga, T. and Bracken, W., The effects of antioxidants on skin tumor initiation and aryl hydrocarbon hydroxylase, *Cancer Res.,* 37, 1631, 1977.
239. Smith, T. L. and Kummerow, F. A., Effect of vitamin E on plasma lipids and atherogenesis in restricted ovulatory chickens, *Atherosclerosis,* 75, 105, 1989.
240. Simon-Schnass, I. and Pabst, H., Influence of vitamin E on physical performance, *Int. J. Vitam. Nutr. Res.,* 58, 49, 1988.
241. Sokol, R. J., Kayden, H. J., Bettis, D. B., Traber, M. G., Neville, H., Ringle, S., Wilson, W. B., and Stump, D. A., Isolated vitamin E deficiency in the absence of fat malabsorption — familial and sporadic cases: characterization and investigation of causes, *J. Lab. Clin. Med.,* 111, 548, 1988.
242. Sparrow, C. P., Doebber, T. W., Diszewski, J., Wu, M. S., Ventre, J., Stevens, K. A., and Chao, Y., Low density lipoprotein is protected from oxidation and the progression of atherosclerosis is slowed in cholesterol fed rabbits by the antioxidant N,N'-diphenyl-*p*-phenylenediamine, *J. Clin. Invest.,* 89, 1885, 1992.
243. Spatz, L. and Bloom, A. D., *Biological Consequences of Oxidative Stress: Implications for Cardiovascular Disease and Carcinogenesis,* Oxford University Press, New York, 1992.
243a. Speer, M. E., Blifeld, C., Rudolph, A. J., Chadda, P., Holbein, M. E. B., and Hittner, H. M., Intraventricular haemorrhage and vitamin E in the very low-birth-weight infant: evidence for efficacy of early intramuscular vitamin administration, *Pediatrics,* 74, 1107, 1984.
244. Stahelin, H. B., Rosel, F., Buess, E., and Brubacher, G., Cancer, vitamins, and plasma lipids: prospective Basel study, *J. Natl. Cancer Inst.,* 73, 1463, 1984.

245. Stahelin, H. B., Gey, K. F., Eichholzer, M., Ludin, E., and Brubacher, G., Cancer mortality and vitamin E status, *Ann. N.Y. Acad. Sci.*, 570, 391, 1989.

246. Stampfer, M. J., Hennekens, C. H., Manson, J. E., Colditz, G. A., Rosner, B., and Willett, W. C., Vitamin E consumption and the risk of coronary disease in women, *N. Engl. J. Med.*, 328, 1444, 1993.

247. Steinberg, D., Parthasarathy, S., Carew, T. E., Khoo, J. C., and Witztum, J. L., Beyond cholesterol. Modifications of low-density lipoprotein that increase its atherogenicity, *N. Engl. J. Med.*, 320, 915, 1989.

248. Steinberg, D., Antioxidants and atherosclerosis: a current assessment, *Circulation,* 84, 1420, 1991.

249. Steinbrecher, U. P., Parthasarathy, S., Leake, D. S., Witztum, J. L., and Steinberg, D., Modification of low density lipoprotein by endothelial cells involves lipid peroxidation and degradation of low density lipoprotein phospholipids, *Proc. Natl. Acad. Sci. U.S.A.*, 83, 3883, 1984.

250. Steinbrecher, U. P., Oxidation of human low density lipoprotein results in derivatization of lysine residues of apolipoprotein B by lipid peroxide decomposition products, *J. Biol. Chem.*, 262, 3603, 1987.

251. Strain, J. J. and Mulholland, C. W., Vitamin C and vitamin E — synergistic interactions in vivo?, in *Free Radicals and Aging,* Emerit, I. and Chance, B., Eds., Birkhauser Verlag, Basel, Switzerland, 1992, 419.

252. Suzuki, Y. J. and Ford, G. D., Mathematical model supporting the superoxide theory of oxygen toxicity, *Free Rad. Biol. Med.*, 16, 63, 1994.

253. Taffe, B. G. and Kensler, T. W., Tumor promotion by a hydroperoxide metabolite of butylated hydroxytoluene, 2,6-di-*tert*-butyl-4-hydroperoxyl-4-methyl- 2,5- cyclohexadienone in mouse skin, *Res. Commun. Clin. Pathol. Pharmacol.*, 61, 291, 1988.

254. Tappel, A. L. and Dillard, C. J., In vivo lipid peroxidation: measurement via exhaled pentane and protection by vitamin E, *Fed. Proc.*, 40, 174, 1981.

255. Tarr, M. and Samson, P., *Oxygen Free Radicals and Tissue Injury,* Birkhauser Verlag, Basel, Switzerland, 1993.

256. Taylor, A., Effect of photoxidation on the eye lens and role of nutrients in delaying cataract, in *Free Raicals and Aging,* Emerit, I. and Chance, B., Eds., Birkhauser Verlag, Basel, Switzerland, 1992, 266.

257. Temple, N. J. and El-Khabib, S. M., Cabbage and vitamin E: their effect on colon tumor formation in mice, *Cancer Lett.*, 35, 71, 1987.

258. Thomas, M. J., Mehl, K. S., and Pryor, W. A., The role of superoxide anion in the xanthine oxidase-induced autoxidation of linoleic acid, *Biochem. Biophys. Res. Commun.*, 83, 927, 1978.

259. Traber, M. G. and Kaydan, H. J., α-Tocopherol as compared with γ-tocopherol is preferentially secreted in human lipoproteins, *Ann. N.Y. Acad. Sci.*, 570, 95, 1989.

260. Traber, M. G., Determinants of plasma vitamin E concentrations, *Free Rad. Biol. Med.*, 16, 229, 1994.

261. Traber, M. G., Sokol, R. J., Burton, G. W., Ingold, K. U., Papas, A. M., Huffaker, J. E., and Kayden, H. J., Impaired ability of patients with familial isolated vitamin E deficiency to incorporate α-tocopherol in lipoproteins secreted by the liver, *J. Clin. Invest.*, 85, 397, 1990.

262. Trevithick, J. R., Robertson, J. McD., and Mitton, K. P., Vitamin E and the eye, in *Vitamin E in Health and Disease,* Packer, L. and Fuchs, J., Eds., Marcel Dekker, New York, 1993, 873.

263. Tuati, D., The molecular genetics of superoxide dismutase in *E. coli, Free Rad. Res. Commun.*, 8, 1, 1989.

264. Uri, N., Mechanism of autoxidation, in *Autoxidation and Antioxidants,* Vol. 1, Lundberg, W. O., Ed., Interscience, New York, 1961, 133.

265. van Kuijk, F. J. G. M., Servanian, A., Handelman, G. J., and Dratz, E. A., A new role for phospholipase A_2: protection of membranes from lipid peroxidation damage, *Trends Biochem Sci.*, 12, 31, 1987.

266. Varma, S. D., Chand, D., Sharma, Y. R., Kuck, J. F., and Richards, R. D., Oxidative stress on lens and cataract formation: role of light and oxygen, *Curr. Eye Res.*, 3, 35, 1984.

267. Varma, S. D., Scientific basis for medical therapy of cataracts by antioxidants, *Am. J. Clin. Nutr.*, 53, 335S, 1991.

268. Verlangieri, A. J. and Bush, M. J., Effects of *d*-alpha-tocopherol supplementation on experimentally-induced primate atherosclerosis, *J. Am. Coll. Nutr.*, 11, 130, 1992.

269. Vigo-Pelfrey, C., *Membrane Lipid Oxidation,* Vol. II, CRC Press, Boca Raton, FL, 1991.

270. Wald, N. J., Thompson, S. G., Densem, J. W., Boreham, J., and Bailey A., Serum vitamin E and subsequent risk of cancer, *Br. J. Cancer*, 56, 69, 1987.

271. Wattenberg, L. W., Chemoprevention of cancer, *Cancer Res.*, 45, 1, 1985.

272. Welsh, A. L., Lupus erythematosus, *Arch. Dermatol.*, 70, 181, 1954.

273. Westlin, W. and Mallanc, K., Does Captopril attenuate reperfusion-induced myocardial dysfunction by scavenging free radicals, *Circulation,* 77 Suppl. 1, 1, 1988.

274. Wheldon, G. H., Bhatt, A., Keller, P., and Hummler, H., Alpha tocopheryl acetate (vitamin E): a long term toxicity and carcinogenicity study in rats, *Int. J. Vitam. Res.*, 53, 287, 1983.

275. Williams, D. M., Lynch, R. E., Lee, G. E., and Cartwright, G. E., Superoxide dismutase in copper deficient swine, *Proc. Soc. Exp. Biol. Med.*, 149, 534, 1975.

276. Williams, G. M., Maeura, Y., and Weisburger, J. H., Simultaneous inhibition of liver carcinogenicity and enhancement of bladder carcinogenicity of N-2-fluorenylacetamide by butylated hydroxytoluene, *Cancer Lett.*, 19, 55, 1983.

277. Williams, R. J., Motteram, J. M., Sharp, C. H., and Gallagher, P. J., Dietary vitamin E and the attenuation of early lesion development in modified Watanabe rabbits, *Atherosclerosis,* 94, 153, 1992.

278. Willingham, A. K., Bolanos, C., Bohannon, E., and Cendella, R. J., The effects of high levels of vitamin E on the progression of atherosclerosis in the Watanabe heritable hyperlipidemic rabbit, *J. Nutr. Biochem.*, 4, 651, 1993.

279. Wiss, O., Bunnell, R. H., and Gloor, U., Absorption and distribution of vitamin E in the tissues, *Vitam. Horm.*, 20, 441, 1962.

280. Witting, L. A., Vitamin E and lipid antioxidants in free-radical initiated reactions, in *Free Radicals in Biology,* Vol. IV, Pryor, W. A., Ed., Academic Press, New York, 1980, 295.

281. Witting, L. A. and Horwitt, M. K., Effect of degree of fatty acid unsaturation in tocopherol deficiency-induced creatinuria, *J. Nutr.*, 82, 19, 1964.

282. Witting, L. A., The oxidation of α-tocopherol during the autoxidation of ethyl oleate, linoleate, linolenate, and arachidonate, *Arch. Biochem. Biophys.*, 129, 142, 1969.

283. Witting, L. A., The effect of antioxidant deficiency on tissue lipid composition in the rat, IV. Peroxidation and interconversion of polyunsaturated fatty acids in muscle phospholipids, *Lipids,* 2, 109, 1967.

284. Witting, L. A., The interrelationship of polyunsaturated fatty acids and antioxidants in vivo, *Prog. Chem. Fats Lipids,* 9, 519, 1970.

285. Wu, T.-W., Hashimoto, N., Au, J-W., Mickle, D. A. G., and Carey, D., Trolox protects rat hepatocytes against oxyradical damage and the ischemic rat liver from reperfusion injury, *Hepatolgy,* 13, 575, 1991.

286. Yamamoto, K., Tajima, K., and Mizatani, T., The acute toxicity of butylated hydroxytoluene and its metabolites in mice, *Toxicol. Lett.*, 6, 173, 1980.

287. Yoshikawa, T., Tanaka, H., and Kondo, M., Effect of vitamin E on adjuvant arthritis in rats, *Biochem. Med.*, 29, 277, 1983.

288. Zigler, J. S. and Hess, H. H., Cataracts in the Royal College of Surgeons rat: evidence for initiation by peroxidation products, *Exp. Eye Res.*, 41, 67, 1985.

289. Zimmer, G. and Evers, J., 2-Mercaptopropionylglycine improves aortic flow after reoxygenation in working rat hearts, *Basic Res. Cardiol.*, 83, 445, 1988.

290. Zweig, J. E., Measurement of superoxide derived free radicals in the reperfused heart, *J. Biol. Chem.*, 263, 1353, 1988.

Chapter 8

SELENIUM: DO WE DARE NEGLECT IT?

John A. Milner

CONTENTS

0-8493-7849-4/95/$0.00+$.50

I. INTRODUCTION

Selenium, first discovered by Jones Jacob Berzelius in 1818, is positioned between arsenic and bromine in the periodic table. It is also positioned in the IVB group of elements and thus shares characteristics with oxygen, sulfur, tellurium, and polonium. Selenium has an atomic number of 34 and has an atomic weight of 78.96. Selenium constitutes a small proportion of the earth's crust, placing it 17th in order of abundance. Biologically, it exists mainly as analogs of the sulfur-containing amino acids, cysteine and methionine. However, several forms of selenium including selenite and selenate are available commercially and frequently used in laboratory investigations. Selenium generally undergoes chemical reduction in biological systems to the -2 oxidation state. The dynamics of selenium metabolism are key to understanding the basis for its essentiality. Furthermore, understanding of the influence of normal selenium intakes during normal conditions should provide insight into the development of rational and effective intervention strategies for aberrant conditions.

II. REQUIREMENTS AND TYPICAL INTAKES

Knowledge of the quantity of selenium needed in the diet to optimize growth and maximize enzymatic activities in humans has been steadily increasing. The daily requirement is largely based on the suggested physiological needs in Chinese men (i.e., 40 μg/day).[127,128] This intake is sufficient to prevent the clinical condition known as Keshan disease. This cardiomyopathy has been characterized in individuals in specific regions of China where selenium intakes are extremely low.[68] Dietary surveys reveal Keshan disease is absent where the food provides approximately 19 and 13 μg selenium per day for men and women, respectively.[128] However, this intake does not appear adequate to optimize the activity of some selenium containing enzymes. For example, the intake needed to maximize the activity of the plasma selenium-containing enzyme, glutathione peroxidase (GPx), is about 40 μg/day for men weighing approximately 60 kg.[67,127] While the present RDA of 70 and 55 μg/day for adult men and women, respectively, is based on the aforementioned information and takes into consideration differences in body size and possible individual variations in requirements, it does not address needs to minimize risk of certain diseases or needs during disease conditions.

Assuming the criteria for estimating minimal needs for prevention of Keshan disease are adequate and appropriate, individuals residing in countries with relatively selenium-rich soils can generally meet requirements by eating typical diets. Although this may be the case in the U.S., the intakes of traditional diets in some areas of China, New Zealand, and Scandinavia may not be adequate because of the poor selenium content of the soil. Several dietary factors, including exposure to heavy metals, are known to influence selenium needs. The impact of these environmental and dietary factors on the adequacy of selenium in diets consumed worldwide remains to be adequately evaluated.

In all species, reproducing females and their offspring appear to be particularly vulnerable to inadequate selenium intake. This vulnerability is associated with enhanced needs during periods of growth. General acceptance of this need is demonstrated by the use of oral and parenteral selenium preparations worldwide to prevent and treat nutritional muscular dystrophy and other selenium deficiency syndromes in a variety of reproducing animals.[8] With the exception of marked selenium deficiency, neither age nor the blood selenium concentration during pregnancy appears to have a marked effect on weight of the offspring or the duration of pregnancy. However, this does not necessarily mean that demands for selenium have been met, since growth and GPx activity may not be sensitive indicators of adequate body levels of this trace element. The intake of selenium in children is known to vary considerably throughout the world.[54] The physiological significance of such wide variations in selenium intake remains to be determined but may be significant given selenium's involvement in a number of physiological processes.

The selenium content of human milk depends on the geographic location of the lactating woman and probably reflects the maternal intake of locally grown foods.[27] Interestingly, up to 18% of the selenium consumed may be excreted in milk.[74] However, all selenium sources are not equally effective in increasing milk selenium concentrations.[74,77] When selenium was provided in the form of selenomethionine, during the first 8 weeks after parturition, milk selenium concentrations increased significantly. This was not the case when an isomolar amount of selenium in the form of selenium yeast was given.[77] This source of selenium resulting from the growth of yeast in the presence of supplemental selenium likely represents several selenium species that are not limited to selenoamino acids. The reason for the differential partitioning of selenium remains to be determined. Furthermore, it remains to be determined if this added selenium provides any selective advantage for nursing.

Not surprisingly, selenium needs increase during gestation and lactation in production and laboratory animals.[8,107] The National Research Council's recommendation of 0.1 µg selenium per gram of diet for the growing rat appears to be inadequate to meet the needs during pregnancy or lactation.[107] Lactating women are also frequently observed to have depressed plasma selenium concentrations compared to their nonlactating counterparts.[66] This reduction may reflect either physiological changes resulting from lactation or depressed maternal selenium stores. McGuire et al.[77] examined these possibilities while testing the impact of selenomethionine (2.7 µmol Se) or selenium-enriched yeast (2.9 µmol) supplements on the selenium status of lactating and nonlactating postpartum women. Although these women had customary intakes of approximately 1.3 µmol selenium per day, plasma selenium in unsupplemented lactating women decreased significantly during the fourth to eighth week after parturition, again supporting the belief by some that during these taxing times the intake of selenium even in the U.S. may be less than optimal. A similar decline in nonlactating women was not observed; this suggests that lactation was indeed causing these changes. In their studies, selenomethionine, but not selenium yeast supplements, increased plasma selenium during this period. Thus, the form of selenium may also be a significant factor influencing blood selenium concentrations and presumably selenium needs in human beings. At present an additional 20 µg of dietary selenium is recommended beyond the 55 µg (0.70 µmol) suggested for nonpregnant, nonlactating women to cover the amount of selenium typically secreted in milk.[95] It remains to be determined if this intake is adequate for long-term health of the reproducing woman and her offspring.

While intakes of 50 to 140 µg/day are adequate to prevent classical deficiency syndromes in humans, they may not be adequate to influence the incidence and severity of a number of diseases including cancer. The possibility that larger intakes of selenium may have health promoting properties has raised considerable debate on "adequate" vs. "optimal" intake. Future research must address this issue of "optimal" intakes while minimizing risk of toxicity. An important issue is what determination (s) is/are appropriate for establishing the minimum selenium needs.

III. ASSESSING SELENIUM STATUS

Wide variation in the selenium status of individuals is recognized throughout the world. Populations or groups of individuals with less than adequate intakes are more numerous than previously thought. The development of methods to adequately assess the selenium status remains of paramount importance. Blood selenium measurements have been questioned as a reliable index of actual selenium status. A review of human blood selenium concentrations reveals marked differences in the apparent status of individuals. A relationship was found to be highly dependent on the country where the individual resided.[31] Diplock concluded that the preferred indexes of human selenium status are concentrations of the element in blood, or plasma, and/or serum and the level of activity of GPx in erythrocytes or in plasma. Blood selenium concentrations at about 100 ng/ml are needed to achieve maximum GPx activity.[114] Until more refined techniques for assessment are available, the use of blood measurements appears the most appropriate and reliable biomarkers. Nevertheless, blood values reflect absorption, utilization, and excretion. Thus, a decrease in blood values may not necessarily signal a deficiency but adjustments in homeostasis.

Measurements of selenium and/or GPx in specific blood cells may provide a more sensitive method to evaluate the selenium status of an individual. Platelet selenium concentrations are recognized to be extremely responsive to selenium intakes.[99] Bibow et al.[11] contrasted the response of whole blood, serum and platelets to supplemental wheat selenium in healthy Norwegian females. The daily intake of 60 μg selenium significantly increased platelet, serum, and whole blood selenium concentrations. Although platelet selenium concentrations reflected the total intake, a simple linear relationship was not evident. In another recent study, Thomson et al.[114] examined the influence of providing selenium supplements daily for 32 weeks on blood cells and plasma indicators of selenium status in New Zealand women aged 18 to 23 years. Selenium supplementation raised platelet and erythrocyte GPx activity, and also the selenium concentration and activity of GPx in whole blood and plasma. Although selenomethionine was more effective in raising blood selenium concentrations than selenate, both were equally effective in raising GPx activities in whole blood, erythrocytes, and plasma; this indicates a similar bioavailability. However, selenate raised platelet GPx activities to a greater extent than did selenomethionine; cells may therefore vary in their sensitivity to the source of selenium. Thus, recent studies demonstrate that differences in sensitivity of blood cells exist and that the form of selenium provided does influence the response. Difficulties in isolating platelets may limit the usefulness of these cells to assess selenium status except under experimental conditions. However, as indicated below, the involvement of platelets in prostaglandin biosynthesis warrants that additional attention be given to their use as a sensitive biomarker of selenium nutriture.

Other biological materials may also reflect dietary selenium intakes and corresponding status. Toenail selenium concentration may be a useful indicator of human selenium status. Ovaskainen et al.[89] investigated the association between toenail selenium concentration and selenium intake in 166 urban men aged 55 to 69 years. Analysis of covariance revealed that the best predictors of toenail selenium concentration were selenium intake from supplements and food. The merit of using a single toenail sample to reflect long-term intake/ exposure was evaluated by Garland et al.[41] Reproducibility of toenail analysis over a six-year period made with paired specimens collected in 1982 to 1983 and 1988 from 127 women in the U.S. yielded a Spearman correlation coefficient of 0.48. Thus, under some circumstances toenail selenium concentrations may serve as a useful biomarker of selenium status.

Urinary selenium concentrations may be another indicator of selenium status, in as much as the kidney appears important in the homeostatic regulation of selenium. Dietary selenium intake and daily urinary selenium excretion have been found to correlate well in several populations throughout the world.[100] Selenium excretion between 20 to 200 μg/day is not associated with deficiency or toxicity symptoms. However, several factors may influence the excretion of selenium. Lower excretion is frequently reported in children, elderly people, and pregnant women, possibly reflecting lower intakes or increased demands during these periods of life. Furthermore, cancer patients also frequently have lower urinary concentrations, possibly reflecting poor intake or enhanced needs. Exposure to heavy metals is recognized to increase urinary selenium losses. The merit of using urinary selenium as a biomarker of selenium status is probably limited to experimental conditions, but may be useful in an initial evaluation of intake extremes.

IV. INADEQUATE INTAKES

A. IN ANIMALS

The essentiality of selenium for animals was first supported by the observations of Schwartz and Foltz.[105] Since this early observation, numerous investigators have demonstrated that selenium is a naturally occurring trace element essential to the health of mammalian and avian species. Lower intakes are characterized by a variety of symptoms, many of which are related to alterations in the cardiac and muscular systems. Diseases that are widely recognized for their responsiveness to supplemental selenium[117] include necrotic liver degeneration in rats, mice, rabbits, and turkeys; infertility in ewes; unthriftiness in cattle and sheep; poor hair development in pigs and horses; poor feather development in chickens; exudative diathesis in chickens; and pancreatic atrophy and fibrosis in chickens.

The etiology of selenium responsive diseases is probably complex and dependent upon the intake of several nutrients.[117] Deficiencies in animals resulting from pure selenium deficiency are likely rare and probably are limited to laboratory studies that can utilize extreme conditions. However, several factors may affect the occurrence of selenium deficiency diseases including intakes of S-containing amino acids, antagonist such as heavy metals, and various prooxidant substances including iron compounds, oxygen, ozone, and various drugs.[47] Many of the selenium responsive syndromes probably involve a combined deficiency of several nutrients including vitamin E.[117] Most, if not all, symptoms of selenium deficiencies in animals can be corrected by administrations of pharmacological quantities of vitamin E (Van Vleet and Ferrans, 1992). The interrelationships among selenium, sulfur, and vitamin E are particularly intriguing since they are known to influence cellular oxidation-reduction status.

B. IN HUMANS

In humans inadequate selenium is associated with the incidence of a cardiomyopathy called Keshan disease.[43,68] This disease, which is endemic to certain areas of China, is characterized by severe deterioration and multiple focal necrosis of the heart. Blood selenium concentrations and GPx activities are extremely low in the afflicted individual. However, these markedly depressed blood values do not appear to be the sole determinant of this disease. Similar to deficiency syndromes in animals, the intake or lack of intake of several other dietary constituents may accentuate the development of this cardiac myopathy.[43,44] Nevertheless, providing selenium fortified table salt has been shown to be effective in substantially reducing the incidence of Keshan disease.[22] Thus, it appears that increased intakes of selenium can under some circumstances modulate imbalances in other dietary nutrients and/or compensate for exposure to nutrient antagonists.

Selenium inadequacy may also arise from the use of specialized formulas for specific clinical situations. Selenium is not routinely included in total parenteral nutrition solution. Thus, patients receiving prolonged nutrition intervention are at risk of developing selenium inadequacy including the precipitation of fatal cardiomyopathy. Selenium supplementation has been shown to restore plasma and erythrocyte GPx to normal values even in those with short bowels and using clinical preparations. Rannem et al.[94] proposed that to avoid depletion all patients who receive long-term parenteral nutrition because of short bowel syndrome should receive at least 100 µg sodium selenite per day.

Inadequate selenium intake can also occur in individuals with inborn errors of metabolism because of the type of diets consumed.[9] For example, individuals with phenylketonuria frequently have reduced serum selenium concentrations.[25] Yannicelli et al.[130] found that four months of selenium supplementation (50 µg/day) was effective in normalizing plasma selenium concentrations and dramatically improve hair length, growth, and color in a child with biotin-nonresponsive propionic acidaemia who had received a propiogenic, amino acid-restricted diet. Thus, special attention is warranted to insure that adequate selenium is provided to all individuals who consume synthetic diets or diets with limited variety.

Inadequate selenium nutriture has been proposed to be a factor in poor adaptation to the aging process. Several reports suggest that the selenium status of the elderly is typically lower than that of younger populations.[33] Lower selenium status may reflect a number of factors, including reduced food intake or changes in utilization. Depressed selenium levels are frequently attributed to changes in the free radical population. Since enhanced formation of free radicals may be a key factor in the aging process,[108] it seems logical that selenium may play a significant role. Aerobic cells are known to contain various amounts of three principal antioxidant enzymes: superoxide dismutase, catalase, and GPx. A depression in one or more of these enzymes may enhance free radical concentrations and enhance the aging process, at the same time causing the arrest of cell mitosis and leading to cell death. Of these three enzymes, GPx may be the most efficient in limiting free radical generation. Yet a depression in the activity of these enzymes does not totally explain the aging process.[96,108] Instead, the rates of oxidants that are generated may be a more significant predictor of the rates of aging than are the levels of antioxidant defenses, including GPx.[96]

Selenium deficiency is common in patients infected with the human immunodeficiency virus and may contribute to the development of cardiomyopathy.[9] Kavanaugh-McHugh et al.[57] have reported that a five-year old boy with congenital human immunodeficiency virus infection developed cardiomyopathy that was responsive to selenium supplementation. Supplementation with several nutrients, including selenium, for malnourished patients with acquired immunodeficiency is justifiable in many circumstances and may reduce the complications associated with this diseased state.

V. SELENIUM PROTEINS

Selenium is believed to exert its biological activity largely through it participation in the activity of selenoproteins. During the last decade remarkable progress has been made in the recognition of the structure and function of several selenoproteins. The field of selenium biochemistry greatly stimulated in 1986 with the discovery that genes that encode the selenoproteins GPx and bacterial formate dehydrogenase contain each an TGA codon within their coding sequence.[12,13] This codon directs insertion of selenium in the form of selenocysteine into a growing polypeptide. Consequently, selenocysteine may truly be the 21st amino acid. Co-translational insertion of selenocysteine into the polypeptide chain and the existence of a tRNA molecule for selenocysteine emphasize the essentiality of this system. The discovery that tRNASec has its own special translation factor that delivers it to the translating ribosome has added additional excitement to this already flourishing area of investigation.

Changes in mRNA levels appear to be primarily involved in the regulation of the individual selenoproteins during selenium inadequacy. Although factors that affect these mRNA levels have not been completely characterized, a drop in mRNA does not always coincide with a decrease in transcription rate. For example, Baker et al.[6] found using nuclear run-on studies that the rate of GPx-specific mRNA synthesis was not different between nuclei from selenium-replete and selenium-deficient liver cells. Thus, differential transcription rates do not appear to explain metabolic defects created by selenium deficiency and suggest instead that stabilization of mRNA occurs in selenium replete cells. Since selenium deficiency generally decreases GPx mRNA levels by about 60%, while enzyme activity decreased by 93%, both co- and/or posttranslational control mechanisms may be involved in the regulation of this enzyme. It remains to be determined if similar sites for regulation occur in the other identified selenoproteins. Overall, changes in degradation of mRNA levels for selenoproteins may be the key to explain some of the complications arising from selenium inadequacy.

Selenium is known to influence the steady-state levels and distributions of two tRNA isoacceptors involved in the insertion of selenocysteine into protein, in response to certain UGA codons. Diamond et al.[29] demonstrate an increase in the levels of these isoacceptors in rats fed a selenium-adequate diet, as well as a shift in the relative distribution of tRNA. Both selenocysteine tRNAs differed only by ribose 2'-O-methylation of 5-methylcarboxymethyluridine that occurs in the wobble position of the anticodon. The role of methylation of the wobble nucleotide remains to be determined.

To date, several selenoproteins have been characterized in mammalian tissues.[20] Similar to GPx, evidence exists that the selenium moiety in these selenoproteins is incorporated into the protein molecule by the selenocysteinyl-tRNA. Again, this tRNA recognizes the specific UGA codons in mRNAs to insert selenocysteine into the primary structure. Several of these selenoproteins have recently been reviewed by Zachara[132] and Burk and Hill.[20] A brief discussion of these recognized selenoproteins is included below.

Although selenium deficiency causes a decrease in most selenoproteins, a uniform drop in all is not common. Thus, some selenoproteins may be of greater importance in maintaining or sustaining the organism. The regulation and interrelationships of these selenoproteins are a complex process that is incompletely understood. Recent advances in molecular biology offer exciting opportunities to unravel the mysteries associated with the formation of the various selenoproteins and to elucidate their physiological importance. New selenoproteins may well be discovered in the future and shed new light on the physiological significance of this trace element. Evidence for the existence of these proteins and their tissue specificity continues to accumulate at staggering rates.

A. CELLULAR GLUTATHIONE PEROXIDASE

Cellular glutathione peroxidase (GPx) was the first enzyme recognized as a selenoprotein.[98] This tetrameric protein is composed of four identical subunits each containing one atom of selenium. Prohaska and Sunde[93] found that gender and species were determinants of GPx activity, mRNA level, and selenium concentration. The possible involvement of this enzyme in the protection of cells from damage caused by products of oxidative reactions and the regulation of prostaglandin biosynthesis raises intriguing questions about its physiological importance. Interestingly, the selenoorganic compound ebselen, 2-phenyl-1,2-benzisoselenazol-3(2H)-one, has been reported to mimic enzymatic activity.[34,106] The ability of ebselen to quench free radical and singlet oxygen has been used in model experiments with liposomes, microsomes, isolated cells, and organs to show that benefits occur by minimizing an oxidative challenge.

Nevertheless, considerable controversy exists on the exact role of GPx in mammalian tissues. It is possible that depressed GPx activity and the resulting impairment in peroxide metabolism may account for some of the biochemical and clinical changes caused by selenium deficiency. Although this selenoprotein is sensitive to selenium inadequacy, at least in liver and some other tissues, there is little *in vivo* evidence to show that a depression in the activity of this enzyme leads to enhanced free radical generation. The lack of a response in free radical production may reflect changes induced in other enzymes involved in oxidation-reduction reactions to compensate for the depression in GPx. Since GPx contains a significant fraction of the body selenium, a decrease in its synthesis may also serve another function. It may provide selenium needed for the synthesis of other selenoproteins that are possibly more important for survival. Could it be possible that the primary function of GPx is to serve as a reservoir for selenium? The answer may depend not only on the intake of selenium but also on the tissue in question. In brain, there appears to be a sequestration of selenium and a conservation of GPx activity during selenium deprivation,[18] suggesting that in this tissue GPx needs to be retained. Different patterns of selenoprotein expression between liver and brain emphasize the tissue specificity of changes in selenium homeostasis. Additional attention needs to be given to the impact of selenium deprivation or exaggerated intakes on tissues other than the liver. Because increased selenium intake may minimize the risk of chronic diseases, there is ample justification to examine tissues other than liver.

B. PLASMA OR EXTRACELLULAR GLUTATHIONE PEROXIDASE

Plasma GPx, also referred to as extracellular GPx, has a tetrameric form with identical subunits and with one atom of selenium per subunit. It is a glycosylated protein and is distinct from the cellular enzyme. Yet, both enzymes catalyze the reduction of hydrogen peroxide and a variety of organic hydroperoxides by utilizing glutathione.

Avissar et al.[4] have reported that patients with renal failure who were on dialysis and nephrectomized patients had reduced plasma GPx activities. A similar relationship between plasma GPx and kidney function was observed in the rat.[4] Kidney transplantation markedly increased plasma GPx activity. Hybridization studies with rat kidney slices revealed that only proximal tubular epithelial cells and parietal epithelial cells of Bowman's capsule contained extracellular GPx transcripts. These results strongly suggest that kidney proximal tubular cells are the main source for plasma or extracellular GPx.

Previous studies[5] revealed that about 90% of human milk GPx activity was precipitated by anti-plasma GPx-immunoglobulin G. Thus, most, if not all, milk GPx is due to the plasma selenoprotein form of the enzyme. Factors regulating the release of this enzyme from the kidney and its passage into the milk remain to be determined.

C. PHOSPHOLIPID HYDROPEROXIDE GLUTATHIONE PEROXIDASE

A third GPx, called phospholipid hydroperoxide glutathione peroxidase (PHGPx), is a monomeric, membrane-associated enzyme that contains one atom of Se per mole of protein. This enzyme destroys esterified lipid hydroperoxides. Sunde et al.[111] isolated and sequenced a full-length cDNA clone for PHGPx (Genbank accession number L12743) from a pig blastocyst cDNA library. Use of this clone in Northern blot analysis revealed that PHGPx mRNA levels were marginally affected by selenium deficiency, whereas GPx mRNA levels were decreased by about 90% in the same preparations.[111] Maintenance of this enzyme may be one explanation for the limited evidence of oxidative damage during selenium deficiency. On the other hand, PHGPx, by regulating the tone of endogenous hydroperoxides,[123] governs the activity of leukocyte 5-lipoxygenase. Future studies dealing with the regulation of this intriguing enzyme appear justified.

D. TYPE I IODOTHYRONINE 5′-DEIODINASE

The fourth known mammalian selenoenzyme is a type I iodothyronine 5′-deiodinase that catalyzes the deiodination of L-thyroxine to the biologically active hormone 3,3′,5-triiodothyronine. It is a monomeric enzyme and contains one atom of Se per mole of protein. Reduced activity of this enzyme may explain the impairment in thyroid hormone metabolism caused by selenium deficiency.[1-3,24,131] Impaired thyroid hormone metabolism may account for the decrease in growth and resistance to cold stress caused by prolonged selenium deficiency. A depression in the conversion of thyroxine (T_4) to the more metabolically active 3,3′,5-triiodothyronine (T_3) during selenium inadequacy is consistent with this overall hypothesis.

Type I 5′-deiodinase activities appear to be under homeostatic control and are not further increased by exaggerated selenium intakes. The dietary selenium requirement for normal deiodinase activity is lower than it is for adequate GPx activity.[10,116] Vadhanavikit and Ganther[116] reported that providing approximately 0.05 mg Se per kg diet was sufficient for normal deiodinase activity in the liver and approximately 0.01 mg Se per kg for normal activity in the thyroid. Thyroid tissue appears to have priority over liver when the selenium intake is limited. A cellular hierarchy of selenite incorporation for Type I 5′-deiodinase over GPx has been observed in the porcine kidney epithelial cells LLC-PK1.[59] Regulation of the expression of Type I 5′-deiodinase by selenium occurs both transcriptionally and posttranscriptionally.[59]

Meinhold et al.[80] examined the effects of selenium deficiency over a period of three generations and during a combined selenium and iodine deficiency on rat hepatic and cerebrocortical iodothyronine deiodinases and on circulating thyroid hormone levels. Selenium deficiency markedly decreased hepatic type I iodothyronine 5′- and 5-deiodinase, while iodine depletion only marginally decreased type I activity. Cerebrocortical type II 5′-deiodinase was decreased in selenium deficient, iodine-replete rats. The five- to sixfold increase in cerebrocortical type II 5′-deiodinase in iodine-deficient rats was not reversed by additional selenium deficiency. Cortex type III 5-deiodinase was modestly decreased in all animals consuming insufficient selenium. Maintenance of increased cerebrocortical type II deiodinase in iodine-depleted animals is independent of selenium supply.[81] Further studies are necessary to clarify whether the weak, but repeatedly confirmed, decrease of cortex type III deiodinase is the direct effect of selenium deficiency or the indirect consequence of the multilevel changes in thyroid hormone metabolism.

The overall significance of prolonged selenium deficiency on thyroid metabolism is not completely understood. Meinhold et al.[80] reported that long-term selenium deficiency had only limited effects on serum T_4 and T_3 levels. Administration of 100 µg selenium per day as selenomethionine to 8 euthyroid females prone to develop thyroid dysfunction did not decompensate thyroid hormone synthesis of these subjects.[97] The lack of any effect in subjects with subtle thyroid hormone synthesis defect may be due to the fact that these subjects had a sufficient selenium dietary intake before selenium supplementation and an only marginally reduced dietary iodine intake.

E. SELENOPROTEIN P

Selenoprotein P, a fifth known selenoprotein, is a glycosylated, monomeric protein containing ten atoms of selenium per molecule. The function of this protein is also not known, but may play a role in selenium transport or be connected with a protective activity against free radicals. Deagen et al.[26] have reported that most of the selenium in rat plasma was associated with selenoprotein P, but not when the intake of selenomethionine was high. Competitive binding assays have also revealed that selenoprotein P binds differentially to tissues (brain > kidney > testes > liver). Specific binding to these tissues from rats increased with increasing amounts of dietary selenium. Binding does appear to be saturable. Wilson and Tappel[125] detected a 134 kDa complex that likely serves as the membrane receptor for selenoprotein P.

F. FATTY ACID BINDING PROTEIN

A selenoprotein weighing about 14 kDa (SLP-14) also has been isolated and partially characterized from mouse mammary glands.[7] This protein belongs to the family of fatty acid-binding proteins, as virgin mouse mammary gland expressed a protein homologous to the adipocyte lipid binding protein, whereas pregnant and lactating mouse mammary glands expressed a protein highly homologous to mouse heart fatty acid-binding protein.[7]

G. SELENOPROTEIN W

Selenite treatment is also known to induce the formation of a low molecular weight selenocysteine-containing protein in rat muscle.[120] These proteins have masses of about 9.5 kDa and contain about 0.92 g atoms of selenium per g mol of protein. The function and regulation of selenoprotein W remain to be determined.

VI. SELENIUM AND OXIDATIVE STRESS

As indicated earlier, selenium is required for activity of glutathione peroxidase and thus the regulation of free radicals. Interest in free radical events has stimulated speculation that a disorder in their concentration may be involved in a number of disease states. The control of free radicals depends on the integrity of an enzymatic system that requires adequate intake of several nutrients, including selenium.[30] When selenium intakes are low, active oxygen metabolites may proliferate. This increase could result in damage to DNA, proteins, and polyunsaturated phospholipids. While damage to any of these may be lethal, peroxidation of polyunsaturated phospholipids might also disrupt membranes and lead to profound changes in the cell.[15]

Support for the concept that selenium can reduce oxidative damage comes from several sources. Lii and Hendrich[70] found that hepatocytes from rats fed adequate amounts of selenium were more effective in increasing glutathione disulfide than those prepared from rats fed a selenium inadequate diet. This difference became even more apparent following exposure to the oxidative stressors, t-butyl hydroperoxide and menadione. Nevertheless, the effects of selenium on oxidative stress must be considered in relationship to other nutrients. Chen and Tappel[21] examined the effects of the combination of vitamin E, selenium, and beta-carotene on oxidative damage to rat heart, kidney, lung, and spleen by measurement of the production of oxidized heme proteins during spontaneous and prooxidant-induced (bromotrichloromethane) oxidation. Dietary supplements of all of these antioxidants had strong protective effects against oxidative damage to heme proteins during the early stages of spontaneous and bromotrichloromethane-induced oxidation. Synergism of multiple antioxygenic nutrients against oxidative damage also was evident.

Other dietary factors may also influence the ability of selenium to modify free radical generation. Using ESR spin-trapping techniques, Kadiiska et al.[55] found that copper intake modified the capacity of dietary selenium and vitamin E to protect against lipid peroxidation. Interestingly, either vitamin E or selenium was sufficient to prevent the formation of radical adducts resulting from excessive copper intake. Collectively, these studies suggest that selenium adequacy can influence the ability of cells to withstand oxidative stress. However, selenium's importance must be considered in terms of a host of environmental and dietary factors.

VII. SELENIUM AND IMMUNITY

Selenium appears to influence all components of the immune system. The development and expression of nonspecific, humoral, and cell-mediated responses are all influenced by dietary selenium intake.[58,109] The intake of selenium on the immune system is known to be highly dependent on how much of this trace element is consumed or administered, as well as on the intake of several other nutrients. The mechanism(s) whereby selenium affects the immune system remain(s) speculative, but may relate to changes in peroxidase activity. This in turn will affect peroxide concentrations, changes in cellular levels of reduced glutathione and H_2Se, and/or changes in cell membrane thiols.

Selenium deficiency inhibits resistance to microbial and viral infections, changes in neutrophil function, and antibody production. As a result, the proliferation of T and B lymphocytes, in response to mitogens, is reduced as is cytodestruction by T lymphocytes and natural killer cells.[28,58] The suppression of antibody production, and possibly other alterations in the immune response, caused by selenium deficiency, is generally magnified by a simultaneous vitamin E deficiency. Unlike vitamin E, selenium restriction causes mainly a depression in polymorphonuclear cell function.

Selenium supplementation at moderate levels has been shown to stimulate the function of neutrophils, and generally to overcome the effects of selenium deficiency described above. Selenium supplementation also enhances the ability of a host to reject transplanted malignant tumors. Experiments using animal models have demonstrated a positive relationship between selenium status and resistance against infections. Harvima et al.[48] examined the effect of selenium supplementation (400 μg/day for six weeks as selenium yeast) on skin and blood selenium content, on skin GPx activity and on various chemical and immunological parameters of blood and skin in seven psoriatic patients. GPx activity in normal and psoriatic skin remained unchanged during the experiment. Nevertheless, a slight but statistically significant increase in the number of CD4+ T-cells was observed in the reticular dermis of the psoriatic lesions, whereas the number of CD8+, CD11c+, and CD1+ cells was not altered. This study suggests that selenium may be able to modulate the immunological mechanism of psoriatic lesions by increasing the number of CD4+ T-cells.

Part of the effect of selenium on the immune system may relate to its ability to regulate the concentrations of hydroperoxides. Modulation of cellular hydroperoxide levels is considered one of the important physiological mechanisms regulating the synthesis of prostaglandins and leukotrienes in mammalian cells. The role of selenium-containing enzymes on the formation of lipoxygenase metabolites was recently examined by Weitzel and Wendel.[123] Basophilic leukemia cells from selenium-deficient rats had less than 1% GPx activity of controls and about 35% phospholipid hydroperoxide-glutathione peroxidase activity of controls. Stimulation of these selenium deficient cells released eightfold more lipoxygenase metabolites compared to controls. Addition of selenium to these cells restored phospholipid hydroperoxide-glutathione peroxidase activity within eight hours, whereas glutathione peroxidase restoration required about seven days. Interestingly, the restoration of phospholipid hydroperoxide-glutathione peroxidase activity was accompanied by normal leukotriene metabolism. Weitzel and Wendel studies[123] also revealed that injection of selenium into rats substantially increased leukocyte phospholipid hydroperoxide-glutathione peroxidase activity and reduced the formation of lipoxygenase metabolites. These data, therfore, provide evidence that phospholipid hydroperoxide-glutathione peroxidase activity may be a selenium dependent enzyme that governs the activity of leukocyte 5-lipoxygenase by regulating endogenous hydroperoxides.

Eskew et al.[35] investigated the ability of selenium to regulate arachidonic acid metabolism in polymorphonuclear leukocytes derived from the lung of endotoxin-challenged rats. Selenium deficiency had no significant effect on lavage fluid levels of thromboxane B2, leukotriene B4 or leukotriene C4. Vitamin E deficiency, however, led to a significant increase in leukotriene B4, with no effect on thromboxane B2. In contrast, selenium deficiency resulted in a significant increase in the release of thromboxane B2 by polymorphonuclear leukocytes. The increase in thromboxane B2 release was seen in both *in vitro*-stimulated and nonstimulated polymorphonuclear leukocytes.

Alterations in the immune response by selenium may also relate to modulation of the respiratory burst in phagocytic cells. In platelets GPx probably acts as a scavenger of the peroxides generated during the burst of arachidonic acid metabolism. This scavenging inhibits the biosynthesis of both thromboxane A2 and lipoxygenase products, but does not appear to alter prostacyclin biosynthesis.[91] Platelet GPx activation caused by selenium supplementation was found to parallel an enhancement of platelet aggregation threshold values for arachidonic acid and a progressive increase in blood clotting time that was unmodified by aspirin.

VIII. SELENIUM AND DISEASES

Research in human medicine and nutrition continues to be devoted to the possibility of using selenium for the prevention or treatment of a variety of degenerative diseases.[83,86,104]

A. SELENIUM AND HEART DISEASE

As already discussed, severe selenium deficiency is known to result in a cardiomyopathy known as Keshan disease. Similar disorders have been observed in individuals who are on parenteral feeding for long periods. Lockitch et al.[73] have recently reported on a 17-year old female who died after a cardiac arrest secondary to septic shock; the pathological diagnosis was that of cardiomyopathy due to prolonged selenium deficiency.

Although limited in number, some epidemiological studies have suggested a relationship between low serum selenium concentrations and the risk of cardiovascular disease.[88] Shifts in peroxide concentrations and shifts in eicosanoids have been proposed to account for this relationship. On the other hand, Bukkens et al.[19] found no association between selenium status and gender, age, serum total-, low density lipoprotein (LDL)-, and high density lipoprotein (HDL)-cholesterol, systolic and diastolic blood pressure, alcohol intake, or body mass index.

While epidemiological data may not consistently show a relationship between selenium and heart disease, some recent laboratory investigations raise interesting possibilities about selenium as a modifier of the risk of heart disease.[112] In these studies the influence of selenium on the toxicity of oxidized low density lipoprotein (LDLox) was examined. LDLox is believed to be an important contributor to endothelial cytodamage and atherogenesis. The investigators found that LDLox caused lethal damage to bovine aortic endothelial cells *in vitro.* Growth of these cells without added selenium lowered the activity of GPx and phospholipid hydroperoxide GPx and increased their sensitivity to oxidative injury induced by t-butyl hydroperoxide, liposomal cholesterol hydroperoxides, and LDLox. Preincubation of LDLox with GSH and Ebselen (a selenoperoxidase mimetic) dramatically reduced the peroxide content of these cells and restored their resistance to LDLox-induced damage. These results demonstrate that the selenoperoxidases may play an important role in the cellular defense against oxidized low density lipoprotein. Presumably this involves detoxifying lipid hydroperoxides and thereby preventing iron-catalyzed decomposition to damaging free radical intermediates.

Selenium likely influences factors involved in the risk of cardiac disease in other ways. Ueki et al.[115] found that sodium selenate, as well as insulin, increased lipoprotein lipase activity in isolated rat fat pads in a time- and dose-dependent manner. The effect of selenate was highly dependent on the calcium concentration of the incubation medium. Dibutyryl cyclic AMP, 3-isobutyl-1-methylxanthine, carbonyl cyanide m-chlorophenylhydrazone, tunicamycin, and monensin all inhibited the effect of selenate on the LPL activity to various degrees. Their results suggest that selenate increases LPL activity via amiloride- and monensin-sensitive processes, involving Ca^{+2} mobilization resulting from a rapid increase in the inositol 1,4,5-trisphosphate content in fat pads.

B. SELENIUM AND CANCER

The complexities of lifestyles and dietary habits not withstanding, there are compelling reasons to believe that a variety of essential nutrients can modify carcinogenesis in humans. Furthermore, there is sufficient parallelism between controlled animal studies and human behavior that responses in laboratory settings may signal true benefits of several nutrients as modifiers of the cancer process.[15,87] Both epidemiological and laboratory investigations provide evidence for the anticarcinogenic effects of selenium. The increasing recognition of selenium as a viable dietary anticarcinogenic agent[51,83,104,110] has not always been appreciated. Early investigations actually suggested that selenium might promote cancer development.[85] Based upon this study and other limited data, selenium was labelled as a suspect carcinogen. In a 1975 IARC review[50] of selenium and selenium-containing compounds, it was concluded, "The available data provide no suggestion that selenium is carcinogenic in man." Nevertheless, even today a number of selenium compounds are marketed with a warning label that indicates the substance may be a carcinogen.

1. Epidemiological Studies

Several epidemiological studies support the belief that selenium consumption is inversely correlated with cancers at a variety of sites.[17,42,60] Schamberger and Willis[101] were among the first to report that an inverse relationship existed between cancer death rates and the selenium levels in forage plants and presumed greater selenium intakes. Hardell et al.[46] examined plasma selenium and GPx in erythrocytes in a case-control study encompassing 441 cases with breast cancer and 191 controls with benign breast disease. No difference in mean serum selenium levels between cases and controls receiving supplementary selenium was seen. If, however, only those individuals were considered who received no selenium supplements (278 cases and 135 controls), a preventive effect was found with increasing selenium. This finding was significant among women 50-years old or more, with a Mantel–Haenszel odds ratio of 0.16 for individuals with serum selenium >1.21 µmol/L. Also for subjects with serum selenium in the range 1.00 to 1.21 µmol/L, a significant preventive effect was seen. For women under 50-years of age there was no significant preventive effect. Glutathione peroxidase in erythrocytes did not correlate well with serum selenium and was not a marker for the risk of breast cancer.

The association between toenail selenium and lung cancer was investigated in a cohort study of diet and cancer among 120,852 Dutch men and women aged 55 to 69 years.[118] After 3.3 years of follow-up, 550 incident cases of lung carcinoma were detected. Toenail selenium data were available for 370 lung cancer cases and 2459 members of a randomly selected subcohort. The rate ratio of lung cancer for subjects in the highest compared to the lowest quintile of toenail selenium, after controlling for age, gender, smoking, and education, was 0.50 (95% confidence interval, 0.30 to 0.81), with a significant inverse trend across quintiles ($p = 0.006$). The results of this study support an inverse association between selenium status and lung cancer and suggest a modification of the effect of selenium by the antioxidants beta-carotene and vitamin C.

Krishnaswamy et al.[61] examined the selenium nutriture of oral and esophageal cancer patients. The mean selenium level in oral cancer patients was 102.6 ng/ml and in esophageal cancer 103.3 ng/ml, while in the matched controls it was 117.5 and 116.2 ng/ml, respectively. Relative risk estimates were 3.16 ($p < 0.02$) and 16.0 ($p < 0.01$) in oral and esophageal cancer patients, respectively. Risk appeared to increase with selenium levels below 115 ng/ml.

The effects of vitamin and mineral supplementation on cancer incidence and mortality were recently examined in an intervention study conducted in Linxian, China.[69] This area is known to have one of the highest mortality rates from esophageal/gastric cancer. Among those receiving beta-carotene/vitamin E/selenium supplementation, total mortality was reduced by 9% and cancer mortality by 13%. Gastric cancer mortality was significantly reduced by 20%, while mortality from other cancers was reduced by 19%.

Risk of cancer also appears to be inversely related to blood selenium levels.[16,17] Bratakos et al.[14] recently examined the selenium status of cancer patients in Greece and found a strong and significant inverse correlation between the concentration of selenium in blood, urine, or hair and the presence of newly diagnosed cancers. However, the reduction in selenium concentrations may relate to changes in dietary habits of these individuals and be a secondary complication of the progression of the disease. Nevertheless,

Broghamer et al.[16] found that increased blood selenium concentrations (>180 ng/ml) were associated with tumors that remained confined to the region of origin, had fewer distant metastases, showed a reduced number of primary neoplasms, and displayed a decreased frequency of tumor recurrence. However, the biological behavior of all tumors, particularly reticuloendothelial, does not appear related to blood selenium concentrations.[17]

It must be emphasized that not all studies provide support for a protective effect of selenium against cancer.[32,119] These inconsistencies could be due to lack of a true protective effect, or to methodological problems in assessing dietary intake.

2. Laboratory Studies

Selenium supplementation has also been found to reduce the incidence and total tumor number in laboratory animals treated with a variety of chemical carcinogens.[23,51-53,72,113,124] It appears to be effective in counteracting the carcinogenicity of 3-methyl-4-dimethyl-aminoazobenzene, 2-acetylamino-fluorene, diethylnitrosamine, aflatoxin, 7,12-dimethylben(a)anthracene, benzopyrene and 3-methylcholanthrene. However, it is less effective against dimethylhydrazine, azoxymethane, methylazoxymethanol, *bis*(2-oxopropyl) nitrosamine, 1-methyl-1-nitrosourea and *N*-methyl-*N*-nitro-nitrosoguanidine. As might be expected if enough studies are performed, there is also limited evidence that selenium may even increase tumors in some cases. Evidence for this effect is seen with the incidence of pancreatic carcinomas following treatment with *bis*(2-oxopropyl) nitrosamine and esophageal cancer in hamsters treated with methylnitrosurea. Nevertheless, the majority of studies support the anticarcinogenic effects of selenium. The effectiveness of selenium has been observed with both direct and indirect carcinogens, although inhibition appears to be slightly more effective with compounds that require metabolic activation.

The ability of selenium to inhibit tumors resulting from such a wide range of carcinogens suggests a general mechanism that is not limited to a specific tissue. Numerous studies demonstrate that both phase I and II enzymes are modified by supplemental selenium. In many cases these are accompanied by a reduction in the binding of the carcinogen to the DNA of the target tissue.[71]

Considerable debate has centered on the impact of selenium deficiency on cancer risk. Ip and Sinha[51] showed that selenium-deficient rats fed a high fat diet had a slightly higher incidence of mammary tumors following dimethylbenz(a)anthracene (DMBA) treatment than rats supplemented with 0.1 ppm selenite. Nevertheless, epidemiological data do not support that selenium deficiency is associated with enhanced cancer risk in humans. Rather, most of the available information suggests that high selenium intake is associated with a reduction in cancer risk.

The quantity of selenium required to elicit an anticarcinogenic response is generally 20 to 40 times that required to prevent classic deficiency symptoms.

Thus, the protective functions cannot be solely attributed to the action of GPx. Instead, selenium appears to operate by several mechanisms, depending on the quantity and chemical form of selenium provided.[104] It must be emphasized that the method used to study chemically induced carcinogenesis may necessitate that large intakes of selenium are needed to observe a significant effect. Long-term studies with low intakes of selenium are needed adequately to evaluate the minimum quantity needed to reduce cancer risk in experimental animals.

How the form of selenium influences the cancer process has not been extensively examined. Limited evidence suggests that organic selenium compounds such as selenomethionine may be slightly less effective on a molar basis than selenite. However, the quantity of selenium employed and variation in tumor incidence in most studies make it difficult to demonstrate major differences. Recent evidence suggests that there is a difference between the chemopreventive effect exacted by dietary selenium in the form of 1,4-phenylenebis(methylene) selenocyanate (p-XSC) or in the form of selenite in connection with the induction of lung tumor by the tobacco-specific 4-(methylnitrosamino)-1-(3-pyridyl)-1-butanone (NNK).[34] Although neither form altered body weights of mice, pXSc significantly inhibited lung tumor multiplicity. In contrast, sodium selenite had no protective effect against induction of these chemically induced tumors.

Selenium may also work in combination with several other compounds to markedly inhibit tumor incidence. Providing supplemental selenium in combination with difluoromethylornithine, an inhibitor of ornithine decarboxylase, was found to selectively inhibit distal colon tumors in rats treated with dimethylhydrazine to a greater degree than either provided alone.[75] Inoue et al.[49] investigated the inhibitory effects of vitamin A, selenium, butylated hydroxytoluene, and their combinations on tongue carcinogenesis induced by 4-nitroquinoline-1-oxide in Sprague-Dawley rats. After four months of administration of 4-nitroquinoline-1-oxide, a wide range of lesions from hyperplasia to early invasive carcinoma was seen. The lesions were fewer and the carcinomas were less advanced in the rats given vitamin A, selenium, and butylated hydroxytoluene. However, the inhibitory effect of combined chemopreventives was not always superior to that of a single agent.

Generally, selenium appears to be equally effective in inhibiting the initiation and promotion stages of carcinogenesis.[52] Thompson and Becci[113] reported that selenium had the greatest effect on the early promotion phases of carcinogenesis. More recent studies with DMBA suggest that about half of the anticarcinogenic effects of selenium can be explained by alterations in the initiation phase of carcinogenesis.[72] Alterations in carcinogen metabolism, presumably by alterations in phase I and II enzymes, are associated with protection of DNA against carcinogen-induced damage.

Several studies have shown that selenium inhibits the *in vitro* and *in vivo* growth of several transplantable tumors.[38] The ability of selenium to inhibit tumor cell growth is known to be dependent upon plating density, length of selenium incubation, the form of selenium used and the specific cell line examined. Clear differences in the ability of selenium to inhibit tumor cells have been reported.[38,45,63,78,84,122] Recent evidence suggests that part of the differences between cells may relate to their ability to regulate glutathione concentrations[39,62,63] and alter specific proteins.[39,79] Selenium appears to inhibit the replication of tumor viruses and the activation of oncogenes by similar mechanisms.[103,104]

Selenium may also offer some advantages when provided in conjunction with more classical chemotherapeutic treatments. Administration of sodium selenite has been reported to reduce the nephrotoxicity of the antitumorigenic agent *cis*-diaminedichloroplatinum (II) (cisplatin). The protection provided by sodium selenite against cisplatin-induced nephrotoxicity was without influence on the systemic availability of cisplatin and total platinum.[121]

C. OTHER DISEASES

Several diseases and disorders display spatial patterns that suggest the involvement of selenium.

1. Kaschin–Beck Disease

Fu and Zhang[40] studied the effects of cereals from a region where Kaschin–Beck's disease is endemic. Their results indicated that feeding rats with low-selenium cereals from this region decelerated fibrillogenesis of type II collagen, reduced fibril stability and diameter. When cereals from this region were supplemented with selenium, these pathologic changes were partially corrected.

2. Diabetes

In a study[56] to determine whether antioxidant therapy improves the prognosis of the diabetic late syndrome, patients received 600 mg of alpha lipoic acid, 100 µg of selenium (sodium selenite) daily or 1200 IE of D-alpha-tocopherol for 3 months. Those receiving the antioxidant supplements had lower serum concentrations of substances that react with thiobarbituric acid. Symptoms of distal symmetric neuropathy also improved. These results provide evidence that oxidative stress may play a promoting role in the complications of diabetes and that adjuvant therapy with antioxidants may be beneficial.

3. Arthritis

Selenium is involved in several metabolic pathways that are relevant to rheumatic diseases. As indicated previously, experimental and clinical investigations suggest that selenium can modulate the inflammatory and immune responses. While patients suffering from inflammatory rheumatic diseases frequently have lower selenium concentrations, the absolute selenium content does not correlate with the severity of the disease.[90] Conceivably moderate supplementation, by preventing imbalances, might enhance host defense mechanisms. The true impact of selenium on arthritis has not been adequately examined.

4. Cystic Fibrosis

The effect of supplemental selenium (2.8 µg of sodium selenite per kg of body weight per day) was examined in 27 patients with cystic fibrosis.[92] After an interval of two months, treatments of the two groups were interchanged (crossed-over) for another five-month period. During the study, selenium concentrations in plasma decreased in patients that received the placebo treatment and increased during selenium intake. This study suggests the existence of a fragile equilibrium exists in patients with cystic fibrosis.

5. Malaria

Murine malaria appears to be a useful experimental model for investigating interrelationships of selenium and vitamin E.[65] Experiments in mice reveal that vitamin E deficiency protects against the parasite, especially in conjunction with peroxidizable fat, such as fish or linseed oils. Selenium deficiency, on the other hand, has little or no protective effect against the parasite. The practical utility of pro-oxidant diets in combating human malaria remains to be determined.

6. Sudden Infant Death

It is possible that low selenium status could cause immunosuppression and be an etiologic factor in Sudden Infant Death.[37,76] However, Lemke et al.[64] were unable to find evidence of low selenium serum concentrations deficiency in SID victims.

IX. TOXICITY

The earliest written report of selenium poisoning, also known as selenosis, may be the description by Marco Polo of a necrotic hoof disease of horses.[82] By the 1930s, it was becoming abundantly clear that excessive exposure to selenium was toxic in many birds and animals. The degree of toxicity depended on several factors including the chemical species of selenium, the animal species, and the route of administration.[82,117] Soluble salts, including sodium selenite and sodium selenate, are among the more toxic compounds. Selenium in the form of seleno-amino acids (selenomethionine and selenocysteine) as found in grains and other foods is only moderately toxic when compared to the higher toxicity of soluble salts. This may be due to the widespread incorporation of the seleno-amino acids into cellular proteins in the place of their sulfur amino acid counterparts. Relatively insoluble forms, such as elemental selenium, sodium selenide, selenium disulfide, and diphenyl selenide are among the least toxic of the selenium compounds. Generally, toxicity is substantially less when selenium is given orally rather than parenterally.

Despite recent concerns about the availability of selenium as a dietary supplement and as an environmental contaminant, toxicity in humans is relatively rare. A few cases of selenosis are known to have occurred from industrial accidents, and one episode involved the ingestion of superpotent selenium supplements.[36] Chronic selenosis is essentially unheard of in the U.S. This rarity may be related to the typical diversity of the American diet. Nevertheless, selenosis can occur in humans following chronic consumption of excess selenium, as occurs in China's Enshi county, probably due to the extremely high selenium content of the soil and food in the region. Although there were no detectable abnormalities in liver or heart of these individuals, other symptoms were evident.[129] These symptoms were typically found in individuals consuming about 910 μg selenium per day and individuals with blood selenium concentrations of about 1.05 mg/L. Overall, observations made in this select population suggest that a daily intake of 750 to 850 μg selenium may pose little toxicity. Nevertheless, Yang et al.[129] suggest that since other variable factors may influence toxicity, a daily intake of 400 μg selenium might constitute a safe daily maximum. Even this intake is about three times that typically consumed in the U.S.

Growing public interest in selenium as a dietary supplement and the occurrence of environmental selenium contamination serve to emphasize the need for recognizing the manifestations of selenium toxicity. Morphological changes in fingernails are recognized as an early characteristic of excessive selenium exposure. These pathological nails occurred frequently in adults, infrequently in teenagers, and not at all in young children.[129] Garlic odor of breath and sweat associated with volatile selenium metabolites also is a common feature associated with excessive exposure. Severe irritations of the respiratory system, metallic taste in mouth, abnormal formation in the nose, including signs of rhinitis, lung edema, and brancho-pneumonia, are frequently observed following excessive exposure. Other signs primarily identified in animals include lethargy, excessive salivation, vomiting, dyspnea, muscle tremors, and respiratory distress.[47,117] Pathological findings in animals following acute or chronic exposure to excess selenium include congestion of the liver and kidney, fatty degeneration, and focal necrosis of the liver, endocarditis, and myocarditis.

The mechanism by which excess selenium brings about symptoms of toxicity remains largely unknown. Yan and Spallholz[126] tested several selenium compounds for their abilities to generate superoxide by the oxidation of glutathione and other thiols in the absence and presence of cells of the human mammary tumor cell line HTB123/DU4475. Free radical generation was measured by lucigenin- or luminol-amplified chemiluminescence. In the presence of mammary tumor cells, lucigenin-dependent chemiluminescence was observed from the reactions of selenite and selenocysteine with glutathione that were 5 and 23 times greater than their respective reactions with glutathione in the absence of tumor cells. The enhanced chemiluminescence generated by selenite and selenocysteine in the presence of the tumor cells was also suppressed by superoxide dismutase, catalase and GPx. These data suggest that a free radical, the superoxide anion (O^{2-}), and H_2O_2 are produced from the reaction of selenite and selenocysteine with glutathione. These free radical reactions may account for the toxicity of selenite and selenocystine *in vitro*. Spallhoz[110] provides strong evidence that selenium is toxic owing to its prooxidant catalytic activity to produce superoxide, hydrogen peroxide, and possibly other cascading oxyradicals. It is possible that part of the anticancer effects of selenium relate to its ability to alter prooxidant status.

X. SUMMARY AND CONCLUSIONS

Selenium is an amazing trace element. It has survived many challenges to its merit in the diet of animals and humans. Given the many physiological functions that seem to involve selenium, the future of selenium research remains extremely bright. In particular, advances in the identification and characterization of several selenoproteins are likely to improve the respect gained by this element for maintaining health. As far as the dietary consumption of selenium is concerned, it seems prudent to consume, at a minimum, the RDA for selenium. Enhancing the intake of foods rich in selenium, as true for many fish and grain products, will not only increase the intake of this essential nutrient, but may also reduce the risk of some of the most dreaded diseases faced by human beings.

REFERENCES

1. Arthur, J. R., Nicol, F., and Beckett, G. J., Selenium deficiency, thyroid hormone metabolism, and thyroid hormone deiodinases, *Am. J. Clin. Nutr.,* 57, 236S, 1993.
2. Arthur, J. R., Nicol, F., and Beckett, G. J., The role of selenium in thyroid hormone metabolism and effects of selenium deficiency on thyroid hormone and iodine metabolism, *Biol. Trace Elem. Res.,* 33, 37, 1992.
3. Arthur, J. R., The role of selenium in thyroid hormone metabolism, *Can. J. Physiol. Pharm.,* 69, 1648, 1991.
4. Avissar, N., Ornt, D. B., Yagil, Y., Horowitz, S., Watkins, R. H., Kerl, E. A., Takahashi, K., Palmer, I. S., and Cohen, H. J., Human kidney proximal tubules are the main source of plasma glutathione peroxidase, *Am. J. Physiol.,* 266, C367, 1994.
5. Avissar, N., Slemmon, J. R., Palmer, I. S., and Cohen, H. J., Partial sequence of human plasma glutathione peroxidase and immunologic identification of milk glutathione peroxidase as the plasma enzyme, *J. Nutr.,* 121, 1243, 1991.
6. Baker, R. D., Baker, S. S., LaRosa, K., Whitney, C., and Newburger, P. E., Selenium regulation of glutathione peroxidase in human hepatoma cell line Hep3B, *Arch. Biochem. Biophys.,* 304, 53, 1993.
7. Bansal, M. P. and Medina, D., Expression of fatty acid-binding proteins in the developing mouse mammary gland, *Biochem. Biophys. Res. Commun.,* 191, 61, 1993.
8. Beale, A. M., Fasulo, D. A., and Craigmill, A. L., Effects of oral and parenteral selenium supplements on residues in meat, milk and eggs, *Rev. Environ. Contam. Toxicol.,* 115, 125, 1990.

9. Bedwal, R. S., Nair, N., Sharma, M. P., and Mathur, R. S., Selenium — its biological perspectives, *Med. Hypoth.*, 41, 150, 1993.
10. Behne, D. and Kyriakopoulos, A., Effects of dietary selenium on the tissue concentrations of type I iodothyronine 5′-deiodinase and other selenoproteins, *Am. J. Clin. Nutr.*, 57, 310S, 1993.
11. Bibow, K., Meltzer, H. M., Mundal, H. H., Paulsen, I. T., and Holm, H., Platelet selenium as indicator of wheat selenium intake, *J. Trace Elem. Electrol. Health Dis.* 7, 171, 1993.
12. Bock, A., Forchhammer, K., Heider, J., and Baron, C., Selenoprotein synthesis: an expansion of the genetic code, *Trends Biochem. Sci.*, 16, 463, 1991.
13. Bock, A., Forchhammer, K., Heider, J., Leinfelder, W., Sawers, G., Veprek, B., and Zinoni, F., Selenocysteine: the 21st amino acid, *Mol. Microbiol.*, 5, 515, 1991.
14. Bratakos, M. S., Vouterakos, T. P., and Ioannou, P. V., Selenium status of cancer patients in Greece, *Sci. Total Environ.*, 92, 207, 1990.
15. Borek, C., Free-radical processes in multistage carcinogenesis, *Free Rad. Res. Commun.*, 12-13, 745, 1976.
16. Brogharmer, W. L., McConnell, K. P., Grimaldi, M., and Blotchy, A. J., Relationship between serum selenium levels and patients with carcinoma, *Cancer*, 37, 1384, 1976.
17. Brogharmer, W. L., McConnell, K. P., Grimaldi, M., and Blotchy, A. J., Serum selenium and reticuloendothelial tumors, *Cancer*, 41, 1462, 1978.
18. Buckman, T. D., Sutphin, M. S., and Eckhert, C. D., A comparison of the effects of dietary selenium on selenoprotein expression in rat brain and liver, *Biochim. Biophys. Acta*, 1163, 176, 1993.
19. Bukkens, S. G., de Vos, N., Kok, F. J., Schouten, E. G., de Bruijn, A. M., and Hofman A., Selenium status and cardiovascular risk factors in healthy Dutch subjects, *J. Am. Coll. Nutr.*, 9, 128, 1990.
20. Burk, R. F. and Hill, K. E., Regulation of selenoproteins, *Annu. Rev. Nutr.*, 13, 65, 1993.
21. Chen, H. and Tappel, A. L., Protection of heme proteins by vitamin E, selenium, and beta-carotene against oxidative damage in rat heart, kidney, lung and spleen, *Free Rad. Res. Commun.*, 19, 183, 1993.
22. Cheng, Y. Y. and Qian, P. C., The effect of selenium-fortified table salt in the prevention of Keshan disease on a population of 1.05 million, *Biomed. Environ. Sci.*, 3, 422, 1990.
23. Clayton, C. C. and Baumann, C. A., Diet and azo tumors: effect of diet during a period when the dye is not fed, *Cancer Res.*, 9, 575, 1949.
24. Corvilain, B., Contempre, B., Longombe, A. O., Goyens, P., Gervy-Decoster, C., Lamy, F., Vanderpas, J B., and Dumont, J. E., Selenium and the thyroid: how the relationship was established, *Am. J. Clin. Nutr.*, 57, 244S, 1993.
25. Darling, G., Mathias, P., O'Regan, M., and Naughten, E., Serum selenium levels in individuals on PKU diets, *J. Inherit. Metab. Dis.*, 15, 769, 1992.
26. Deagen, J. T., Butler, J. A., Zachara, B. A., and Whanger, P. D., Determination of the distribution of selenium between glutathione peroxidase, selenoprotein P, and albumin in plasma, *Ann. Biochem.*, 208, 176, 1993.
27. Debski, B., Finley, D. A., Picciano, M. F., Lonnerdal, B., and Milner, J., Selenium content and glutathione peroxidase activity of milk from vegetarian and nonvegetarian women, *J. Nutr.*, 119, 215, 1989.
28. Dhur, A., Galan, P., and Hercberg, S., Relationship between selenium, immunity and resistance against infection, *Comp. Biochem. Physiol.-C: Comp. Pharm. Toxicol.*, 96, 271, 1990.
29. Diamond, A. M., Choi, I. S., Crain, P. F., Hashizume, T. Pomerantz, S. C., Cruz, R., Steer, C. J., Hill, K. E., Burk, R. F., McCloskey, J. A., et al., Dietary selenium affects methylation of the wobble nucleoside in the anticodon of selenocysteine tRNA([Ser.]Sec.), *J. Biol. Chem.*, 268, 14215, 1993.
30. Diplock, A. T., Antioxidant nutrients and disease prevention: an overview, *Am. J. Clin. Nutr.*, 53, 189S, 1991.

31. Diplock, A. T., Indexes of selenium status in human populations, *Am. J. Clin. Nutr.,* 57, 256S, 1993.

32. Dorgan, J. F. and Schatzkin, A., Antioxidant micronutrients in cancer prevention, *Hematol.-Oncol. Clin. North Am.,* 5, 43, 1991.

33. Dubois, F., Teby, A., Belleville, F., Nabet, P., and Paysant, P., Common values of serum selenium in a population in Eastern France, *Ann. Biol. Clin.,* 48, 28, 1990.

34. el-Bayoumy, K., Upadhyaya, P., Desai, D. H., Amin, S., and Hecht, S. S., Inhibition of 4-(methylnitrosamino)-1-(3-pyridyl)-1-butanone tumorigenicity in mouse lung by the synthetic organoselenium compound, 1,4-phenylenebis(methylene) selenocyanate, *Carcinogenesis,* 14, 1111, 1993.

35. Eskew, M. L., Zarkower, A., Scheuchenzuber, W. J., Hildenbrandt, G. R., Scholz, R. W., and Reddy, C. C., Increased thromboxane A2 synthesis by rat lung neutrophils during selenium deficiency, *Prostaglandins,* 46, 319, 1993.

36. Fan, A. M. and Kizer, K. W., Selenium, Nutritional, toxicologic, and clinical aspects. *West. J. Med.,* 153, 160, 1990.

37. Foster, H. D., The iodine-selenium connection: its possible roles in intelligence, cretinism, sudden infant death syndrome, breast cancer and multiple sclerosis, *Med. Hypoth.,* 40, 61, 1993.

38. Fico, M. E., Poirier, K. A., Watrach, A., Watrach, M., and Milner, J. A., Differential effects of selenium on normal and nonneoplastic mammary cells, *Cancer Res.,* 46, 3384, 1986.

39. Frenkel, G. D., Walcott, A., and Middleton, C., Inhibition of RNA and DNA polyerases by the product of the reaction of selenite with reduced glutathione, *Mol. Pharmacol.,* 31, 112, 1987.

40. Fu, Z. H. and Zhang, S. Y., Effects of cereals from Kaschin–Beck's disease endemic area on fibrillogenesis in vitro of cartilage type II collagen in rats, *Chin J. Pathol.,* 27, 77, 1993.

41. Garland, M. M., Morrism J. S., Rosner, B. A., Stampfer, M. J., Spate, V. L., Baskett, C. J., Willett, W. C., and Hunter, D. J., Toenail trace element levels as biomarkers: reproducibility over a 6-year period, *Cancer Epidem. Biomarkers Prevent.,* 2, 493, 1993.

42. Garland, M., Willett, W. C., Manson, J. E., and Hunter, D. J., Antioxidant micronutrients and breast cancer, *J. Am. Coll. Nutr.,* 12, 400, 1993.

43. Ge, K. and Yang, G., The epidemiology of selenium deficiency in the etiological study of endemic diseases in China, *Am. J. Clin. Nutr.,* 57, 259S, 1993.

44. Ge, L. Y., Effects of low calcium on myocardial necrosis of Keshan disease by food, *Chin. J. Pathol.,* 22, 133, 1993.

45. Greeder, G. A. and Milner, J. A., Factors influencing the inhibitory effect of selenium on mice inoculated with Ehrlich Ascites tumor cells, *Science,* 209, 825, 1980.

46. Hardell, L., Danell, M., Angqvist, C. A., Marklund, S. L., Fredriksson, M., Zakari, A. L., and Kjellgren, A., Levels of selenium in plasma and glutathione peroxidase in erythrocytes and the risk of breast cancer, A case-control study, *Biol. Trace Elem. Res.,* 36, 99, 1993.

47. Harr, J. R. and Muth, O. H., Selenium poisoning in domestic animals and its relationship to man, *Clin. Toxicol.,* 5, 175, 1972.

48. Harvima, R. J., Jagerroos, H., Kajander, E. O., Harvima, I. T., Aalto, M. L., Neittaanmaki, H., Naukkarinen, A., Kantola, M., Miettinen, U. K., and Horsmanheimo, M., Screening of effects of selenomethionine-enriched yeast supplementation on various immunological and chemical parameters of skin and blood in psoriatic patients, *Acta Dermato-Vener.,* 73, 88, 1993.

49. Inoue, I., Yamamoto, Y., Ito, T., and Takahashi, H., Chemoprevention of tongue carcinogenesis in rats, *Oral Surg. Oral Med. Oral Path.,* 76, 608, 1993.

50. International Agency for Research on Cancer (IARC), IARC Monographs on the evaluation of carcinogenic risk of chemical to man, 9, 245, 1993.

51. Ip, C. and Sinha, D. E., Anticarcinogenic effect of selenium in rats treated with dimethylbenz(a)anthracene and fed different levels and types of fat, *Carcinogenesis,* 2, 435, 1981.

52. Ip, C., Factors influencing the anticarcinogenic efficacy of selenium in dimethylbenz(a)anthracene induced mammary tumorigenesis in rats, *Cancer Res.*, 41, 2682, 1981.
53. Jacobs, M. M., Selenium inhibition of 1,2-dimethyl hydrazine induced colon carcinogenesis, *Cancer Res.*, 43, 1646, 1983.
54. Jaffe, W., Selenium, an essential and toxic element, Latin American data, *Arch. Latinoam. Nutr.*, 42, 90, 1992.
55. Kadiiska, M. B., Hanna, P. M., Jordan, S. J., and Mason, R. P., Electron spin resonance evidence for free radical generation in copper-treated vitamin E- and selenium-deficient rats: in vivo spin-trapping investigation, *Mol. Pharmacol.*, 44, 222, 1993.
56. Kahler, W., Kuklinski, B., Ruhlmann, C., and Plotz, C., Diabetes mellitus — a free radical-associated disease. Results of adjuvant antioxidant supplementation, *Zeits. Gesamte Innere Med. Ihre Grenzgebiete*, 48, 223, 1993.
57. Kavanaugh-McHugh, A. L., Ruff, A., Perlman, E., Hutton, N., Modlin, J., and Rowe, S., Selenium deficiency and cardiomyopathy in acquired immunodeficiency syndrome, *J. Parenteral Enteral Nutr.*, 15, 347, 1991.
58. Kiremidjian-Schumacher, L. and Stotzky, G., Selenium and immune responses, *Environ. Res.*, 42, 277, 1987.
59. Kohrle, J., The trace components — selenium and flavonoids — affect iodothyronine deiodinases, thyroid hormone transport and TSH regulation, *Acta Med. Aust.*, 1, 13, 1992.
60. Knekt, P., Aromaa, A., Maatela, J., Alfthan, G., Aaran, R. K., Hakama, M., Hakulinen, T., Peto, R., and Teppo, L., Serum selenium and subsequent risk of cancer among Finnish men and women, *J. Natl. Cancer Inst.*, 82, 864, 1990.
61. Krishnaswamy, K., Prasad, M. P., Krishna, T. P., and Pasricha, S. A., Case control study of selenium in cancer, *Indian J. Med. Res. Sect. A Infect. Dis.*, 98, 124, 1993.
62. Kuchan, M. J. and Milner, J. A., Involvement of cellular sulphydryls in the selenite-mediated growth inhibition of canine mammary tumor cells in culture, *Cancer Res.*, 52, 1091, 1992.
63. Kuchan, M. J. and Milner, J. A., Influence of intracellular glutathione on selenite-mediated growth inhibition of canine mammary tumor cells, *Cancer Res.*, 52, 1091, 1992.
64. Lemke, R., Schafer, A., and Makropoulos, W., Postmortem serum selenium concentrations and their possible etiological role in sudden infant death (SID), *Forensic Sci. Int.*, 60, 179, 1993.
65. Levander, O. A., Selenium and sulfur in antioxidant protective systems: relationships with vitamin E and malaria, *Proc. Exp. Biol. Med.*, 200, 255, 1992.
66. Levander, O. A., Moser, P. B., and Morris, V. C., Dietary selenium intake and selenium concentrations of plasma, erythrocytes, and breast milk in pregnant and postpartum lactating and nonlactating women, *Am. J. Clin. Nutr.*, 46, 694, 1987.
67. Levander, O. A., Scientific rationale for the 1989 recommended dietary allowance for selenium, *JADA*, 91, 1572, 1991.
68. Li, G. S., Wang, F., Kang D., and Li, C., Keshan disease: an endemic cardiomyopathy in China, *Hum. Pathol.*, 16, 602, 1985.
69. Li, J. Y., Li, B., Blot, W. J., and Taylor, P. R., Preliminary report on the results of nutrition prevention trials of cancer and other common diseases among residents in Linxian, China, *Chin. J. Pathol.*, 15, 165, 1993.
70. Lii, C. K. and Hendrich, S., Selenium deficiency suppresses the S-glutathiolation of carbonic anhydrase III in rat hepatocytes under oxidative stress, *J. Nutr.*, 123, 1480, 1993.
71. Liu, J. Z. and Milner, J. A., Age, dietary selenium and quantity of 7,12-dimethylbenz(a)anthracene influence the in vivo occurrence of rat mammary DNA adducts, *J. Nutr.*, 122, 1361, 1992.
72. Liu, J. Z., Gilbert, K., Parker, H. M., Haschek, W. M., and Milner, J. A., Inhibition of 7,12-dimethylbenz(a)anthracene-induced mammary tumors and DNA adducts by dietary selenite, *Cancer Res.*, 51, 4613, 1991.

73. Lockitch, G., Taylor, G. P., Wong, L. T., Davidson, A. G., Dison, P. J., Riddell, D., and Massing, B., Cardiomyopathy associated with nonendemic selenium deficiency in a Caucasian adolescent, *Am. J. Clin. Nutr.,* 52, 572, 1990.

74. Maus, R. W., Martz, F. A., Belyea, R. L., and Weiss, M. F., Relationship of dietary selenium to selenium in plasma and milk from dairy cows, *J. Dairy Sci.,* 63, 532, 1980.

75. McGarrity, T. J. and Peiffer, L. P., Selenium and difluoromethylornithine additively inhibit DMH-induced distal colon tumor formation in rats fed a fiber-free diet, *Carcinogenesis,* 14, 2335, 1993.

76. McGlashan, N. D., Low selenium status and cot deaths, *Med. Hypoth.,* 35, 311, 1991.

77. McGuire, M. K., Burgert, S. L., Milner, J. A., Glass, L., Kummer, R., Deering, R., Boucek, R., and Picciano, M. F., Selenium status of lactating women is affected by the form of selenium consumed, *Am. J. Clin. Nutr.,* 58, 649, 1992.

78. Medina, D., Morrison, D., and Oborn, C. J., Selenium retention and inhibitory of cell growth in mouse mammary epithelial cell in vitro, *Biol. Trace Elem. Res.,* 8, 19, 1985.

79. Morrison, D. G., Dishart, M. K., and Medina, D., Intracellular 58kd selenoprotein levels correlate with inhibition of DNA synthesis in mammary epithelial cells, *Carcinogenesis,* 9, 1801, 1988.

80. Meinhold, H., Campos-Barros, A., Walzog, B., Kohler, R., Muller, F., Behne, D., Kohrle, J., Oertel, M., and Gross M., Selenium supply regulates thyroid function, thyroid hormone synthesis and metabolism by altering the expression of the selenoenzymes Type I 5'-deiodinase and glutathione peroxidase, *Thyroid,* 4, 17, 1992.

81. Meinhold, H., Campos-Barros, A.,Walzog, B., Kohler, R., Muller, F., and Behne, D., Effects of selenium and iodine deficiency on type I, type II and type III iodothyronine deiodinases and circulating thyroid hormones in the rat, *Exp. Clin. Endocrinol.,* 101, 87, 1993.

82. Mihajlovic, M., Selenium toxicity in domestic animals. Glas - Srpska Akademija Nauka i Umetnosti, Odeljenje Medicinskih Nauka. 42, 131, 1992.

83. Milner, J. A., Effect of Se on virally induced and transplantable tumor models, *Fed. Proc.,* 44, 2568, 1985.

84. Nano, J. L., Czerucka, D., Menguy, F., and Rampal, P., Effect of selenium on the growth of three human colon cancer cell lines, *Biol. Trace Elem. Res.,* 20, 31, 1989.

85. Nelson, A. A., Fitzhugh, O. G., and Calvery, H. O., Liver tumors following cirrhosis by selenium in rats, *Cancer Res.,* 3, 230, 1943.

86. Neve, J., Physiological and nutritional importance of selenium, *Experientia,* 47, 187, 1991.

87. Newberne, P. M. and Locniskar, M., Roles of micronutrients in cancer prevention: recent evidence from the laboratory, *Prog. Clin. Biol. Res.,* 346, 119, 1990.

88. Oster, O. and Prellwitz, W., Selenium and cardiovascular disease, *Biol. Trace Elem. Res.,* 24, 91, 1990.

89. Ovaskainen, M. L., Virtamo, J., Alfthan, G., Haukka, J., Pietinen, P., Taylor, P. R., and Huttunen, J. K., Toenail selenium as an indicator of selenium intake among middle-aged men in an area with low soil selenium, *Am. J. Clin. Nutr.,* 57, 662, 1993.

90. Peretz, A. M., Neve, J. D., and Famaey, J. P., Selenium in rheumatic diseases, *Semin. Arth. Rheum.,* 20, 305, 1991.

91. Perona, G., Schiavon, R., Guidi, G. C., Veneri D., and Minuz P., Selenium dependent glutathione peroxidase: a physiological regulatory system for platelet function, *Thromb. Haemo.,* 64, 312, 1990.

92. Portal, B., Richard, M. J., Ducros, V., Aguilaniu, B., Brunel, F., Faure H., Gout, J. P., Bost, M., and Favier, A., Effect of double-blind crossover selenium supplementation on biological indices of selenium status in cystic fibrosis patients, *Clin. Chem.,* 39, 1023, 1993.

93. Prohaska, J. R. and Sunde, R. A., Comparison of liver glutathione peroxidase activity and mRNA in female and male mice and rats, *Comp. Biochem. Physiol.-B: Comp. Biochem.,* 105, 111, 1993.

94. Rannem, T., Ladefoged, K., Hylander, E., Hegnhoj, J., and Jarnum, S., Selenium depletion in patients on home parenteral nutrition. The effect of selenium supplementation, *Biol. Trace Elem. Res.,* 39, 81, 1993.
95. U.S. Department of Agriculture, Recommended Dietary Allowances, Tenth Ed., National Academy Press, Washington, D.C., 1989.
96. Remacle, J., Michiels, C., and Raes, M., The importance of antioxidant enzymes in cellular aging and degeneration, *EXS,* 62, 99, 1992.
97. Roti, E., Minelli, R., Gardini, E., Bianconi, L., Ronchi, A., Gatti, A., and Minoia, C., Selenium administration does not cause thyroid insufficiency in subjects with mild iodine deficiency and sufficient selenium intake, *J. Endocrinol. Invest.,* 16, 481, 1993.
98. Rotruck, J. T., Pope, A. L., Ganther, H. E., Swanson, A. B., Hafeman, D. G., and Hoekstra, W. G., Selenium: biochemical role as a component of glutathione peroxidase, *Science,* 179, 558, 1973.
99. Sando, K., Hoki, M., Nezu, R., Takagi, Y., and Okada A., Platelet glutathione peroxidase activity in long-term total parenteral nutrition with and without selenium supplementation, *J. Parenteral Enteral Nutr.,* 16, 54, 1990.
100. Sanz Alaejos, M. and Diaz Romero, C., Urinary selenium concentrations, *Clin. Chem.,* 39, 2040, 1993.
101. Schamberger, R. J., and Willis, C. E., Selenium distribution and human cancer mortality, *CRC Crit. Rev. Lab. Sci.,* 2, 211, 1971.
102. Schrauzer, G. N., White, D. H., and Schneider, C. J., Cancer mortality correlation studies III. Statistical association with dietary selenium intakes, *Bioinorg. Chem.,* 7, 23, 1977.
103. Schrauzer, G. N. and Ishmael, D., Effect of selenium and of arsenic on the genesis of spontaneous mammary tumors in inbred C_3H mice, *Ann. Clin. Lab. Sci.,* 4, 411, 1974.
104. Schrauzer, G. N., Selenium, Mechanistic aspects of anticarcinogenic action, *Biol. Trace Elem. Res.,* 33, 51, 1992.
105. Schwartz, K. A. and Foltz, C. M., Selenium as an integral part of factor 3 against dietary necrotic liver degeneration, *J. Am. Chem. Soc.,* 79, 3292, 1957.
106. Sies, H., Ebselen, a selenoorganic compound as glutathione peroxidase mimic, *Free Rad. Biol. Med.,* 14, 313, 1993.
107. Smith, A. M. and Picciano, M. F., Evidence for increased selenium requirement for the rat during pregnancy and lactation, *J. Nutr.,* 116, 1068, 1986.
108. Sohal, R. S. and Orr, W. C., Relationship between antioxidants, prooxidants, and the aging process, *Ann. N.Y. Acad. Sci.,* 663, 74, 1992.
109. Spallholz, J. E., Boylan, L. M., and Larsen, H. S., Advances in understanding selenium's role in the immune system, *Ann. N.Y. Acad. Sci.,* 587, 123, 1990.
110. Spallholz, J. E., On the nature of selenium toxicity and carcinogstatic activity, *Free Rad. Biol. Med.,* 17, 45, 1994.
111. Sunde, R. A., Dyer, J. A., Moran, T. V., Evenson, J. K., and Sugimotom M., Phospholipid hydroperoxide glutathione peroxidase: full-length pig blastocyst cDNA sequence and regulation by selenium status, *Biochem. Biophys. Res. Commun.,* 193, 905, 1993.
112. Thomas, J. P., Geiger, P. G., and Girotti, A. W., Lethal damage to endothelial cells by oxidized low density lipoprotein: role of selenoperoxidases in cytoprotection against lipid hydroperoxide- and iron-mediated reactions, *J. Lipid Res.,* 34, 479, 1993.
113. Thompson, J. H. and Becci, P. J., Selenium inhibition of N-methyl 1-mitrosourea induced mammary carcinogenesis in the rat, *J. Natl. Cancer Inst.,* 45, 1299, 1980.
114. Thomson, C. D., Robinson, M. F., Butler, J. A., and Whanger, P. D., Long-term supplementation with selenate and selenomethionine: selenium and glutathione peroxidase (EC 1.11.1.9) in blood components of New Zealand women, *Brit. J. Nutr.,* 69, 577, 1993.
115. Ueki, H., Ohkura, Y., Motoyashiki, T., Tominaga, N., and Morita, T., Increase in lipoprotein lipase activity in isolated rat adipose tissue by selenate, *Biol. Pharm. Bull.,* 16, 6, 1993.
116. Vadhanavikit, S. and Ganther, H. E., Selenium requirements of rats for normal hepatic and thyroidal 5'-deiodinase (type I) activities, *J. Nutr.,* 123, 1124, 1993.

117. Van Vleet, J. F. and Ferrans, V. J., Etiologic factors and pathologic alterations in selenium-vitamin E deficiency and excess in animals and humans, *Biol. Trace Elem. Res.,* 33, 1, 1992.

118. van den Brandt, P. A., Goldbohm, R. A., van't Veer, P., Bode, P., Dorant, E. Hermus, R. J., and Sturmans, F., A prospective cohort study on selenium status and the risk of lung cancer, *Cancer Res.,* 53, 4860, 1993.

119. van Noord, P. A., Maas, M. J., van der Tweel, I., and Collette, C., Selenium and the risk of postmenopausal breast cancer in the DOM cohort, *Breast Cancer Res. Treat.,* 25, 11, 1993.

120. Vendeland, S. C., Beilstein, M. A., Chen, C. L., Jensen, O. N., Barofsky, E., and Whanger, P. D., Purification and properties of selenoprotein W from rat muscle, *J. Biol. Chem.,* 268, 17103, 1993.

121. Vermeulen, N. P., Baldew, G. S., Los, G., McVie, J. G., and De Goeij, J. J., Reduction of cisplatin nephrotoxicity by sodium selenite. Lack of interaction at the pharmacokinetic level of both compounds, *Drug Metab. Disp.,* 21, 30, 1993.

122. Watrach, A. M., Watrach, M. A., Milner, J. A., and Poirier, K. A., Inhibition of human breast cancer cells by selenium, *Cancer Lett.,* 25, 41, 1984.

123. Weitzel, F. and Wendel, A., Selenoenzymes regulate the activity of leukocyte 5-lipoxygenase via the peroxide tone, *J. Biol. Chem.,* 268, 6288, 1993.

124. Whanger, P. D., Selenium in the treatment of heavy metal poisoning and chemical carcinogenesis, *J. Trace Elem. Electro. Health Dis.,* 6, 209, 1992.

125. Wilson, D. S. and Tappel, A. L., Binding of plasma selenoprotein P to cell membranes, *J. Inorg. Biochem.,* 51, 707, 1993.

126. Yan, L. and Spallholz, J. E., Generation of reactive oxygen species from the reaction of selenium compounds with thiols and mammary tumor cells, *Biochem. Pharm.,* 45, 429, 1993.

127. Yang, G., Zhu, L. Z., Liu, S. J., Gu, L. Z., Qian, P. C., Huang, J. H., and Lu, M. O., Human selenium requirements in China, in *Proc. 3rd Int. Symp. Selenium Biol. Med.,* Combs, G. F. Jr., Spallholz, J. E., Levander, O. A., and Oldfield, J. E., Eds., AVI Publishing, Westport, 1987, 589.

128. Yang, G., Ge, K., Chen, J., and Chen, X., Selenium-related endemic diseases and the daily selenium requirement of humans, *World Rev. Nutr. Diet.,* 55, 98, 1988.

129. Yang, G., Yin, S., Zhou, R., Gu, L., Yan, B., Liu, Y., and Liu Y., Studies of safe maximal daily dietary Se-intake in a seleniferous area in China, Part II. Relation between Se-intake and the manifestation of clinical signs and certain biochemical alterations in blood and urine, *J. Trace Elem. Electro. Health Dis.,* 3, 123, 1989.

130. Yannicelli, S., Hambidge, K. M., and Picciano M. F., Decreased selenium intake and low plasma selenium concentrations leading to clinical symptoms in a child with propionic acidaemia, *J. Inher. Metab. Dis.,* 15, 261, 1992.

131. Yoshida, M., Changes in serum thyroid hormone levels and urinary ketone body excretion caused by a low selenium diet or silver loading in rats, *J. Trace Elem. Electro. Health Dis.,* 7, 25, 1993.

132. Zachara, B. A., Mammalian selenoproteins, *J. Trace Elem. Electro. Health Dis.,* 6, 137, 1992.

Chapter 9

ANTIOXIDANTS AND ATHEROSCLEROSIS

I. Jialal, Scott M. Grundy, and S. Devaraj

CONTENTS

I. INTRODUCTION

An increased level of plasma low density lipoprotein (LDL) cholesterol constitutes a major risk factor for premature atherosclerosis. Evidence continues to accumulate in support of the hypothesis that the oxidative modification of LDL is a key step in the genesis of the atherosclerotic lesion. The mechanism(s), however, by which LDL promotes the development of the early fatty streak lesion remains to be elucidated. Dietary micronutrients with antioxidant properties, such as ascorbate, alpha tocopherol and beta carotene, levels of which can be manipulated by dietary measures without generally resulting in side effects, could provide a safe approach in inhibiting LDL oxidation and thereby preventing the progression of atherosclerosis. This article will focus on the proposed role of oxidized LDL in atherosclerosis, the available sources of dietary antioxidants, and the mechanisms by which antioxidant nutrients can affect the process. Finally, the evidence supporting a role of dietary antioxidants in atherosclerosis prevention will be discussed.

II. LDL OXIDATION AND ATHEROSCLEROSIS

The earliest and most common atherosclerotic lesion is the fatty streak, which consists of subendothelial aggregates of foam cells, which are mainly of macrophage origin. Fatty streaks may regress. Alternatively, they may progress into fibrous plaques, which represent the characteristic lesions of advancing atherosclerosis. The major cell type of the fibrous plaque is the smooth muscle cell. Fibrous plaques may undergo calcification, necrosis, hemorrhage, ulceration or thrombosis to form a complex lesion, which is most often associated with clinical atherosclerosis.

LDL may play a role at several steps in atherogenesis, but the precise mechanism by which LDL promotes the development of the lipid-laden foam cells in the fatty streak lesion remains to be elucidated. Uptake of cholesterol by way of the classical LDL receptor cannot result in appreciable cholesterol accumulation, because the LDL receptor is subject to feedback inhibition by the cholesterol contained in the cell.[5] The macrophage scavenger receptor, however, can recognize the LDL modified by acetylation.[55] This can result in substantial accumulation of cholesterol and in the formation of foam cells in the macrophages. This is because the scavenger receptor is not subject to regulation by the cellular cholesterol content.

The most plausible and biologically relevant modification of the LDL particle appears to be due to oxidation. The free radical peroxidation of lipids results in numerous structural changes, all of which depend on a common initiating event, namely, the peroxidation of polyunsaturated fatty acids on LDL. Even in a cell-free environment, LDL can be oxidatively modified in the presence of transition metal ions, such as iron and copper.[77] Further, the major cells of the arterial wall — endothelial cells, smooth muscle cells, and macrophages — can oxidatively modify LDL *in vitro*.[5,50,69] Both types of oxidized LDL are taken up more avidly by macrophages than native LDL via the scavenger receptor mechanism. The characteristics of oxidized LDL are listed in Table 1. The reduction in polyunsaturated fatty acids is accompanied by an

TABLE 1
Characteristics of Oxidized LDL

Reduction in polyunsaturated fatty acids
Increase in lipid peroxides
Increase in negative charge of apo B-100*
Increase in oxysterol content
Increase in lysolecithin content
Fragmentation of apo B-100
Reduced uptake by LDL receptor
Increased uptake by macrophage scavenger receptor

* apo B-100 is the major apolipoprotein present in the LDL particle.

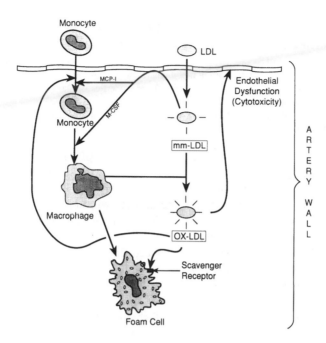

FIGURE 1. Schema depicting the relationship between oxidized LDL and the genesis of the fatty streak lesion. (From Jialal, I. and Grundy, S. M., *Ann. N. Y. Acad. Sci.,* 669, 237, 1992. With permission.)

increase in lipid peroxides and aldehydes.[16,36] Cholesterol in LDL can be oxidized to oxysterols, mainly 7-ketosterol.[70] The lecithin content of LDL decreases upon oxidation, resulting in an increase in lysolecithin content.[69] Extensive oxidative modification of LDL results in derivatization of lysine residues on apolipoprotein B (apo B) by lipid hydroperoxides or aldehydes such as malondialdehyde, 4-hydroxynonenal and hexanal, thus increasing the negative charge on LDL.[48] These changes in apo B lead to decreased LDL uptake by the scavenger receptor of the macrophage.[69]

The biological effects of oxidized LDL may contribute to initiation and progression of the atherosclerotic process (Figure 1). Ox-LDL is a potent chemoattractant for the circulating monocytes, but not neutrophils.[38] In the early phase of oxidation, mild oxidation of LDL results in the formation of minimally modified LDL(MM-LDL) in the subendothelial space. Once formed, MM-LDL may be able to induce the endothelium to express adhesion molecules for monocytes and to secrete monocyte chemotactic protein-1 (MCP-1) and macrophage colony stimulating factor (M-CSF). These events result in the monocyte binding to the endothelium and subsequent migration of the monocyte into the subendothelial space. There, MM-LDL promotes differentiation into macrophages, via M-CSF, which in turn, modify MM-LDL into a more oxidized form. This Ox-LDL can then be processed by way of the scavenger

TABLE 2
Evidence for the *In Vivo* Existence of Oxidized LDL (Ox-LDL)

Antibodies to Ox-LDL immunostain in rabbit atherosclerotic lesions
LDL isolated from aortic atherosclerotic lesions have properties similar to LDL
Autoantibodies in plasma of humans and rabbits react with Ox-LDL
Antioxidants like BHT, DPPD, probucol, and vitamin E prevent progression of atherosclerosis
    in animal models

receptor mechanism, thus leading to accumulation of cholesterol esters.[58] As Ox-LDL is a potent inhibitor of macrophage motility, it may also promote retention of macrophages in the arterial wall. Products of LDL oxidation are cytotoxic and this cytotoxicity may be important in inducing endothelial cell dysfunction and in promoting the evolution of the fatty streak into a more complex and advanced lesion.

Ox-LDL may be responsible for reduced fibrinolysis in blood vessels and may also promote procoagulant activity by inducing expression of tissue factor.[12] It has been shown that PAI-1 levels are increased in coronary heart disease.[24] Ox-LDL causes endothelial cells in culture to increase PAI-1 synthesis and secretion in a dose-dependent fashion.[43] Also it inhibits nitric oxide production; this, in turn, could promote vasoconstriction.[74]

Several lines of evidence can be cited in support of the *in vivo* existence of oxidized LDL (Table 2). A modified form of LDL that has many of the physical, chemical, and biological properties of Ox-LIL occurs in arterial lesions. For example, oxidatively modified and fragmented apo B has been isolated from the plasma of normal subjects and from patients with atherosclerosis.[45] Also, antibodies against epitopes on Ox-LDL recognize material in atherosclerotic lesions, but not in normal arteries; circulating antibodies against epitopes of Ox-LDL have been demonstrated in the plasma of Watanabe heritable hyperlipidemic (WHHL) rabbits and humans.[23,80] The presence of autoantibodies against Ox-LDL has been positively correlated[65] with the progression of atherosclerosis, as manifested by carotid artery stenosis. Also, it was recently shown that the susceptibility of LDL to oxidation varied with the severity of coronary atherosclerosis, as evaluated by angiography.[62] Finally, antioxidants such as probucol, alpha tocopherol, BHT or DPPD, have been shown to decrease the degree of oxidation and the extent of the atheromatous lesions in animal models of atherosclerosis.[7] Hence, the role of dietary micronutrients with antioxidant properties assumes great significance, particularly because these can be manipulated by dietary means without inducing side effects.

III. ANTIOXIDANTS AND LDL OXIDATION

Aerobic metabolism leads to the generation of reactive oxygen species. Interception is the main line of defense against oxidative damage and is brought about by antioxidants. In a theoretical sense, an antioxidant can be defined as "any substrate that, when present at low concentrations compared to those of an oxidizable substrate, significantly inhibits or delays oxidation of that substrate."[67] Our major objective is to review the data concerning the effects of antioxidants on LDL oxidation and accordingly, the effect of probucol, alpha tocopherol, ascorbate, carotenoids, flavonoids, and ubiquinol-10 on LDL oxidation; the development of atherosclerosis will also be discussed.

Most antioxidants that have been tested in animal models are chemical compounds — probucol, butylated hydroxytoluene (BHT) and diphenyl phenylenediamine (DPPD). Although BHT and DPPD are effective in the prevention of atherosclerosis in animals, their toxicity limits the use in humans.[26,57] BHT in doses over 1% of the diet can cause hepatic and renal dysfunction, while DPPD is a mutagen.

A. PROBUCOL

Probucol, a lipid-soluble *bis*-tertiary butyl phenol, is a potent antioxidant and hypocholesterolemic agent.[30] It has been shown to reduce the progression of atherosclerosis in rabbits[42] and to reduce the extent of lipoprotein oxidation in diabetic rats.[8] In humans, probucol decreased the susceptibility of LDL to oxidation.[31] Cristol et al.,[10] in a randomized placebo-controlled study, showed that probucol treatment for four months increased the lag phase of LDL oxidation. Probucol pretreatment of endothelial cells protects them against oxidative stress induced by oxidized LDL. Probucol also inhibits interleukin-1 release from macrophages.[2] Since this cytokine may stimulate smooth muscle cell proliferation, this effect of probucol may be antiatherogenic in nature. Probucol enhances reverse cholesterol transport by increasing concentrations of cholesterol ester transfer protein and apo E.[47] However, probucol-treated subjects showed a significant drop in HDL cholesterol. Probucol also has an elimination half life of 47 days[57] and prolongs the Q-T interval. The latter may predispose some patients to ventricular fibrillation. These effects militate against the use of probucol as an antioxidant for prevention of atherosclerotic disease in the clinical setting.

Given the toxicity of BHT and DPPD and the potential side effects of probucol, dietary antioxidant supplementation may be a better approach to prevent atherosclerosis.

B. ALPHA TOCOPHEROL

Alpha tocopherol, the most active and the most abundant isomer of the vitamin E family, is the principal lipid-soluble antioxidant in tissues and plasma. It is also the predominant antioxidant in the LDL particle.[17] Alpha tocopherol, a chain-breaking antioxidant, traps peroxyl free radicals. Several studies[11,29] have associated low alpha tocopherol levels with the development of atherosclerosis. Subsequently, in a cross-sectional study of 16 European populations, a significant inverse correlation was found between alpha tocopherol levels and mortality from coronary artery disease.[22] A recent study[63] has shown an inverse correlation between plasma vitamin E levels and the risk of angina pectoris. Vitamin E supplementation has been shown to reduce the risk of coronary artery disease in men and women,[64,68] but not in middle aged Finnish smokers, who were receiving 50 mg/d alpha tocopherol for five years.[75] Conceivably, the failure in the Finnish study can be attributed to the long period during which the study population was at risk and the relatively late time point when supplementation was initiated. Moreover, the dose of vitamin E given might have been too low to inhibit LDL oxidation. Data from some animal studies have also shown that dietary alpha tocopherol can retard the progression of atherosclerosis.[29,77,78]

Alpha tocopherol has also been shown to inhibit LDL oxidation *in vitro*. Esterbauer et al.[15] have reported that increasing the alpha tocopherol content of LDL *in vitro* prolonged the lag phase of LDL oxidation. Vitamin E supplementation has also reduced the susceptibility of LDL to *in vitro* oxidation.[35,58] Dieber-Rotheneder et al.[11] showed that lag phase was prolonged by three weeks of alpha tocopherol supplementation with concomitant increase in LDL alpha tocopherol levels.[11] A 12-week placebo-controlled randomized study from our laboratory that focused on the time course of LDL oxidation also showed a significant prolongation of the lag phase, with a reduction in the rate of oxidation.[33] Alpha tocopherol levels correlated significantly with both lag phase and oxidation rate. A further study, in which subjects received alpha tocopherol for only seven days, showed a similar effect.[58] Also, it was recently reported that by decreasing LDL oxidation in normal volunteers, alpha tocopherol prevented the cytotoxic effects of Ox-LDL on endothelial cells.[3] The relative effects of natural and synthetic alpha tocopherol on LDL oxidation are however unclear until dose response studies are conducted. Nevertheless, all these studies show that alpha tocopherol supplementation seems to increase the lag phase of oxidation and to decrease the rate of oxidation.

Alpha tocopherol may have additional benefits for cardiovascular disease. Alpha tocopherol, alone or in combination with ascorbate and beta-carotene, has been shown to reduce platelet adhesion.[28,66] Physiological levels of alpha tocopherol also inhibit smooth muscle proliferation and protein kinase C activity.[54] Low dose supplementation with alpha tocopherol preserves endothelium-dependent vasodilation in hypercholesterolemic rabbits.[41]

C. ASCORBATE

Ascorbate (vitamin C) is a water-soluble, chain-breaking antioxidant. It appears to be the most effective antioxidant in plasma reacting with superoxide, hydroxyl radicals, and singlet oxygen. It also regenerates alpha tocopherol from the chromanoxyl radical form.[55] In plasma incubated with a water-soluble radical initiator,[17] ascorbic acid was the most powerful antioxidant.

Low plasma and tissue levels of ascorbate have been identified as a risk factor for atherosclerosis. Plasma ascorbate and coronary disease mortality have been shown to be inversely correlated.[13,21] Moreover, the levels of ascorbate in atherosclerotic aortas are lower than in control vessels.[69] Smokers, diabetics and patients with coronary artery disease[9,14,60] all have lower levels of plasma ascorbate. Also, a recent study suggests that there is an inverse relationship between vitamin C intake and both cardiovascular disease and mortality.[36] It therefore seems that low ascorbate levels contribute to an increase in LDL oxidation and atherogenesis.

Jialal et al.[18] have shown that physiological levels of ascorbate can inhibit LDL oxidation brought about by copper or cultured human monocyte-derived macrophages. By preventing LDL oxidation, ascorbate blocked subsequent uptake and degradation by the macrophage scavenger receptor pathway. Ascorbate also appears to protect the endogenous antioxidants in LDL (beta-carotene, alpha and gamma tocopherol) from copper-catalyzed oxidation, whereas probucol failed to show such a protective effect. In addition, ascorbate can also inhibit oxidation by activated neutrophils or U937 cells;[25,35] both systems lack transition metal catalysts. Thus, ascorbate possibly scavenges free radicals before they can reach the LDL. Moreover, dietary supplementation with ascorbate prevented LDL oxidation, induced by acute cigarette smoking.

D. CAROTENOIDS

Carotenoids are a group of plant pigments that comprise more than 600 heterogenous compounds with conjugated double bonds. Carotenoids, in addition to being potent quenchers of singlet oxygen, display significant radical trapping behavior. Beta-carotene, an important hydrophobic member of the carotenoid family, is carried in the blood, primarily by LDL, and is bound to the hydrophobic core of the LDL particle. Like other carotenoids, beta carotene is an effective singlet oxygen quencher and antioxidant, particularly at low oxygen pressures.[6]

The relationship of beta-carotene to atherosclerosis is still being explored. The occurrence of angina seems lower when beta-carotene intake is increased.[63] Preliminary data from the Physicians Health Study[20] have shown that over a five-year period, beta-carotene supplementation significantly reduced all major vascular events in male physicians. Also, smokers who are more prone to atherosclerosis have lower beta-carotene levels than nonsmokers.[4] A European multicenter trial[40] indicated that individuals with lower adipose beta-carotene had a greater risk of myocardial infarction.

It is tempting to speculate that the beneficial effect of beta-carotene is due to its inhibitory effect on LDL oxidation. Both Esterbauer et al.[16] and Reaven et al.[61] have shown that carotenoids provide auxiliary antioxidant defenses with respect to LDL, after alpha tocopherol. An important point for *in vitro* testing is the varying solubility of beta-carotene in different solvents. Jialal et al. reported that properly dissolved beta-carotene can inhibit LDL oxidation induced by copper or macrophages.[38] Recent studies show that beta-carotene could reduce LDL and Lp(a) oxidation[50] and trans beta-carotene is more effective than a mixture of trans and cis isomers.[44] Preincubation of co-cultures of endothelial cells and smooth muscle cells with beta-carotene prevented LDL modification and its induction of monocyte transmigration.[51] Also, Princen et al.[58] have shown that beta-carotene produced a small but significant increase in the lag time of copper-catalyzed LDL oxidation. This laboratory also has observed such an effect in normal volunteers.[19] However, the effect of a supplement containing alpha tocopherol, beta-carotene and ascorbic acid, was almost entirely due to alpha tocopherol.[1,32,61] Beta-carotene, therefore, seems to have only a minor effect in inhibiting LDL oxidation.

E. FLAVONOIDS

Flavonoids are a class of plant-derived phenylbenzopyrone derivatives with antioxidant properties. Several studies, using different flavonoids, such as morin, rutin, catechin, quercetin, ficetin, and gossypetin have shown that these compounds inhibit *in vitro* copper-catalyzed, ultraviolet-induced and macrophage-mediated LDL oxidation.[46,52,53] However, their mechanism of action is still unclear. Substitution of the flavone nucleus by hydroxyl groups may be important for their antiatherogenic action. Pharmacokinetic studies, focusing on whether flavonoids partition into LDL, are needed to help determine whether these compounds can act as antioxidants and thereby help reduce the incidence of atherosclerosis.

F. UBIQUINOL-10

Ubiquinol-l0 (the reduced form of coenzyme Q10) is an effective, lipid-soluble chain-breaking antioxidant that reacts faster during peroxidation than alpha tocopherol. It protects LDL from oxidation in two types of situations, where oxidation is either due to aqueous peroxy radicals or to lipid-phase peroxyl radicals.[72,73] Supplementation of 3 persons with 300 mg/day ubiquinol-10 for 11 days produced a fourfold increase in plasma and LDL ubiquinol-10 and reduced the susceptibility of LDL to oxidation.[48] The effects of ubiquinol-10 in more physiological LDL oxidation systems needs to be investigated.

IV. SOURCES OF ANTIOXIDANTS

Both epidemiological evidence and basic research can thus be cited in support of the possibility, that antioxidants, especially alpha tocopherol and ascorbic acid, have a protective effect on atherogenesis. Hence, it is important to know dietary sources of antioxidants and their content. This knowledge will then make it possible to specify the recommended daily allowance of these micronutrients in the diet, keeping in mind the labile nature of the antioxidants, as a result of which they may be lost in food processing or cooking. Table 3 gives the recommended dietary intake of these antioxidants and Table 4 summarizes the sources of major antioxidants, vitamin E, C, and beta-carotene.

TABLE 3
Dietary Antioxidants

Antioxidant	Current Recommendation
Beta-carotene	No recommended RDA, but 60 mg (10,000 IU) could meet daily requirements
Vitamin C	60 mg
Vitamin E	8–10 IU

TABLE 4
Sources of Major Dietary Antioxidants

Major Dietary Antioxidants	Food Sources
Vitamin C	Citrus fruits such as oranges, grapefruit, lemon, cantaloupe; green vegetables such as broccoli, green peppers and cabbage; strawberries and raspberries; small amounts are found in milk, meat and cereals
Beta-carotene	Carrots, squash, pumpkin, sweet potato; leafy green vegetables like spinach, dandelion greens and mustard greens; fruits such as cantaloupe and papaya
Vitamin E	Rich sources are grains (wheat germ, soybean, corn), nuts (almonds, peanuts); vegetable oils (safflower, sunflower); seeds (cotton seed); spinach and pasta

The richest sources of alpha tocopherol in the U.S. diet are the common vegetable oils (such as soybean, cottonseed, corn, and safflower) and products made from them (e.g., margarine and shortening). Wheat germ and nuts are high in vitamin E. Meat, fish, animal fats, and most fruits and vegetables contain little vitamin E, whereas green leafy vegetables supply appreciable amounts of this nutrient. The recommended dietary allowance for alpha tocopherol is 10 mg/day for men and 8 mg/day for women. An adequate level of vitamin E in the diet implies that the ratio of alpha tocopherol to polyunsaturated fatty acids in the tissues protects the lipids from peroxidation, permits normal physiological function, and allows for individual variations of lipids in the tissues.

Vitamin C is generally present in high quantities in vegetables and fruits, e.g., green and red peppers, broccoli, spinach, tomatoes, potatoes, strawberries, oranges, and other citrus fruits. Meat, fish, poultry, eggs, and dairy products contain smaller amounts. Ascorbic acid in the U.S. food is provided almost entirely by foods of vegetable origin — 38% by citrus fruits, 16% by potatoes, and 32% from other vegetables. The recommended dietary allowance for men and women is 60 mg/day. Cigarette smokers have low levels of ascorbate and it is recommended that regular cigarette smokers ingest at least 100 mg of vitamin C daily. During pregnancy, the concentration of vitamin C in the plasma decreases and a 10 mg/day increment in the maternal vitamin supplement is recommended.

Biologically active carotenoids are present in large quantities in carrots, green leafy vegetables such as spinach, broccoli, fruits such as apricots, cantaloupe, watermelon, and prunes.

The studies cited in this review provide increasing evidence linking antioxidants to better health. Although clinical trials are needed to establish the role of antioxidant nutrients in the prevention of atherosclerosis, the results of the studies in this article clearly point to the significant role played by antioxidants in preventing atherogenesis. However, the optimum dosages of these nutrients necessary to afford protection against LDL oxidation and the long-term effects of high dosage antioxidant supplementation need to be examined in greater detail. Until the benefits of supplementation have been established by clinical trials, it seems best to recommend obtaining antioxidants from dietary sources.

REFERENCES

1. Abbey, M., Nestel, P. J., and Baghurst, P. A., Antioxidant vitamins and low density lipoprotein oxidation, *Am. J. Clin Nutr.,* 58, 525, 1993.
2. Akeson, A., Woods, C., Mosher, L., Thomas, C., and Jackson, R., Inhibition of IL-1 expression in THP-1 cells by probucol and tocopherol, *Atherosclerosis,* 86, 261, 1991.
3. Belcher, J. D., Balla, J., Jacobs, D. R., Gross, M., Jacob, H. S., and Vercelloti, G. M., Vitamin E, LDL and endothelium: brief oral vitamin supplementation prevents oxidized LDL-mediated vascular injury in vivo, *Arterioscler. Thromb.,* 13, 1779, 1993.
4. Bolton Smith, C., Casey, C. E., Gey, X. F., Smith, W. C. S., and Tunstall-Pedoe, H., Antioxidant vitamin intake assessed using a food frequency questionnaire: correlation with biochemical status in smokers and non-smokers, *Brit. J. Nutr.,* 65, 337, 1991.
5. Brown, M. S. and Goldstein, J. L., Lipoprotein metabolism in the macrophage, *Ann. Rev. Biochem.,* 52, 223, 1983.
6. Burton, G. W. and Ingold, K. U., An unusual type of lipid antioxidant, *Science,* 224, 569, 1984.
7. Carew, T. E., Schwenke, D. C., and Steinberg, D., Antiatherogenic effect of probucol unrelated to its hypocholesterolemic effect: evidence that antioxidants in vivo can selectively inhibit low density lipoprotein degradation in macrophage-rich fatty streaks and slow the progression of atherosclerosis in Watanabe heritable hyperlipidemic rabbit, an animal model for familial hypercholerterolemia, *Proc. Natl. Acad. Sci. U.S.A.,* 84, 5928, 1987.
8. Chisolm, G. M. and Morel, D. W., Lipoprotein oxidation and cytotoxicity. Effect of probucol on streptozotocin-treated rats, *Am. J. Cardiol.,* 62, 20B, 1988.
9. Chow, C. K., Thacker, R. R., Changchit, C., Bridges, R. B., Rehm, S. R., Humble, J., and Turbok, J., Lower levels of vitamin C and carotenes in plasma of cigarette smokers, *J. Am. Coll. Nutr.,* 3, 305, 1986.
10. Cristol, L. S., Jialal, I., and Grundy, S. M., Effect of low dose probucol therapy on LDL oxidation and plasma lipoprotein profile in male volunteers, *Atherosclerosis,* 97, 11, 1992.
11. Dieber-Rotheneder, M., Puhl, H., Waeg, G., and Esterbauer, H., Effect of oral supplementation with d-alpha tocopherol on the vitamin E of human low density lipoproteins and resistance to oxidation, *J. Lipid Res.,* 32, 1325, 1991.

12. Drake, T. A., Hanani, K., Fei, H., Lavi, S., and Berliner, J. A., Minimally oxidized low density lipoprotein induces tissue factor expression in cultured human endothelial cells, *Am. J. Path.,* 138, 601, 1991.

13. Dubick, M., Hunter, G., Casey, S., and Keen, C., Aortic ascorbic acid, trace elements and superoxide dismutase activity in human aneurysmal and occlusive diseases, *Proc. Soc. Exp. Biol. Med.,* 184, 138, 1987.

14. Enstrom, J. E., Kanim, L. E., and Klein, M. A., Vitamin C intake and mortality among a sample of United States population, *Epidemiology,* 3, 194, 1992.

15. Esterbauer, H., Dieber-Rotheneder, M., Streigl, G., and Waeg, G., Role of vitamin E in preventing the oxidation of low density lipoprotein, *Am. J. Coll. Nutr.,* 53, 314S, 1991.

16. Esterbauer, H., Dieber-Rotheneder, M., Waeg, G., Streigl, G., and Jurgens, G., Biochemical, structural and functional properties of oxidized low density lipoprotein, *Chem. Res. Toxicol.,* 3, 77, 1990.

16a. Esterbauer, H., Jurgens, G., Quenhenberger, O., and Koller, E., Autoxidation of human low density lipoprotein: loss of polyunsaturated fatty acids and vitamin E and generation of aldehydes, *J. Lipid Res.,* 28, 495, 1987.

17. Esterbauer, H., Dieber-Rotheneder, M., Waeg, G., Puhl, H., and Tatzber, F., Endogenous antioxidants and lipoprotein oxidation, *Biochem. Soc. Transac.,* 18, 1059, 1990.

17a. Frei, B., England, L., and Ames, B. N., Ascorbate is an outstanding antioxidant in human blood plasma, *Proc. Natl. Acad. Sci. U.S.A.,* 86, 6377, 1989.

18. Frei, B., Ascorbic acid protects lipids in human plasma and low density lipoprotein against oxidative damage, *Am. J. Clin. Nutr.,* 54, 1113S, 1991.

19. Fuller, C. J., Kent, R., Cristol, S., and Jialal, I., Effect of beta carotene supplementation on LDL oxidation in healthy subjects, *FASEBJ,* 7(Abstr.), A796, 1993.

20. Gaziano, J. M., Manson, J. E., Ridker, P. M., Buring, J. E., and Hennekens, C. H., Beta carotene therapy for chronic stable angina, *Circulation,* 82, 102, 1990.

21. Gey, K. F., Brubacher, G. B., and Stahlein, H. B., Plasma levels of antioxidant vitamins in relation to ischemic heart disease and cancer, *Am. J. Clin. Nutr.,* 45, 1368, 1987.

22. Gey, K. F., Puska, P., Jordan, P., and Moser, U., Inverse correlation between vitamin E and mortality from ischemic heart disease in cross-cultural epidemiology, *Am. J. Clin. Nutr.,* 53, 326, 1992.

23. Haberland, M. E., Fong, D., and Cheng, L., Malondialdehyde-altered protein occurs in atheroma of Watanabe heritable hyperlipidemic rabbits, *Science,* 241, 215, 1988.

24. Hamsten, A., De faire, U., Walldius, G., Dahlen, G., Szamosi, A., Landou, C., Blomback, M., and Wiman, B., Plasminogen activator inhibitor in plasma: risk factor for recurrent myocardial infarction, *Lancet,* I, 3, 1987.

25. Harats, D., Ben Naim, M., Debach, Y., Hollander, G., Havivi, E., Stein, O., Stein, Y., Effect of vitamin C and E supplementation on susceptibility of plasma lipoproteins to peroxidation induced by acute smoking, *Atherosclerosis,* 85, 47, 1990.

26. Hirose, M., Shibata, M., Hagiwara, A., Imaida, K., and Ito, N., Chronic toxicity of butylated hydroxytoluene in Wistar rats, *Food Cosmet. Toxicol.,* 19, 147, 1981.

27. Jacobs, M., Plane, F., and Bruckdorfer, K. R., Native and oxidized low density lipoproteins have different inhibitory effects on endothelium-derived relaxing factor in the rabbit aorta, *Br. J. Pharmacol.,* 100, 21, 1990.

28. Jandak, J., Steiner, M., and Richardson, P. D., Alpha-tocopherol, an effective inhibitor of platelet adhesion, *Blood,* 73, 141, 1989.

29. Janero, D. R., Therapeutic potential of vitamin E in the pathogenesis of spontaneous atherosclerosis, *Free. Rad Biol. Med.,* 11, 129, 1991.

30. Jialal, I. and Scaccini, C., Antioxidants and atherosclerosis, *Curr. Opin. Lipidol.,* 3, 324, 1992.

31. Jialal, I. and Grundy, S. M., Preservation of the endogenous antioxidants in low density lipoprotein by ascorbate but not probucol during oxidative modification, *J. Clin. Invest.,* 87, 597, 1991.

32. Jialal, I. and Grundy, S. M., Effect of dietary supplementation with alpha tocopherol on the oxidative modification of low density lipoprotein, *J. Lipid Res.,* 33, 899, 1992.
33. Jialal, I. and Scaccini, C., Antioxidants and atherosclerosis, *Curr. Opin. Lipidol.,* 3, 324, 1992.
34. Jialal, I. and Grundy, S. M., Effect of combined supplementation with alpha tocopherol, ascorbate and beta carotene on low density lipoprotein oxidation, *Circulation,* 88, 2780, 1993.
35. Jialal, I. and Grundy, S. M., Influence of antioxidant vitamins on LDL oxidation, *Ann. N.Y. Acad. Sci.,* 669, 237, 1992.
36. Jialal, I., Vega, G. L., Grundy, S. M., Physiologic levels of ascorbic acid inhibit the oxidative modification of low density lipoprotein, *Atherosclerosis,* 82, 185, 1990.
37. Jialal, I., Freeman, D. A., and Grundy, S. M., Varying susceptibility of different low density lipoproteins to oxidative modification, *Arterioscler. Thromb.,* 11, 482, 1991.
38. Jialal, I., Norkus, P., Cristol, L., and Grundy, S. M., Beta carotene inhibits the oxidative modification of low density lipoprotein, *Biochem. Biophys. Acta,* 1086, 134, 1991.
39. Jurgens, G., Hoff, H. F., and Chisolm, G. M., Modification of human serum low density lipoprotein by oxidation-characterization and pathophysiological implications, *Chem. Phys. Lipids,* 45, 315, 1987.
40. Kardinaal, A. F. M., Kok, F. J., Ringstad, J., Gomez-Arcena, J., Mazaev, V. P., Kohlmeler, L., Martin, B. C., Aro, A., Kark, J. D., Delgado-Rodriguez, M., Riemersma, R. A., Van Veer, P., Multunen, J. K., and Martin-Moreno, J. M., Antioxidants in adipose tissue and risk of myocardial infarction: the EURAMIC study, *Lancet,* 342, 1379, 1993.
41. Keaney, J. F., Gaziano, J. M., Xu, A., Frei, B., Curran-Celentano, J., Shwaery, G. T., Loscalzo, J., and Vita, A., Low dose alpha-tocopherol improves and high dose alpha-tocopherol worsens endothelial vasodilator function in cholesterol-fed rabbits, *Clin. Invest.,* 93, 844, 1994.
42. Kita, T., Nagano, Y., Yokode, M., Ishii, X., Kume, N., Oshima, A., Yoshida, H., and Kawai, C., Probucol prevents the progression of atherosclerosis in Watanabe heritable hyperlipidemic rabbit, an animal model for familial hypercholesterolemia, *Proc. Natl. Acad. Sci. U.S.A.,* 84, 5928, 1987.
43. Latron, Y., Chautan, M., Anfosso, F., Alessi, M. C., Nalbone, G., Lafort, H., and Juhan-Vague, I., Stimulating effect of oxidized low density lipoproteins on plasminogen activator inhibitor-1 synthesis by endothelial cells, *Artenoscler. Thromb.,* 11, 1821, 1991.
44. Lavy, A., Ben Amotz, A., and Aviram, M., Preferential inhibition of LDL oxidation by the all trans isomer of beta carotene in comparison with 9-cis beta carotene, *Eur. J. Clin. Chem. Clin. Biochem.,* 31, 83, 1993.
45. Lecomte, E., Artur, Y., Chancerelle, Y., and Herbeth, B., Adducts to, and fragmentation of apolipoprotein B from human plasma, *Clin. Chim. Acta,* 218, 39, 1993.
46. Mangiapane, H., Thompson, J., Salter, A., Brown, S., Bell, D. G., White, D., The inhibition of the oxidation of low density lipoprotein by catechin, a naturally occurant flavenoid, *Biochem. Pharmacol.,* 43, 445, 1992.
47. McPherson, R., Hogue, M., Milne, R. W., Tall, A. R., and Marcel, T. L., Increase in plasma cholesteryl ester transfer protein during probucol treatment: relation to changes in high density lipoprotein composition, *Arteriosclerosis,* 11, 476, 1991.
48. Mohr, D., Bowry, V. W., and Stocker, R., Dietary supplementation wlth coenzyme Q10 results in increased levels of ubiquinol-10 within circulating lipoproteins and increased resistance of human low density lipoprotein to the initiation of lipid peroxidation, *Biochim. Biophys. Acta,* 1126, 247, 1992.
49. Morel, D. W., Hessler, J. R., and Chisolm, G. M., Low density lipoprotein cytotoxicity induced by free radical peroxidation of lipid, *J. Lipid Res.,* 24, 1070, 1983.
50. Naruszewicz, M., Selinger, E., and Davignon, J., Oxidative modification of lipoprotein (a) and the effect of beta carotene, *Metabolism,* 41, 1215, 1992.

51. Navab, M., Imes, S. S., Hama, S. Y., Hough, G. P., Ross, L. A., Bork, R. W., Valente, A. J., kBerliner, J. A., Drinkwater, J. C., Laks, H., and Fogelman, A. M., Monocyte transmigration induced by modification of low density lipoprotein in cocultures of human arterial wall cells is due to induction of monocyte chemotactic protein 1 synthesis and is abolished by high density lipoprotein, *J. Clin. Invest.,* 88, 2039, 1991.

52. Negre-Salvaytre, A., Alomar, Y., Troly, M., and Salvaytree, R., Ultraviolet-treated lipoprotein as a model system for the study of the biological effects of lipid peroxides of culture cells, *Biochim. Biophys. Acta,* 1096, 291, 1991.

53. Negre-Salvayre, A. and Salvayre, R., Quercitin prevents the cytotoxicity of oxidized LDL on lymphoid cell lines, *Free Rad. Biol. Med.,* 12, 101, 1992.

54. Ozer, N. K., Palozza, P., Boscoboinik, D., and Azzi, A., D-alpha tocopherol inhibits low density lipoprotein induced proliferation and protein kinase C activity in vascular smooth muscle cells, *FEBS Lett.,* 322, 307, 1993.

55. Packer, J. E., Slater, T. F., and Willson, R. L., Direct observation of a free radical interaction between vitamin E and vitamin C, *Nature (London),* 278, 737, 1979.

56. Parthasarathy, S. and Rankin, S. M., Role of oxidized low density lipoprotein in atherogenesis, *Prog. Lipid Res.,* 92(31), 127, 1992.

57. *Physicians Desk Reference, 44th ed.,* Medical Economics Company, Oradell, NJ, 1990.

58. Princen, H. M. G., Van Poppel, G., Vogelezang, C., Bukytenhek, R., and Kok, F. J., Supplementation with vitamin E but not beta carotene in vivo protects low density lipoprotein from lipid peroxidation in vitro: effect of cigarette smoking, *Arterioscler. Thromb.,* 12, 554, 1992.

59. Quinn, M. T., Parthasarathy, S., and Steinberg, D., Endothelial cell-derived chemotactic activity for mouse peritoneal macrophages and the effects of modified forms of low density lipoprotein, *Proc. Natl. Acad. Sci. U.S.A.,* 82, 5949, 1985.

60. Ramirez, J. and Flowers, N., Leucocyte ascorbic acid and its relationship to coronary artery disease in man, *Am. J. Clin. Nutr.,* 33, 2079, 1980.

61. Reaven, P. D., Khouw, A., and Beltz, W. F., Parthasarathy, S., and Witztum, J. L., Effect of dietary antioxidant combinations in humans: protection of LDL by vitamin E but not by beta carotene, *Arterioscler. Thromb.,* 13, 590, 1993.

62. Regnstrom, J., Nilsson, J., Tornvall, P., Landou, C., and Hamsten, A., Susceptibility to low density lipoprotein oxidation and coronary atherosclerosis in man, *Lancet,* 339, 1183, 1992.

63. Riemersma, R., Wood, D., McIntyre, C., Elton, R., Gey, K., and Oliver, M., Risk of angina pectoris and plasma concentrations of vitamins A, C, E and carotene, *Lancet,* 337, 1, 1991.

64. Rimm, E. B., Ascherio, A., Willett, W. C., Giovannucci, E. L., and Stampfer, M. J., Vitamin E supplementation and risk of coronary artsery disease among men, *Circulation,* 86, I-463, 1992.

65. Salonen, J. T., Yla-Herttuala, S., Yamamoto, R., Butler, S., Korpela, H., Salonen, R., Nyyssonen, X., Palinski, W., and Witztum, J. L., Auto-antibody against oxidized LDL and progression of carotid atherosclerosis, *Lancet,* 339, 883, 1992.

66. Salonen, J. T., Salonen, R., Rinta Kiikas, Kuukka, M., Korpela, H., Alfthan, G., Kantola, M., and Schalch, W., Effects of antioxidant supplementation on platelet function: a randomized pair-matched, placebo-controlled, double blind trial in men with low antioxidant status, *J. Clin. Nutr.,* 53, 1222, 1991.

67. Sies, H., Stahl, W., and Sundquist, A. R., Antioxidant functions of vitamins: vitamins E and C, beta carotene and other carotenoids, *Ann. N.Y. Acad. Sci.,* 669, 7, 1992.

68. Stampfer, M. J., Manson, J. E., Colditz, G. A., Speizer, F. E., Willet, W. C., and Hennekens, C. H., A prospective study of vitamin E supplementation and risk of coronary disease in women, *Circulation,* 86, I-463, 1992.

69. Stankova, L., Riddle, M., Larned, J., Burry, K., Menashe, D., Hart, J., and Bigley, R., Plasma ascorbic acid concentrations and blood cell dehydroascorbate transport in patients with diabetes mellitus, *Metobolism,* 33, 347, 1984.

70. Steinbrecher, U. P., Parthasarathy, S., Leake, D. S., Witztum, J. L., and Steinberg, D., Modification of low density lipoprotein by endothelial cells involves lipid peroxidation and degradation of low density lipoprotein phospholipids, *Proc. Natl. Acad. Sci. U.S.A.,* 81, 3883, 1984.
71. Steinbrecher, U. P., Zhang, H., and Lougheed, M., Role of oxidatively modified LDL in atherosclerosis, *Free Rad. Biol. Med.,* 9, 155, 1990.
72. Stocker, R., Bowry, V. W., and Frei, B., Ubiquinol-10 protects human low density lipoprotein more efficiently against lipid peroxidation than does alpha tocopherol, *Proc. Natl. Acad. Sci. U.S.A.,* 88, 1646, 1991.
73. Suarna, C., Hood, R. L., Dean, R. T., and Stocker, R., Comparative antioxidant activity of tocotrienols and other natural lipid-soluble antioxidants in a homogenous system, and in rat and human lipoproteins, *Biochim. Biophys. Acta,* 1166, 163, 1993.
74. Tanner, F. C., Noll, G., Boulanger, C. M., and Luscher, T. F., Oxidized low density lipoproteins inhibit relaxations of porcine coronary arteries: role of scavenger receptor and endothelium-derived nitric oxide, *Circulation,* 83, 2012, 1991.
75. The Alpha tocopherol, Beta carotene Cancer Prevention Study Group, The effect of vitamin E and beta carotene on the incidence of lung cancer and other cancers in male smokers, *N. Engl. J. Med.,* 330, 1029, 1994.
76. Van Hinsbergh, V. W. M., Scheffer, M., Havekes, L., and Rempen, H. J. M., Role of endothelial cells and their products in the modification of low density lipoproteins, *Biochem. Biophys. Acta,* 878, 49, 1986.
77. Verlangieri, A. J. and Buxh, M. J., Effect of d-alpha tocopherol supplementation on experimentally induced primate atherosclerosis, *J. Am. Coll. Nutr.,* 11, 131, 1992.
78. Williams, R. J., Motteram, J. M., Sharp, C. H., and Gallagher, P. J., Dietary vitamin E and the attenuation of early lesion development in modified Watanabe rabbits, *Atherosclerosis,* 94, 153, 1992.
79. Witztum, J. L. and Steinberg, D., The role of oxidized LDL in atherogenesis, *J. Clin. Invest.,* 88, 1785, 1991.
80. Yla-Herttuala, S., Palinski, W., Rosenfield, M., Parthasarathy, S., Carew, T. E., Butler, S., Witztum, J., and Steinberg, D., Evidence for the presence of oxidatively modified LDL in atherosclerotic lesions of rabbit and man, *J. Clin. Invest.,* 284, 1086, 1989.

INDEX

A

Adjuvant therapy, in cancer prevention, 68–83
Advertising, 32
Aequorin, 143
Agricultural production, 30–31
Alcohol, osteoporosis and, 126
Allopurinol, 182
Alpha tocopherol, 233–234
American dietary patterns, trends in, 2–37
American Dietetic Association, 58
Amino acids, restriction in, 73–75
　cancer risk, relationship to, 73–75
Antioxidant consumption, trends in, 23–30
　antioxidant supplements, change in intake of, 26
　antioxidant vitamins, 23–24
　β-carotene, 25
　carotenoids, 23
　dietary intake surveys, 27
　dietary patterns, 27–28
　dietary recommendations, 23
　food additive antioxidants, 25–26
　Food Additives Survey, 24–25
　food supply data, 23–24
　generally recognized as safe (GRAS), 24
　National Health Interview Survey, 25–27
　serum antioxidant levels, 28–29
　vitamin A, 24–25, 28, 30
　vitamin C, 23–26, 28–30
　vitamin E, 23–26
Antioxidant requirement, 165
Antioxidant vitamins, 23–24, 175
Antioxidants, 229–238
　alpha tocopherol, 233–234
　ascorbate, 234–235
　carotenoids, 235–236
　flavonoids, 236
　LDL oxidation and, 232–236
　probucol, 233
　sources of, 236–238
　ubiquinol-10, 236
Aortic lesion development, 179
Apolipoproteins, 91
Arachidonic acid metabolism, 213
Arthritis, 182–183, 218–219
Ascorbate, 234–235
Ascorbic acid, 170–171
Asparagine, 74

Assessment methods, 11–14
　dietary intake surveys, 12
　food composition data, 10–11
　food frequency questionnaires (FFQs), 13
　food records or diaries, 13
　food supply surveys, 11–12
　24-hour recalls, 12–13
　household food consumption, 13
　questions of comparability, 13–14
　recommended dietary allowances (RDAs), 12
　serving size estimations, 11
Atherogenesis, 91, 230
Atherosclerosis, 89, 99, 177–180, 229–238
　antioxidants and, 229–238
　epidemiology of, 179–180
　LDL oxidation and, 232–236
Atrial natriuretic factor, 142

B

β-Carotene, 25, 179–181, 211, 215–216, 236–237
BHA, 168, 172–173, 175
BHT, 168, 172–173, 175, 179, 233
Bias issues, 8–10
Blood cholesterol levels, 23
Blood pressure, calcium intake and, 147–149
Blood selenium concentrations, 202, 204, 216
Bone, biology of, 119–124
　bone destruction, 120
　bone formation, 120
　cortical bone, 120
　trabecular bone, 120
Bone calcium, 114, 116, 119
　deposition, 114, 116
　pool, 119
　resorption rates, 116
Bone destruction, 120
Bone formation, 120
Bone mineral content, 115
Bone salts, 119
Breast Cancer Dietary Intervention (BCDI), 48–49
Bypass surgery, 181

C

Cachexia, 75
Caffeine, osteoporosis and, 126

243